VASCULAR ENDOTHELIUM:
MECHANISMS OF CELL SIGNALING

NATO Science Series

A Series presenting the results of activities sponsored by the NATO Science Committee.
The Series is published by IOS Press and Kluwer Academic Publishers in conjunction with the NATO Scientific Affairs Division.

General Sub-Series

A Life Sciences	IOS Press
B Physics	Kluwer Academic Publishers
C Mathematical and Physical Sciences	Kluwer Academic Publishers
D Behavioural and Social Sciences	Kluwer Academic Publishers
E Applied Sciences	Kluwer Academic Publishers
F Computer and Systems Sciences	IOS Press

Partnership Sub-Series

1 Disarmament Technologies	Kluwer Academic Publishers
2 Environmental Security	Kluwer Academic Publishers
3 High Technology	Kluwer Academic Publishers
4 Science and Technology Policy	IOS Press
5 Computer Networking	IOS Press

The Partnership Sub-Series incorporates activities undertaken in collaboration with NATO's Partners in the Euro-Atlantic Partnership Council - countries of the CIS and Central and Eastern Europe - in Priority Areas of concern to those countries.

NATO-PCO-DATA BASE

The NATO Science Series continues the series of books published formerly in the NATO ASI Series. An electronic index to the NATO ASI Series provides full bibliographical references (with keywords and/or abstracts) to more than 50 000 contributions from international scientists published in all sections of the NATO ASI Series.
Access to the NATO-PCO-DATA BASE is possible in two ways:
- via online FILE 128 (NATO-PCO-DATA BASE) hosted by ESRIN,
Via Galileo Galilei, I-00044 Frascati, Italy;
- via CD-ROM "NATO-PCO-DATA BASE" with user-friendly retrieval software in English, French and German (© WTV GmbH and DATAWARE Technologies Inc., 1989).
The CD-ROM of the NATO ASI Series can be ordered from PCO, Overijse, Belgium.

Series A: Life Sciences - Vol. 308   ISSN: 1387-6686

Vascular Endothelium: Mechanisms of Cell Signaling

Edited by

John D. Catravas

Vascular Biology Center
Medical College of Georgia
Augusta, GA, USA

Allan D. Callow

Boston University Medical Center
Vascular Biology Research Laboratory
Boston, MA, USA

and

Una S. Ryan

AVANT Immunotherapeutics, Inc.
Needham, MA, USA

IOS
Press

Ohmsha

Amsterdam • Berlin • Oxford • Tokyo • Washington, DC

Published in cooperation with NATO Scientific Affairs Division

Proceedings of the NATO Advanced Study Institute on
Vascular Endothelium: Mechanisms of Cell Signaling
Knossos, Crete, Greece
20-29 June 1998

ISBN 90 5199 443 5 (IOS Press)
ISBN 4 274 90280 3 C3047 (Ohmsha)

Publisher
IOS Press
Van Diemenstraat 94
1013 CN Amsterdam
Netherlands
fax: +31 20 620 3419
e-mail: order@iospress.nl

Distributor in the UK and Ireland
IOS Press/Lavis Marketing
73 Lime Walk
Headington
Oxford OX3 7AD
England
fax: +44 1865 75 0079

Distributor in the USA and Canada
IOS Press, Inc.
5795-G Burke Center Parkway
Burke, VA 22015
USA
fax: +1 703 323 3668
e-mail: iosbooks@iospress.com

Distributor in Germany
IOS Press
Spandauer Strasse 2
D-10178 Berlin
Germany
fax: +49 30 242 3113

Distributor in Japan
Ohmsha, Ltd.
3-1 Kanda Nishiki-cho
Chiyoda-ku, Tokyo 101
Japan
fax: +81 3 3233 2426

Preface

This monograph contains the contributions to the NATO Advanced Study Institute on *"Vascular Endothelium: Mechanisms of Cell Signaling"* which took place in Crete, Greece from June 20–29, 1998. This was the sixth in the series of NATO-supported ASIs in selected specific areas of endothelial cell biology, which began in 1988. Over the past decade, these ASIs have combined clinical with basic scientists and renowned experts with novices in the field, in an attractive setting conducive to dissemination of knowledge, high quality discussions and exchange of ideas.

This, as did previous ASIs, reflects the work of several people. As Co-Directors, we have been particularly fortunate to benefit from the expert advice of the International Organizing Committee, which included Alberto Mantovani (Milan) and Magdi Yacoub (London). Their insightful suggestions were the principal force that enabled us to formulate a successful scientific program. In addition, we are grateful to the tireless work of the Local Organizing Committee that included Stelios Orfanos, Panayotis Behrakis, Michael Maragoudakis, Dimitris Kremastinos and Nikos Behlitzanakis. We are also indebted to Jim Parkerson, Connie Snead and Michael Theodorakis for volunteering their time and help during the preparations for the conference. To Lydia Argyropoulos, we are indebted for making sure, once again, that all hotel, food and beverage, travel and transport arrangements were executed in a timely and orderly manner and for providing her problem-solving expertise for the duration of the ASI. A very special thanks to Joanna Daglis, the ASI coordinator, for her efficient, solicitous and pleasant demeanor, before as well as during the ten days of the conference, as well as for her meticulous work in the preparation of this volume.

We wish to acknowledge the generous contribution of T-Cell Sciences, Inc. and Texas Biotechnology Corporation. Their support was germane to the success of the ASI.

John Catravas (Augusta)
Allan Callow (Boston)
Una Ryan (Needham)

List of Participants

Tove Andersson
Department of Biochemistry and
Biotechnology
Royal Institute of Technology, KTH
Teknikringen 34
Stockholm S-100 44
SWEDEN

Moshe Arditi M.D.
Department of Pediatrics
Cedars Sinai Medical Center, Room 4310
8700 Beverly Blvd
Los Angeles CA 90048
USA

Nicholaos Bachlitzanakis M.D.
Venizelio General Hospital
Heraklion Crete
GREECE

Olga Bandman M.D.
Incyte Pharmaceuticals
3174 Porter Drive
Palo Alto CA 94304
USA

Abdul I. Barakat Ph.D.
Department of Mechanical and
Aeronautical Engineering
University of California, Davis
One Shields Avenue
Davis CA 95616
USA

Omar Benzakour Ph.D.
Thrombosis Research Institute
Manresa Road
Chelsea London SW3 6LR
UNITED KINGDOM

Kare Berg M.D., Ph.D.
Institute of Medical Genetics
University of Oslo
Ulleval University Hospital
PO Box 1036
Blindern Oslo N-0315
NORWAY

Bradford C. Berk M.D., Ph.D.
University of Rochester Medical Center
Box 679
601 Elmwood Avenue
Rochester NY 14642
USA

Richard Bogle M.B., Ph.D.
The National Hospital for Neurology and
Neurosurgery
19 Barnfield Close
Earlsfield London SW17 0AU
UNITED KINGDOM

Ruth E. Bundy BSc., MSc.
Cardiothoracic Surgery
NHLI
Harefield Hospital
Hill End Road
Harefield Middlesex UB9 6JH
UNITED KINGDOM

Anne Burke-Gaffney Ph.D.
Imperial College
Applied Pharmacology NHLI
Dovehouse Street
London SW3 6LY
UNITED KINGDOM

Allan D. Callow M.D., Ph.D.
Boston University Medical Center
Vascular Biology Research Laboratory
NEB 606
80 East Concord Street
Boston MA 02118-2396
USA

John D. Catravas Ph.D.
Vascular Biology Center
Medical College of Georgia
CB-3602A
Augusta GA 30912-2500
USA

Adrian Chester Ph.D.
Cardiothoracic Surgery, Imperial College
NHLI, Heart Science Center
Harefield Hospital
Harefield Middlesex UB9 6JH
UNITED KINGDOM

Shawn G. Clark Ph.D.
Department of Pharmacology & Toxicology
Medical College of GA
CB-3501
Augusta GA 30912-2300
USA

Benjamin G. Cocks Ph.D.
Functional Biology
Incyte Pharmaceuticals
3174 Porter Drive
Palo Alto CA 94304
USA

Valerie Cullen BSc.
Department of Pharmacology
University College Dublin
Foster Avenue
Blackrock Co. Dublin
IRELAND

Patrizia d' Alessio M.D., Ph.D.
Biochimie Pharmacologique et Metabolique
Faculty de Medecine, Necker Enfants-
Malades
INSERM UNITE 75
156, rue de Vaugirard
Paris 75015
FRANCE

Flip G. de Groot Ph.D.
Department of Haematology
Academisch Ziekenhuis Utrecht
University Hospital Utrecht
PO Box 85.500
3508 GA Utrecht
THE NETHERLANDS

Thomas F. Deuel M.D.
Beth Israel Deconess Medical Center
330 Brookline Avenue
Boston MA 02215
USA

Christiana Dimitropoulou Ph.D.
Department of Pharmacology & Toxicology
Medical College of Georgia
Augusta GA 30912-2300
USA

Henrique Sobral do Rosario M.D.
Institute of Biochemistry
Faculty of Medicine of Lisbon
Lisbon
PORTUGAL

Belinda Edmonds BSc.
Department of Haematology/Oncology
The Queen Elizabeth Hospital
28 Woodville Road
Woodville SA 05011
AUSTRALIA

Gerasimos S. Filippatos M.D.
Department of Cardiology
Evangelismos Hospital
28 Doukissis Plakentias Street
Ambelokipi Athens 115 23
GREECE

Frederick W Flitney Ph.D.
Division of Biomedical Sciences
University of St. Andrews
St. Andrews Fife KY16 9TS
UNITED KINGDOM

Bruce A. Freeman Ph.D.
Departments of Anesthesiology, Biochemistry
and Molecular Genetics
University of Alabama at Birmingham
946 THT
619 19th Street South
Birmingham AL 35233-1924
USA

Petra Gehle M.D.
Herzzentrum Leipzing
Russenstrasse 19
Leipzig 04289
GERMANY

Claudia Giampietri Ph.D.
Laboratory of Vascular Pathology
Istituto Dermopatico dell'Immacolata
Via Monti di Creta 104
Roma 00167
ITALY

Ararat D. Giulumian Ph.D.
Vascular Biology Center
Medical College of Georgia
CB-3501
Augusta GA 30912-2500
USA

Constantinos Glynos M.D.
Critical Care Department
Evangelismos Hospital
45-47 Ipsilandou Street
Athens 106 75
GREECE

Haraldur Halldorsson Ph.D.
Department of Pharmacology
P.O. Box 8216
Reykjavik 00128
ICELAND

Nesrin Hasirci M.D.
Chemistry Department
Biomaterials Lab
Middle East Technical University
Ankara 06531
TURKEY

Haroutioun Hassessian Ph.D.
Department of Ophthamology
Guy-Bernier Research Center
Hopital Maisonneuve-Rosemont
Pavillon Maisonneuve
5415 boul. de l'Assomption
Montreal Quebec H1T 2M4
CANADA

Olga Hatzikonti Ph.D.
Department of Pharmacology
University of Patras
Rio Patras 26 110
GREECE

Ginette Sarah Hoare
Cardiothoracic Surgery
Imperial College
NHLI, Heart Science Center
Harefield Hospital
Harefield Middlesex UB9 6JH
UNITED KINGDOM

Erhard Hofer M.D.
Department of Vascular Biology and
Thrombosis Research
University of Vienna
Brunnerstrasse 59
Vienna A-1235
AUSTRIA

E.K. Iliodromitis M.D.
Department of Cardiology and Cardiovascular
Research Unit
Onasio Cardiosurgery Center
356 Syngrou Avenue
Kallithea Athens 176 74
GREECE

Nikos P. Karatzas M.D.
Sismanoglion General Hospital
Maroussi 151 26
GREECE

Panayiotis Katsoris Ph.D.
Lab of Biology, Department of Biology
University of Patras
Rio Patras 26110
GREECE

Alan K. Keenan Ph.D.
Department of Pharmacology
University College Dublin
Foster Avenue
Blackrock Co. Dublin
IRELAND

Nicholas A. Kefalides M.D., Ph.D.
Department of Medicine
Connective Tissue Research Section
University of Pennsylvania School of
Medicine
University City Science Center
3624 Market Street
Philadelphia PA 19104-2614
USA

Siobhan Kelleher BSc.
Department of Pharmacology
University College Dublin
Foster Avenue
Blackrock Co. Dublin
IRELAND

Joseph Khoury Ph.D.
Division of Cardiology
The Sir Mortimer B. Davis - Jewish General
Hospital
Lady Davis Institute
3755 Cote Ste-Catherine
Montreal Quebec H3T 1E2
CANADA

M.A. Konerding M.D.
Johannes Gutenberg-Universität Mainz
Anatomisches Institut
Mikroskopischer Bereich
Becherweg 13
Mainz 55099
GERMANY

D.Th. Kremastinos M.D.
Department of Cardiology and
Cardiovascular Research Unit
Onasio Cardiosurgery Center
356 Syngrou Avenue
Kallithea Athens 176 74
GREECE

David Langleben M.D., FRCP(C)
Department of Medicine
The Sir Mortimer B. Davis - Jewish General
Hospital
Faculty of Medicine, Division of Cardiology
3755 Chemin De La Cote Ste-Catherine
Montreal Quebec H3T 1E2
CANADA

Vangelis G. Manolopoulos Ph.D.
Catholic University of Leuven
Laboratory of Phyciology
Campus Gasthuisberg
Leuven B-3000
BELGIUM

Manolis Maragoudakis
Department of Pharmacology
University of Patras Medical School
Rio Patras 26110, GREECE

Michael E. Maragoudakis Ph.D.
Department of Pharmacology
University of Rio-Patras Medical School
Rio Patras 261 10, GREECE

Nandi Marczin M.D., Ph.D.
Cardiothoracic Surgery
NHLI
Harefield Hospital
Hill End Road
Harefield Middlesex UB9 6JH
UNITED KINGDOM

Diana Mechtcheriakova Ph.D.
Department of Vascular Biology and
Thrombosis Research
Vienna International Research Cooperation
Center
University of Vienna
Brunnerstrasse 59
Vienna A-1235
AUSTRIA

Pier Liugi Meroni M.D.
Alergy & Clinical Immunology
IRCCS Policlinico
University of Milan
Milan
ITALY

Enrique A. Mesri Ph.D.
Department of Medicine
Cornell University Medical College
Division of Hematology-Oncology
Room C-609
1300 York Avenue
New York NY 10021
USA

Carine Michiels Ph.D.
Laboratory of Biochemistry and Cellular
Biology
Facultés Universitaires
Notre Dame de la Paix
rue de Bruxelles
Namur 05000
BELGIUM

Marta Muzio Ph.D.
Department of Immunology
Instituto di Richercher "Mario Negri"
Via Eritrea 62
Milano 20157
ITALY

Suzanne Oparil M.D.
Department of Medicine
University of Alabama at Birmingham
Division of Cardiovascular Disease Vascular
Biology and Hypertension Program
1034 Zeigler Research Building
703 South 19th Street
Birmingham AL 35294-0007
USA

Stylianos E. Orfanos M.D., Ph.D.
Critical Care Department
University of Athens Medical School
Evangelismos General Hospital
45-47 Ipsilandou St
Athens 10676
GREECE

Lily Papadimitriou Ph.D.
Department of Pharmacy
University of Patras
Lab of Molecular Pharmacology
Rio Patras 265 00
GREECE

Stamatis E. Papaioannou Ph.D.
Department of Molecular Pharmacology
University of Patras School of Health
Sciences
Laboratory of Molecular Pharmacology
Rio Patras 261 10
GREECE

Andreas Papapetropoulos Ph.D.
Laboratory for Pharmacology
University of Athens
45-47 Fiddipidou Street
Athens 11527
GREECE

Katerina Pardali
University of Crete, Medical School
Heraklion Crete 71110
GREECE

Jeremy D. Pearson Ph.D.
Biomedical Sciences Division
Kings College London, Vascular Biology
Campden Hill Road
London W8 7AH
UNITED KINGDOM

Charles W. Ritterhaus Ph.D.
AVANT Immunotherapeutics, Inc.
119 Fourth Avenue
Needham MA 02494-2725
USA

Marlene L. Rose M.D.
Department of Surgery NHLI
Imperial College School of Medicine
Heart Science Center
Harefield Hospital
Harefield Middlesex UB9 6JH
UNITED KINGDOM

Joseph W. Rubin M.D., C.M.
Department of Surgery
Medical College of Georgia
1120 15th Street
Augusta GA 30912
USA

Una S. Ryan Ph.D.
AVANT Immunotherapeutics, Inc.
119 Fourth Avenue
Needham MA 02494-2725
USA

Eduardo Salas M.D., Ph.D.
Lacer, SA
Sardnya 350
Barcelona 08015
SPAIN

QingXiang Amy Sang Ph.D.
Department of Chemistry
The Florida State University
Tallahassee FL 32306-4390
USA

Harald Schmidt M.D., Ph.D.
Dept. of Parmacology and Toxicology
Julius-Maximilians
University Wurzburg
Versbacher Str. 9
Wurzburg D-97078
GERMANY

Jan E. Schnitzer M.D.
Department Pathology
Beth Israel Deconess Medical Center
Harvard Medical School
330 Brookline Avenue
Boston MA 02215
USA

Andreina Schoeberlein Stehli Ph.D.
Department of Surgery, Research Division
Raemistrasse 100
Zurich 08091
SWITZERLAND

Tom Scott Ph.D.
Memorial University of Newfoundland
Division of Basic Medical Sciences
St. John's Newfoundland A1B 3V6
CANADA

Mustafa Serteser M.D.
Department of Biochemistry
Akdeniz University, School of Medicine
Antalya 7070
TURKEY

William C. Sessa Ph.D.
Yale University School of Medicine
Boyer Center
295 Congress Avenue
New Haven CT 06536
USA

Nikolaos M. Sitaras M.D., Ph.D.
16 Pilarinou Street
Papagou Athens 156 69
GREECE

Brit B. Sorensen MSc.
Novo Nordisk A/S,
Novo Nordisk Park
Malov DK-2760
DENMARK

Miriam E.J. Taekema-Roelvink Ph.D.
Department of Nephrology
University Hospital Leiden
P.O.Box 9600
2300 RC Leiden
THE NETHERLANDS

Anna Tavridou MSc.
Department of Clinical Biochemistry
The Medical School, Framlintongton Place
Newcastle upon Tyne NE2 4HH
UNITED KINGDOM

Michael J. Theodorakis M.D.
Vascular Biology Center
Medical College of Georgia
Augusta GA 30912-2500
USA

Branko Tomazic Ph.D.
10814 Beech Creek Drive
Columbia M.D. 21044
USA

Victor W.M. van Hinsbergh Ph.D.
Gaubius Laboratory TNO-PG
TNO Prevention and Health
Zernikedreef 9, PO Box 2215
2301 CE Leiden
THE NETHERLANDS

Richard C. Venema Ph.D.
Vascular Biology Center
Medical College of Georgia
Augusta GA 30912-2500
USA

Virginia J. Venema
Vascular Biology Center
Medical College of Georgia
Augusta GA 30912-2500
USA

Christo D. Venkov Ph.D.
Department of Biochemistry
Vanderbilty University School of Medicine
MRB I, Room 670
23rd Avenue South at Pierce Street
Nashville TN 37323-0146
USA

Thierry Vernet Ph.D.
Institut de Biologie Structurale
41 avenue des Martyrs
Grenoble Cedex 1 38027
FRANCE

Irene Virgolini M.D.
Internal Medicine and Experimental Nuclear
Medicine
University of Vienna
Berggasse 4/32
Vienna A-1090
AUSTRIA

Dan Wang M.D., Ph.D.
Department of Nephrology
Nephrologic Laboratory, Afd. 5403
Herlev Hospital
Harlev Ringvej 75
Herlev 02730
DENMARK

Momtaz Wassef Ph.D.
Division of Heart and Vascular Diseases
National Heart, Lung, and Blood Institute
National Institutes of Health, MSC 7956
6701 Rockledge Drive
Bethesda MD 20892
USA

Nabila Wassef Ph.D.
Department of Membrane Biochemistry
Walter Reed Army Institute of Research
Washington DC 20307-5100
USA

David C. West Ph.D.
Department of Immunology
The University of Liverpool
P.O.Box 147
Liverpool L69 3BX
UNITED KINGDOM

Nicholas Wickham FRCPA
Department of Haematology/Oncology
The Queen Elizabeth Hospital
Woodville SA 05011
AUSTRALIA

Joanne Wilson Ph.D.
Department of Immunology
The University of Liverpool
P.O. Box 147
Liverpool L69 3BX
UNITED KINGDOM

Stephen Wilson BSc.
Department of Pharmacology
University College Dublin
Foster Avenue
Blackrock Co. Doublin
IRELAND

Magdi Yacoub FRCS
Department of Surgery NHLI
Imperial College School of Medicine
Heart Science Center
Harefield Hospital
Harefield Middlesex UB9 6JH
UNITED KINGDOM

Vassilis Zannis Ph.D.
Department of Basic Sciences
Division of Medicine
School of Health Sciences
University of Crete
P. O. Box 1398
Heraklion Crete 711 10
GREECE

Hanfang Zhang M.D.
Vascular Biology Center
Medical College of Georgia
CB-3204
Augusta GA 30912-2500
USA

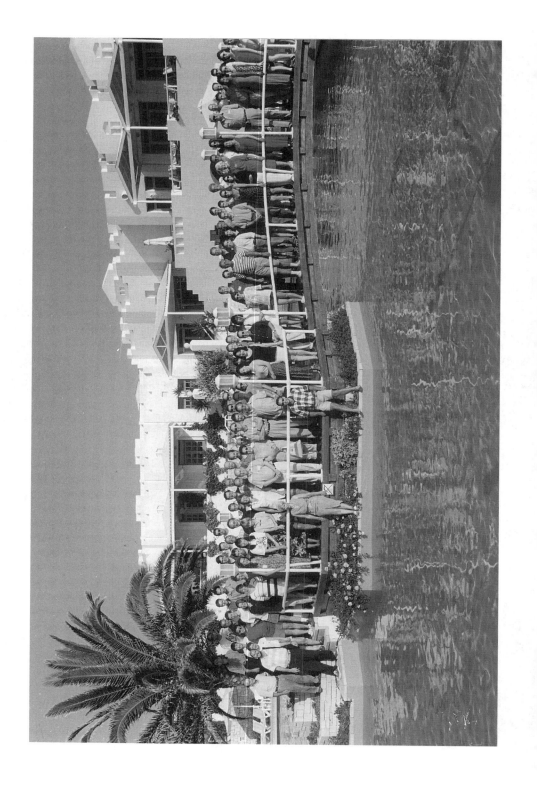

Contents

Part I

Transplantation/Restenosis

Vascular Endothelium: Mechanisms of Cell Signaling
J.D. Catravas et al. (Eds.)
IOS Press, 1999

TRANSCRIPTIONAL REGULATION OF VASCULAR ENDOTHELIAL CELL PROTEINS

Erhard Hofer, Rainer de Martin and Joachim Lipp
Laboratory of Molecular Vascular Biology
at Vienna International Research Cooperation Center
Department of Vascular Biology and Thrombosis Research
University of Vienna
Vienna, Austria

1. Introduction

Vascular endothelium forms a biological interface between circulating blood elements and the subEC and controls the exchange of substances, peptides and immune cells between the blood stream and the various tissues of the body. As such EC (EC) have to respond in a balanced way to a multitude of physiological signals important for maintaining a proper blood flow, providing oxygenation and nutrition of all tissues, fighting microbial infections and inducing growth and regression of blood vessels during wound repair.

To fulfill these functions EC can initiate several distinct, but overlapping and complex programs. For the purpose of this review we want to focus on two main programs of EC, the inflammatory and angiogenic responses. During inflammation EC initiate an immune response resulting in the expression of a number of cell adhesion molecules and cytokines [1, 42] and synthesize prothrombotic proteins such as tissue factor and plasminogen activator inhibitor-1 [20, 68]. In addition, several evidences suggest that anti-apoptotic proteins are generated to protect from excess TNF action [50, 66]. In the second main program, the angiogenic response, EC generate the signals and initiate the synthesis of proteins necessary for growth and migration of the cells leading to invasion of capillaries into the surrounding tissue [4, 58]. Anti- and pro-apoptotic functions are likely to be also important parts of the angiogenic response during sprouting and regression of the vascular network in wound healing.

The different responses are triggered by a large number of different cytokines that activate distinct, in part overlapping functions. Major inducers of the inflammatory response are TNFα, IL-1 and bacterial endotoxins, but additional cytokines such as IL-4, IL-6, IL-8, IL-10, IL-13 as well as IFN-γ, IL-3 and GM-CSF contribute to the process [43, 54]. A major part of these cytokines is produced by activated immune cells such as activated macrophages. The angiogenic response is thought to be mainly triggered by factors of the VEGF, angiopoietin and FGF families [4, 33]. All responses are modulated by cell-cell interactions via specific surface molecules including several forms of integrins, selectins and VE-cadherin [1, 16]. A number of different chemokines and molecules such as nitric oxide appear to play significant roles and influence the processes [42].

Binding of the respective ligands to their specific surface receptors initiates a pattern of cytoplasmic signalling leading to immediate responses such as secretion events and to up-regulation of specific sets of proteins important for the different programs [55]. Up-regulation of these proteins is to a large degree controlled at the transcriptional level, but important posttranscriptional regulation steps have also been described [12, 40]. The purpose of this review is to describe the major transcription factors interacting with regulatory promoter elements found in a number of genes induced by main triggers of the inflammatory and angiogenic response and to define essential signals, proteins and functions which determine these processes.

2. Transcriptional Regulation during Inflammation

2.1. Promoter elements and transcription factors involved

During the inflammatory response leukocytes are recruited from the circulation to the extravascular space. Leukocyte adhesion to activated vascular endothelium is a multistep process of sequential interactions of different classes of adhesion receptors with their respective ligands resulting first in the rolling of leukocytes along the vessel wall followed by firm adhesion and transmigration [1]. The rolling is mediated by the selectins, firm adhesion and diapedesis by members of the immunoglobulin superfamily on the surface of EC. The whole process is initiated following activation of EC by inflammatory mediators leading to the induced expression of specific endothelial-leukocyte adhesion molecules and a variety of activating cytokines such as IL-8 [42]. Transcription of the E-selectin, VCAM-1 and IL-8 genes is strongly up-regulated and transcription of the ICAM-1 gene is also increased [12, 36].

Several laboratories have intensively analyzed the promoter structures of the E-selectin, VCAM-1, ICAM-1 and IL-8 genes mediating this up-regulation [12, 36]. A recurrent feature of these promoters is the occurrence of single or multiple binding sites for the transcription factor NF-κB. The E-selectin promoter contains four positive regulatory domains in the region between -50 and -150 bp, three NF-κB recognition sequences and an element similar to the cAMP response element/activating transcription factor element (CRE/ATF) binding c-JUN/ATF-2 heterodimers [56, 73]. The activation of the VCAM-1 gene (Neish et al. 1995) requires two tandem binding sites for NF-κB located between -50 and -80 bp. Both sites are necessary for the inflammatory transcriptional response. In addition a binding site for the constitutive transcription factor Sp1 is located immediately adjacent 3′ of the NF-κB sites. Another feature of the VCAM-1 promoter is the presence of an interferon regulatory factor-1 (IRF-1) element close to the transcription initiation site which contributes to the inducibility by TNFα. Whereas E-selectin and VCAM-1 expression is normally not detected in resting endothelium ICAM-1 is constitutively expressed, but during the inflammatory response the transcription of the gene is increased. Regulatory elements in the ICAM-1 promoter mediating inflammatory responses are located between -50 and -200 bp [30, 72]. The TNFα response element consists of binding sites for NF-κB and C/EBP. An IFN-γ response element binding p91(STAT1) was also described to occur in this promoter. An example of a strongly up-regulated cytokine gene is the IL-8 gene. The region between -50 and -100bp has been described to be essential for the inflammatory induction and contains NF-κB and NF-IL-6 binding sites. NF-IL-6 belongs to the C/EBP family of transcription factors [26, 36].

In addition to adhesion molecules and cytokines involved in the recruitment of leukocytes the endothelium initiates a prothrombotic program and produces tissue factor and plasminogen activator inhibitor-1 and downmodulates thrombomodulin expression [20, 68, 79]. Tissue factor is a transmembrane glycoprotein with distant structural similarity to the cytokine receptor family and functions as the main cellular activator of the coagulation pathways [20]. It forms a complex with the plasma serine protease factor VII/VIIa which binds and activates factors IX and X. Whereas tissue factor is constitutively produced in cells of the adventitia surrounding blood vessels, it is not normally expressed in EC. Following exposure to endotoxin or inflammatory cytokines, EC rapidly upregulate tissue factor expression. The mechanisms which lead to tissue factor gene upregulation in EC following exposure to inflammatory stimuli have been investigated in some detail [40] by several laboratories including ours. DNAse I footprinting studies of the tissue factor promoter have revealed the occupancy of a number of sites, including NF-κB, AP-1 and Sp1 elements [19, 46]. To investigate the roles of these transcription factor binding sites in tissue factor gene expression reporter genes containing various parts of the tissue factor promoter have been analyzed [46, 53]. Whereas primarily the NF-κB and to some degree also the two AP-1 elements, which are clustered between -140 and -230 of the tissue factor promoter, are involved in the activation of the gene in EC following stimulation with endotoxin, the Sp1 elements are likely required for basal transcription. In case of the plasminogen activator inhibitor-1 promoter no NF-κB sites have been described sofar and the possible transcriptional up-regulation by inflammatory mediators remains still to be defined [68]. The down-modulation of the thrombomodulin gene [79] and of additional genes [Lipp et al., unpublished] constitutes a further interesting question for future studies.

From the data described it appears that the induction of the majority, if not all of the genes induced during the inflammatory response involves the synergistic interaction of NF-κB and a limited number of other transcription factors which bind in a gene-specific way to the individual promoters. In all described cases the deletion of the NF-κB sites from the promoters in reporter gene studies led to a strong decrease or loss of inducibility by inflammatory mediators. In this context it is important that the natural inhibitor of NF-κB, IκBα, is upregulated itself by NF-κB [15]. The promoter of the IκBα gene contains six functional NF-κB sites which differ in their ability to bind various NF-κB subunits [9, 14]. This suggests that NF-κB down-regulates its own activity by upregulation of IκBα after transient activation of target genes has been achieved.

The NF-κB subunits binding to the individual NF-κB sites in the different promoters appear to be heterogenous. Parry and Mackman [52] and our group [46] have reported that the first nucleotide in the NF-κB consensus binding site can determine the subunit specificity of binding. Oligonucleotides with a G in this position bind p50/p65 heterodimers, whereas a C or T in the same position leads to preferential binding of c-Rel/p65 heterodimers. When analyzed in this way it appears that the NF-κB sites in the E-selectin and VCAM-1 promoters are classical p50/p65 binding sites and the corresponding elements in the ICAM-1, IL-8 and tissue factor gene will preferentially bind c-Rel/p65. In some cases the binding of p50 and p65 homodimers has also been described [12]. The understanding of the functional role of this heterogeneity in NF-κB subunit binding will need further investigations.

In combination these data suggest that the various NF-κB dimers must interact cooperatively with a small set of other transcriptional activators to mediate inflammatory transcriptional activation, the various combination of the factors being specific for the individual gene. In addition several lines of evidence indicate that the enhancer regions in these genes involve specific spatial arrangements of transcription factors in combination with other proteins that function as architectural elements to generate higher order complexes. An example of such an architectural protein is the high mobility group protein HMG I(Y) [73]. The binding of HMG I(Y) at multiple sites in the E-selectin promoter bends DNA to increase the binding affinity for NF-κB and ATF-2 and to facilitate the formation of higher order complexes necessary for activation of the basal transcription machinery. Recent evidence implicates in addition the coactivators CREB-binding protein (CBP) and p300 as constituents of these "enhanceosome" complexes. Both CBP and p300 potentiate p65-activated transcription of the E-selectin and VCAM-1 promoters [23].

Multiple cytoplasmic signalling pathways are activated by inflammatory mediators in EC leading to the activation of the respective transcription factors and induction of the genes. Among them are the pathways leading to the nuclear translocation of NF-κB subunits, which will be summarized below, and the activation of c-JUN N-terminal kinase (JNK) as well as p38 kinases leading to transient enhanced phosphorylation of c-JUN, ATF-2 and possibly other transcription factors [56]. It appears however that the pathway leading to the release of NF-κB from its cytoplasmic inhibitor IκB is of primary importance for the inflammatory response. In line with this model are the findings that deletion of the NF-κB sites lead to largely unresponsive promoters [12, 46] and that, as shown by us, overexpression of IκBα in EC can block the induction of inflammatory genes including IL-1, IL-6, IL-8, E-selectin, VCAM-1 and tissue factor as well as prevent induction of leukocyte adhesion and clotting activity by EC [76].

2.2. Signaling pathways leading to NF-κB

During the last year, several groups have identified novel components of the NF-κB signalling pathway in several cell types, resulting in a now contiguous queue of signalling molecules linking cell surface receptors such as the TNFRs and IL-1Rs to those nuclear events mediated through NF-κB. NF-κB is a family of transcription factors consisting of RelA (p65), RelB, c-Rel, NF-κB1 (p50) and NF-κB2 (p52) that form homo- and heterodimers. They regulate, through binding to a decameric sequence motif the expression of, with few exceptions, inducible genes in a variety of cell types [2, 24]. NF-κB family members are regulated through interaction with a family of inhibitory proteins (IκBs) that retain the transcription factor in the cytoplasm by masking of the nuclear localization sequence. The most important breakthrough during the last year was the identification of the IκB kinases that phosphorylate IκBs, leading to their ubiquitinlyation, proteasome-dependent degradation and thus allowing nuclear translocation of NF-κB [18, 45, 57, 75, 81]. Several studies, however, provide evidence that this initial NF-κB signalling pathway may be just an outline of a much more complex situation that includes alternative pathways, modulation by additional components, as well as crosstalk with other signalling pathways.

In the current model of TNFα signalling, binding of TRADD (TNF-receptor associated death domain protein), a death-domain containing protein, to the p55 TNFα receptor 1 generates a platform that allows the recruitment of TRAFs (TNF-receptor associated factors), most importantly TRAF2. At this level, a bifurcation of the signalling pathways occurs, leading on the one hand to activation of NF-κB and on the other hand to the apoptotic response. In regard to NF-κB signalling, TRAF-2 binds NIK (NF-κB inducing kinase), a MAP3K type kinase [41], which in turn binds to and phosphorylates the IκB kinases IKK-1 and -2. IKK-1 and -2 are part of a so-called signalsome, a cytoplasmic complex of approximately 700 kD. Additional components of this signalsome include, besides IκBα, RelA, MEKK-1, MKP-1, as well as two phosphotyrosine containing proteins of unknown identity. It is presently not clear, whether the mere binding of TRAF-2 to NIK is sufficient for propagation of the signal, or whether an additional step for activation of NIK is required. Likewise, neither recruitment of the signalsome to the plasma membrane, nor translocation of (an "activated") TRAF-2 from the receptor complex to the cytosol to meet NIK has been demonstrated, leaving the precise mechanisms of signal propagation unknown.

NIK preferentially activates IKK-1 as compared to IKK-2 through phosphorylation of Ser 176 [38]. This serine (corresponding to Ser 177 in IKK-2) as well as Ser 181 (in IKK-2) was shown to be a regulatory residue essential for IKK activity. Both IKKs, most likely as a heterodimer that is formed through interaction of their leucine zipper domains [75], directly phosphorylate IκBα and IκBβ on their regulatory aminoterminal serine residues (Ser 32 and 36 in IκBα) leading to IκB ubiquitinylation and subsequent proteasome-dependent degradation, thus allowing nuclear translocation of NF-κB. IL-1 signalling involves specific components such as IRAK 1 and 2 as well as TRAF-6 but appears to converge at the level of NIK. There is evidence that an additional modification of p65-NF-κB by phosphorylation of Ser 276 through the catalytic subunit of PKA is required for full transactivation [83].

The described signalling molecules thus constitute a contigous queue from cell surface receptors to NF-κB, though several components of the high molecular weight signalsome complex remain unidentified. However, the mere presence of additional molecules in the complex has led to speculations that they may represent proteins with additional modulating functions on the NF-κB signalling pathway, which would allow either the fine-tuning of NF-κB activity or the integration (crosstalk) of signals from other pathways. Recently, one of these additional components has been cloned using a genetic complementation approach and termed NF-κB Essential Modulator (NEMO) [77]. NEMO is a 48 kD protein that is part of the signalsome and interacts preferentially with IKK-2 possibly through its leucine zipper domain. The functional importance of this protein is demonstrated by impaired NF-κB activation in NEMO deficient cells, concurring with a reduced molecular weight of the signalsome.

Furthermore other IκB kinases have been found and differential phosphorylation of IκBs has been described. IKK-2 is more active as compared to IKK-1 in NF-κB reporter gene assays and IκB kinase assays. It phosphorylates IκBα and IκBβ equally well, whereas IKK-1 phosphorylates Ser 19 of IκBβ rather poorly [48, 75]. In contrast, the catalytic subunit of DNA-dependent protein kinase (DNA-PKcs) phosphorylates Ser 36 of IκBα more efficiently as compared to Ser 32 [39]. DNA-PKcs also phosphorylates Thr 273 in the carboxyterminal PEST region of IκBα, a region that is also a substrate for casein kinase II. The third kinase shown to be capable of phosphorylation of IκBs on their regulatory Ser residues is the product of *ATM*, a gene mutated in *ataxia telangiectasia* (AT) with homology to PI-3 kinase [31]. AT cells show increased sensitivity to radiation and are characterized by constitutive NF-κB activity that cannot be stimulated further. The effect is corrected by a dominant-negative (aminoterminal truncated) IκBα. Fourth, the mitogen-activated 90 kD ribosomal S6 kinase (p90rsk) phosporylates IκBα on Ser 32 and a dominant-negative form of p90rsk can block TPA-stimulated NF-κB activation [63]. Furthermore, a c-Src-dependent pathway (initiated e.g. by bacterial LPS) leads to NF-κB activation via Ras-MEK1/2-ERK1/2-pp90rsk [39], indicating that a distinct, p90rsk dependent NF-κB signalling pathway may be utilized by TPA and LPS.

Together, these findings suggest the possibility of fine-tuning of NF-κB activity through differential phosphorylation of the two aminoterminal Ser residues in IκBα and IκBß through at present four different types of kinases, a number that will most likely increase in the future. In the case that DNA-PKcs and ATM could be demonstrated to be part of the signalsome, the role of this high molecular weight complex as an integration point of different signals that all lead to the common NF-κB response would be further strengthened.

Apart from regulation by serine phosphorylation, tyrosine phosphorylation has been reported as an activation step for IκBα [28]. Treatment of T cells with pervanadate resulted in IκBα proteolysis-independent release of NF-κB. However, the physiological importance of this alternative activation pathway remains to be established.

Some evidences suggest that alternatives to activation by NIK exist. Biochemical purification has revealed the presence of MEKK-1, a kinase of the JNK pathway, in the signalsome complex [37, 45]. Its cognate substrate is MKK4 which in turn activates JNK. This pathway is usually activated by small GTP-binding proteins (e.g., Rac1, Cdc42). In turn, the small GTP-bindig protein Rac1 has been demonstrated to be involved in NF-κB activation as part of a redox-dependent signal transduction pathway. Targets of JNK are c-Jun, ATF-2 and Elk. HTLV-I Tax has been shown to activate NF-κB via binding to MEKK-1 [78]. Thus, at least one additional kinase on the level of NIK can function to activate the IKKs.

It has been described that reactive oxygen species (ROIs) are involved in the activation of NF-κB; generation of ROIs leads to activation, whereas antioxidants (N-acetyl cysteine, pyrrolidine dithiocarbamate) inhibit cytokine stimulation. However, in the now defined signalling pathway there appears to be no obvious role for ROIs and the mechanisms by which ROIs influence the activation of NF-κB still needs to be established.

The emerging TNFα signalling pathway has revealed a connection between NF-κB and apoptosis in terms of NF-κB acting as an antagonist of the apoptotic signal generated by TNFα. NF-κB was proposed to lead to the expression of anti-apoptotic genes that interfere at an early stage with the apoptotic program. Candidate genes include A20 as well as the IAP gene family which is described below. Interestingly, vice versa, anti-apoptotic proteins appear to influence NF-κB: bcl-2, A20 as well as c-IAP1 were shown to inhibit NF-κB activity. Whereas the mechanism of this inhibition by bcl-2 and A20 is not understood, c-IAP1 as well as the related c-IAP2 have been found to be part of the cytoplasmic signalling complex of the TNF-receptors. Thus, additional proteins that are not part of the initially described NIK-IKK1/2-IκB pathway have in part profound modulating properties towards NF-κB activation.

2.3. NF-κB and anti-apoptotic genes

As described above the transcription factor NF-κB has been recognized to be a central mediator of the gene expression in cells induced by pathogens or inflammatory cytokines. Among the many genes upregulated by NF-κB several anti-apoptotic genes were recently detected. It appears that one important aspect of NF-κB function during the inflammatory response of EC is to trigger an anti-apoptotic response and to counteract the induction of apoptosis (or programmed cell death) by the cytokine TNFα [65, 66].

Apoptosis is a regulated process through which unnecessary or harmful cells become eliminated. The apoptotic process is characterized by a succession of cellular events such as chromatin cleavage, organelle breakdown, and fragmentation of cellular contents into vesicles with intact membranes (apoptotic bodies) which are phagocytosed by other cells of the organism. Various stimuli exist that can induce apoptosis, but once initiated, it appears that the apoptotic programme proceeds through a common pathway. Major players of the cell death machinery are a family of proteases, termed caspases, forming a proteolytic cascade [62]. Caspases are present in the cytoplasm as inactive precursors that have to be activated by proteolytic cleavage of carboxy-terminal aspartate residues. Caspases can cleave further downstream target molecules including components of the cytoskeleton, poly(ADP-ribose)-polymerase, DNA fragmentation factor (DFF) p45, and DNA-dependent protein kinase.

Binding of TNFα to TNF-receptors 1 and 2 (TNFR-1/2) can generate two types of signals: one that initiates apoptosis, and one that leads to the activation of NF-κB. Transfer of signals is performed by recruiting different cytoplasmic adaptor proteins that interact with TNFR functional domains. TNFR-1 associated death domain protein (TRADD) interacts with the death domain (DD) of TNFR-1 and mediates both apoptotic and anti-apoptotic pathways. It appears that the two TNFR1-TRADD signalling cascades bifurcate at TRADD, since recruitment of Fas-associating protein with death domain (FADD) or receptor interacting protein (RIP) triggers apoptosis whereas association with TNFR associated factor 2 (TRAF2) activates NF-κB [69, 80].

Several laboratories have now provided evidence that activation of NF-κB and cell death might be connected. In mice lacking p65 (RelA) embryonic lethality is observed, and is most likely caused by extensive apoptosis of liver cells suggesting that in mice NF-κB has a protective role at least during liver development [6]. Fibroblasts and macrophages derived from p65 deficient mice undergo apoptosis when challenged with TNFα, whereas wild type cells survive the treatment [5]. Direct inhibition of NF-κB or of upstream parts of its signalling pathway during TNFα activation results in apoptosis in a variety of cell types originally resistant to TNFα induced apoptosis [67, 70]. In addition, treatment of p65 deficient cells with TNFα did not lead to activation of NF-κB or induction of TNFα responsive genes [5]. Thus, it has been postulated that activation of NF-κB induces the expression of one or several anti-apoptotic genes. Rapid activation of NF-κB in response to an inflammatory stimulus, like TNFα, would be an appropriate mechanism to ensure the prompt expression of anti-apoptotic genes and at the same time would enable the cell to function properly in an inflammatory situation. Several genes that provide partial protection against apoptosis upon constitutive expression have been shown to be induced by TNFα: manganese superoxide dismutase [74], plasminogen activator inhibitor type-2 [35], the bcl-2 homologue A1 [32] and the zinc finger protein A20 [50]. Only in case of A20 NF-κB was identified as one regulator of its expression.

By differential screening for differentially expressed genes in EC activated with inflammatory stimuli we have recently identified inhibitor of apoptosis (iap) gene family members (piap, hiap1, hiap2, and xiap) inducible by TNFα, IL-1, and lipopolysaccharide [65]. Overexpression of IκB, the inhibitor of NF-κB, by recombinant adenovirus suppressed the inducible expression of iap genes and rendered EC sensitive to TNFα-induced apoptosis. This finding indicates that iap gene expression is regulated by NF-κB. The ability of an individual iap gene, namely xiap, to overrule the apoptotic IκB/TNFα effect was tested by co-infection of human EC with recombinant IκB- and xiap-adenovirus vectors. Co-expression of xiap and IκB reduced the percentage of apoptotic cells to background levels obtained in non-infected untreated or TNFα treated cells. Thus, xiap expression is sufficient to prevent EC from TNFα-induced apoptosis [66].

The iap gene family members are distinguished by the presence of up to three BIR (baculovirus inhibitor of apoptosis repeat) motifs. BIR motifs are required, and often sufficient, for the anti-apoptotic function of the iap-related proteins [11]. They are known to act through protein-protein interactions. Members of the IAP proteins appear to interfere with the cell-death triggering cascade at different levels. hIAP1 and hIAP2 can associate with TRAF2 and might participate in the TNFR complex which assembles to mediate NF-κB activation [59, 64]. The same proteins and, in addition, XIAP can bind to and directly inhibit the cell death proteases caspase 3 and 7 [17, 61]. Recently a membrane-associated protein (BRUCE: BIR repeat containing ubiquitin-conjugating enzyme) was identified which combines properties of IAP-like proteins with ubiquitin-conjugating enzymes [27]. Structurally it has an amino-terminally BIR motif and an active ubiquitin-conjugating enzyme domain in the carboxy-terminal part of the protein, suggesting a role in coupling anti-apoptosis pathways to the ubiquitin/proteasome proteolytic machinery. This hypothesis is supported by the observation that the proteasome is required in apoptosis initiated in primary thymocytes by diverse stimuli [25]. The precise functions of IAP proteins or IAP-like proteins in EC is far from being well understood. Angiogenesis and EC migration are additional situations in which a fragile balance between induction of apoptosis and EC survival has to be kept and regulated. It remains to be seen whether IAP proteins or other anti-apoptotic proteins are involved to protect EC from undergoing apoptosis during these processes.

3. Transcriptional Regulation during Angiogenesis

3.1. Angiogenic triggers

Angiogenesis is the sprouting of new capillaries from existing blood vessels [4, 58]. In the adult organism, only transient phases of neovascularization occur in certain physiological processes, for example in the female reproductive cycle, during pregnancy and during wound healing following tissue injuries. The growth and metastasis of malignant tumors depends completely on the induction of *de novo* angiogenesis by the tumor cells. Angiogenesis is a complex multistep process that includes remodelling of the extracellular matrix, migration and proliferation of EC, lumen formation and functional maturation of blood vessels. A multitude of molecules are likely to contribute to these processes, in particular angiogenic growth factors and their receptors on EC such as vascular endothelial cell growth factor (VEGF), basic fibroblast growth factor (bFGF) and the ligands of the Tie receptor family. There is compelling evidence that the angiogenic factor VEGF and its receptor is of central importance for the control of blood vessel growth and differentiation in embryonic development, wound healing and angiogenesis-dependent diseases [4, 33].

VEGF causes a number of pleiotropic effects on EC, the basis of these effects is not yet understood. To date four related angiogenic and endothelial cell-specific growth factors of the VEGF family have been isolated: VEGF-A, VEGF-B, VEGF-C and placental growth factor (PlGF). Three high-affinity tyrosine kinase receptors for VEGF-A, VEGF-C and PlGF have been identified on EC: VEGF receptor-1, encoded by the flt-1 gene, VEGF receptor-2, encoded by the flk-1/KDR gene and VEGF receptor-3, encoded by the Flt-4 gene. Some intracellular signalling pathways triggered by these receptors have recently been described [34]. However, most of the specific endothelial responses mediated by the VEGF receptors, the downstream signal-transduction pathways and the repertoire of genes and proteins induced and activated are still elusive.

3.2. VEGF-regulated genes

In contrast to the inflammatory activation very little is currently known on the mechanisms involved in the induction of genes, such as flt-1 [3], by angiogenic triggers. VEGF receptors are tyrosine kinases and it is likely that these receptors will induce in part signals and genes activated by other growth-promoting factors. However, the signals and genes which differentiate the angiogenic response of EC from the mere induction of cell proliferation and determine the process of capillary formation remain to be defined. We assume that part of the answer may come from an analysis of the repertoire of genes up-regulated by VEGF and the control of their transcription.

We have recently observed that among the genes up-regulated by VEGF is the tissue factor gene suggesting that this gene could be used to investigate transcriptional effects of VEGF and to differentiate the angiogenic signals generated by the VEGF receptor from the inflammatory signals. This finding was based on the recent report that tissue factor is detected on the endothelium of tumor-induced vessels and its expression correlated with the vascularization and malignancy of the tumor [13]. It raised the question whether VEGF produced by tumor cells may trigger tissue factor expression on EC. For these reasons we were interested to understand the molecular mechanisms that would lead to tissue factor induction in EC in response to VEGF.

3.3. Tissue factor is up-regulated by VEGF

Several recent findings suggest that tissue factor may have functions in addition to the activation of the coagulation cascade. This protein has the capacity to transmit intracellular signals [60] and appears to participate in a sofar non-defined way in embryonic blood vessel development [8], metastasis [7, 47] and tumor-associated angiogenesis [21, 82]. In accordance with the assumption that tumor cell-produced VEGF may induce tissue factor expression on tumor vessels, our recent data show that tissue factor expression is induced by VEGF as strongly as by TNFα. However, whereas inflammatory cytokines are known to trigger the tissue factor gene in EC mainly via activation of NF-κB [40, 46, 76], our experiments demonstrated that the mechanisms leading to induction of tissue factor expression by the angiogenic factor VEGF are different from those of inflammatory stimuli and do not involve NFκB [44].

Several independent results indicate that the main factor involved in VEGF-mediated tissue factor expression is the transcription factor EGR-1. Firstly, a VEGF-inducible DNA binding complex was detected with oligonucleotides covering part of a GC-rich region in the tissue factor promoter. This region is separate from the NFκB recognition site and spans several Sp1/EGR-1 overlapping binding sites. In unstimulated EC this element is occupied by Sp1. Supershift data using anti-EGR-1 antibodies clearly showed that the VEGF-inducible complex contains the transcription factor EGR-1. It is intriguing that Sp1 binding to this region decreased substantially and seems to be replaced by EGR-1 upon exposure of the cells to VEGF. Thus, it appears that the induction of the tissue factor gene by VEGF in EC involves the interplay of the zinc-finger transcription factors Sp1 and EGR-1 with the indicated promoter element. Secondly, reporter gene studies confirmed that the VEGF-responsive site is localized within the GC-rich region of tissue factor promoter. Finally, over-expression of full-length EGR-1, but not of an inactive mutant, resulted in trans-activation of the tissue factor promoter comparable to VEGF induction. These findings substantiate the significant role of EGR-1 in VEGF-induced transcriptional regulation of the tissue factor gene in EC.

Our data correlate with observations made *in vivo* showing that vascular EC in a tumor environment express tissue factor and suggest that VEGF secreted by tumor cells can be indeed the cause of elevated levels of tissue factor. This may contribute to the hypercoagulability frequently seen in tumor patients. Alternatively, in the context of vessel formation tissue factor could have additional function(s) independent of its role in triggering coagulation. In this respect, it was demonstrated recently that an interaction of the tissue factor cytoplasmic domain with actin-binding protein 280 supports cell adhesion and migration that may lead to vascular remodelling [51]. It is conceivable that regulated and maybe polarized expression of tissue factor on the basal side of the angiogenic EC could be required in the process of sprouting and/or invasion of capillaries.

3.4. The transcription factor EGR-1

A multitude of data published on EGR-1 supports its central role as a multifunctional transcription factor important for growth and differentiation [22]. EGR-1 mRNA is induced within 15-30 min by a wide range of extracellular signals, including growth factors, and does not require *de novo* protein synthesis. Some data suggest that multiple, independent, possibly additive pathways for the induction of this gene must exist. When EC were treated with a combination of VEGF and TNFα, tissue factor activity was more than additively up-regulated [10 and Mechtcheriakova et al., unpublished data]. However, the specific signalling pathways and their possible cross talk leading to EGR-1 activation in EC still need to be defined. Importantly, EGR-1 is one of only a small number of bifunctional transcription factors that contain both activation and repression domains. Signal-specific posttranslational modification of EGR-1, interaction with other regulating factors and/or presence of a transcription factor inhibitor may activate or repress different target genes in a cell-type specific manner.

In addition to the results discussed above, we have further tested the subcellular localization and expression of EGR-1 protein in EC by immunofluorescence. Its subcellular localization has been described for serum starved fibroblasts following serum stimulation [22, 71]. Using immunostaining, we found that the protein starts to accumulate in the nucleus within 15-30 min, reaches a peak level at about 1 to 2 h, and decreases gradually thereafter within a few hours. The time course of nuclear accumulation is in agreement with its proposed function as the primary inducer of tissue factor by VEGF. Sofar, the mechanisms that mediate rapid egr-1 gene activation by growth factors are only partially understood. Our data suggest the presence of low levels of the protein in the cytoplasm of unstimulated EC. It is not clear at the moment whether that means that low amounts of EGR-1 are continously synthesized in EC in culture or EGR-1 protein could be retained in the cytoplasm in untreated cells.

Although these data clearly show that EGR-1 is important for tissue factor up-regulation it remains to be seen to what extent EGR-1 is a general mediator of the response triggered by VEGF for a number of additional genes involved in the angiogenic process.

4. Therapeutic Aspects

Inflammatory activation of the endothelium can be triggered by infectious agents and/or an imbalanced activation of the cellular and humoral elements of the immune system, e.g. by activated neutrophils, monocytes and lymphocytes, or by immune complexes, complement factors and cytokines leading to activation of the cells. Their interaction with the endothelium can result in acute or chronic endothelial dysfunctions causing inflammation, coagulation and overproliferation of vascular cells. In consequence it can lead to changes in blood flow due to vessel obstruction, dilatation or aneurisma formation. Another important pathological dysfunction is the uncontrolled induction of new capillary growth by tumor cells which is a prerequesite for the growth of solid tumors and their metastases. The vascular endothelium is therefore of central importance to a wide range of human diseases with significant morbidity including several types of local acute and chronic inflammations, atherosclerosis, myocardial infarction, stroke, transplant rejection and cancer.

Defining the key signalling pathways of the inflammatory program including the immune and prothrombotic responses as well as of the angiogenic program of EC is therefore of great importance. It can be assumed that the key regulatory molecules employed in pharmacological screening programs will lead to the isolation of low molecular weight inhibitors to block the essential activatory pathways, e.g. the NF-κB pathway. In addition it could be envisaged that following the development of the proper viral delivery vehicles, naturally inhibitory molecules, e.g. IκB, or dominant negative mutants of signalling enzymes or transcription factors could be used in recombinant viral constructs to prevent endothelial cell activation and to treat the corresponding diseases.

It should be further mentioned, that there is considerable evidence that angiogenesis and chronic inflammation are co-dependent [29]. Inflammatory mediators can also, either directly or indirectly, promote angiogenesis. Angiogenesis, in turn, contributes to inflammatory pathology. It is a relevant point that procedures developed for the treatment of chronic inflammation could also affect angiogenesis and methods developed to target angiogenesis should have benefits for treatment of chronic inflammatory diseases.

5. Concluding Remarks

The work of the last decade demonstrated a remarkable spectrum of responses of EC to a variety of physiological and pathological stimuli. EC are capable to actively interact with leukocytes, to cross-talk with subEC and to initiate complex programs to regulate inflammatory, immune and thrombotic processes. Significant data on the transcriptional mechanisms by which inflammatory mediators such as TNFα, IL-1 or endotoxin induce these programs in EC have been obtained. NF-κB has been defined as a key regulatory molecule, but many open questions, e.g. regarding differential responses to different cytokines and of the fine-tuning of EC activation, remain. Similarly, EC can actively respond to angiogenic triggers, which can be induced by hypoxic conditions, during wound healing or are synthesized by malignant tumor cells, and develop a corresponding angiogenic program resulting in the sprouting of capillaries into the surrounding tissue. Although the main triggers of angiogenesis appear to have been defined recently by molecules such as VEGF and the Tie receptor ligands, the intracellular signals elicited by these factors, the main transcription factors involved and the potential repertoire of induced genes which characterize the angiogenic response are still largely unknown.

Acknowledgements

Our work was supported by the Austrian Science Foundation (SFB05-5, -10 and -12).

References

[1] Albelda SM, Smith CW, Ward PA (1994) Adhesion molecules and inflammatory injury. FASEB J 8:504-512

[2] Baeuerle P (1998) Pro-inflammatory signaling: Last pieces in the NF-κB puzzle? Curr Biology 8:R19-R22

[3] Barleon B, Siemeister G, Martiny Baron G, Weindel K, Herzog C, Marme D (1997) Vascular endothelial growth factor up-regulates its receptor fms-like tyrosine kinase 1 (FLT-1) and a soluble variant of FLT-1 in human vascular EC. Cancer Res 57:5421-5425

[4] Beck L, d'Amore PA (1997) Vascular development: cellular and molecular regulation. FASEB J 11:365-373

[5] Beg AA, Baltimore D (1996) An essential role for NF-kappaB in preventing TNF-alpha-induced cell death. Science 274:782-784

[6] Beg AA, Sha WC, Bronson RT, Ghosh S, Baltimore D (1995) Embryonic lethality and liver degeneration in mice lacking the RelA component of NF-kappa B. Nature 376:167-170

[7] Bromberg ME, Konigsberg WH, Madison JF, Pawashe A, Garen A (1995) Tissue factor promotes melanoma metastasis by a pathway independent of blood coagulation. Proc Natl Acad Sci USA 92:8205-8209

[8] Carmeliet P, Mackman N, Moons L, Luther T, Gressens P, Van Vlaenderen I, Demunck H, Kasper M, Breier G, Evrard P, Muller M, Risau W, Edgington T, Collen D (1996) Role of tissue factor in embryonic blood vessel development. Nature 383:73-75

[9] Cheng Q, Cant CA, Moll T, Hofer-Warbinek R, Wagner E, Birnstiel ML, Bach FH, de Martin R (1994) NF-κB subunit-specific regulation of the IκBα promoter. J Biol Chem 269:13551-13557

[10] Clauss M, Grell M, Fangmann C, Fiers W, Scheurich P, Risau W (1996) Synergistic induction of endothelial tissue factor by tumor necrosis factor and vascular endothelial growth factor: functional analysis of the tumor necrosis factor receptors. FEBS Lett 390:334-338

[11] Clem RJ, Duckett CS (1997) The iap genes: unique arbitrators of cell death. Trends Cell Biol 7:337-339

[12] Collins T, Read MA, Neish AS, Whitley MZ, Thanos D, Maniatis T (1995) Transcriptional regulation of endothelial cell adhesion molecules: NF-kappa B and cytokine-inducible enhancers. FASEB J 9:899-909

[13] Contrino J, Hair G, Kreutzer DL, Rickles FR (1996. In situ detection of tissue factor in vscular endothelial cells: correlation with the malignant phenotype of human breast disease. Nat Med 2:209-15

[14] de Martin R, Holzmüller, H., Hofer, E. and Bach, F. H. (1995) Intron-exon structure of the IκBα-encoding gene. Gene 152:253-255

[15] de Martin R, Vanhove B, Cheng Q, Hofer E, Csizmadia V, Winkler H, Bach FH (1993) Cytokine-inducible expression in EC of an I kappa B alpha-like gene is regulated by NF kappa B. EMBO J 12:2773-2779

[16] Dejana E, Corada M, Lampugnani MG (1995) Endothelial cell-to-cell junctions. FASEB J 9:910-918

[17] Deveraux QL, Takahashi R, Salvesen GS, Reed JC (1997) X-linked IAP is a direct inhibitor of cell-death proteases. Nature 388:300-304

[18] DiDonato JA, Hayakawa M, Rothwarf DM, Zandi E, Karin M (1997) A cytokine-responsive IkappaB kinase that activates the transcription factor NF-kappaB. Nature 388:548-554

[19] Donovan-Peluso M, George LD, Hassett AC (1994) Lipopolysaccharide induction of tissue factor expression in THP-1 monocytic cells. Protein-DNA interactions with the promoter. J Biol Chem 269:1361-1369

[20] Edgington TS, Mackman N, Brand K, Ruf W (1991) The structural biology of expression and function of tissue factor. Thromb Haemost 66:67-79

[21] Folkman J, D'Amore PA (1996) Blood vessel formation: What is its molecular basis? Cell 87:1153-1155

[22] Gashler AL, Swaminathan S, Sukhatme VP (1993) A novel repression module, an extensive activation domain, and a bipartite nuclear localization signal defined in the immediate-early transcription factor Egr-1. Mol Cell Biol 13:4556-4571

[23] Gerritsen ME, Williams AJ, Neish AS, Moore S, Shi Y, Collins T (1997) CREB-binding protein p300 are transcriptional coactivators of p65. Proc Natl Acad Sci USA 94:2927-2932

[24] Ghosh S, May MJ, Kopp EB (1988) NF-kB and Rel proteins: Evolutionary conserved regulators of immune responses. Ann Rev Immunol 16:225-260

[25] Grimm LM, Goldberg AL, Poirier GG, Schwartz LM, Osborne BA (1996) Proteasomes play an essential role in thymocyte apoptosis. EMBO J 15:3835-3844

[26] Harant H, de Martin R, Andrew PJ, Foglar E, Dittrich C, Lindley IJD (1996) Synergistic activation of interleukin-8 gene transcription by all-trans-retinoic acid and tumor necrosis factor-alpha involves the transcription factor NF-kappaB. J Biol Chem 271:26954-26961

[27] Hauser HP, Bardroff M, Pyrowolakis G, Jentsch S (1998) A giant ubiquitin-conjugating enzyme related to IAP apoptosis inhibitors. J Cell Biol 141:1415-1422

[28] Imbert V, Rupec RA, Livolsi A, Pahl HL, Traenckner EB, Mueller Dieckmann C, Farahifar D, Rossi B, Auberger P, Baeuerle PA, Peyron JF (1996) Tyrosine phosphorylation of I kappa B-alpha activates NF-kappa B without proteolytic degradation of I kappa B-alpha. Cell 86:787-798

[29] Jackson JR, Seed MP, Kircher CH, Willoughby DA, Winkler JD (1997) The codependence of angiogenesis and chronic inflammation. FASEB J 11:457-465

[30] Jahnke A, Johnson JP (1994) Synergistic activation of intercellular adhesion molecule 1 (ICAM-1) by TNF-alpha and IFN-gamma is mediated by p65/p50 and p65/c-Rel and interferon-responsive factor Stat1 alpha (p91) that can be activated by both IFN-gamma and IFN-alpha. FEBS Lett 354:220-226

[31] Jung M, Zhang Y, Lee S, Dritschilo A (1995) Correction of radiation sensitivity in ataxia telangiectasia cells by a truncated I kappa B-alpha. Science 268:1619-1621

[32] Karsan A, Yee E, Kaushansky K, Harlan JM (1996) Cloning of human Bcl-2 homologue: inflammatory cytokines induce human A1 in cultured EC. Blood 87:3089-3096

[33] Korpelainen EI, Alitalo K (1998) Signaling angiogenesis and lymphangiogenesis. Cur Opinion Cell Biol 10:159-164

[34] Kroll J, Waltenberger J (1997) The vascular endothelial growth factor receptor KDR activates multiple signal transduction pathways in porcine aortic EC. J Biol Chem 272:32521-32527

[35] Kumar S, Baglioni C (1991) Protection from tumor necrosis factor-mediated cytolysis by overexpression of plasminogen activator inhibitor type-2. J Biol Chem 266:20960-20964

[36] Kunsch C, Lang RK, Rosen CA, Shannon MF (1994) Synergistic transcriptional activation of the IL-8 gene by NF-kappa B p65 (RelA) and NF-IL-6. J Immunol 153:153-164

[37] Lee FS, Hagler J, Chen ZJ, Maniatis T (1997) Activation of the IkappaB alpha kinase complex by MEKK1, a kinase of the JNK pathway. Cell 88:213-222

[38] Ling L, Cao Z, Goeddel DV (1998) NF-kappaB-inducing kinase activates IKK-alpha by phosphorylation of Ser-176. Proc Natl Acad Sci USA 95:3792-3797

[39] Liu L, Kwak Y-T, Bex F, Garcia-Martinez LF, Li X-H, Meek K, Lane WS, Gaynor RB (1998) DNA-dependent protein kinase phosphorylation of IκBα and IκBβ regulates NF-κB DNA binding properties. Mol Cell Biol 18:4221-4234

[40] Mackman N (1995) Regulation of the tissue factor gene. FASEB J 9:883-889

[41] Malinin NL, Boldin MP, Kovalenko AV, Wallach D (1997) MAP3K-related kinase involved in NF-kappaB induction by TNF, CD95 and IL-1. Nature 385:540-544

[42] Mantovani A, Allavena P, Vecchi A, Dejana E, Sozzani S, Introna M (1998) Cytokine regulation of endothelial cell function. In: J. D. Catravas, et al. (ed): Vascular Endothelium, Plenum Press, New York and London, pp 105-134

[43] Mantovani A, Bussolino F, Dejana E (1992) Cytokine regulation of endothelial cell function. FASEB J 6:2591-2599

[44] Mechtcheriakova D, Wlachos A, Holzmüller H, Binder BR, Hofer E (1998) Vascular endothelial cell growth factor-induced tissue factor expression in EC is mediated by EGR-1. submitted

[45] Mercurio F, Zhu H, Murray BW, Shevchenko A, Bennet BL, Li JW, Young DB, Barbosa M, Mann M, Manning A, Rao A (1997) IKK-1 and IKK-2: cytokine-activated IkB kinases essential for NF-kB activation. Science 278:860-866

[46] Moll T, Czyz M, Holzmuller H, Hofer-Warbinek R, Wagner E, Winkler H, Bach FH, Hofer E (1995) Regulation of the tissue factor promoter in EC. Binding of NF kappa B-, AP-1-, and Sp1-like transcription factors. J Biol Chem 270:3849-3857

[47] Mueller BM, Reisfeld RA, Edgington TS, Ruf W (1992) Expression of tissue factor by melanoma cells promotes efficient hematogenous metastasis. Proc Natl Acad Sci USA 89:11832-11836

[48] Nakano H, Shindo M, Sakon S, Nishinaka S, Mihara M, Yagita H, Okumura K (1998) Differential regulation of IkappaB kinase alpha and beta by two upstream kinases, NF-kappaB-inducing kinase and mitogen-activated protein kinase/ERK kinase kinase-1. Proc Natl Acad Sci USA 95:3537-3542

[49] Neish AS, Read MA, Thanos D, Pine R, Maniatis T, Collins T (1995) Endothelial interferon regulatory factor 1 cooperates with NF-kappa B as a transcriptional activator of vascular cell adhesion molecule 1. Mol Cell Biol 15:2558-2569

[50] Opipari AW, Jr., Hu HM, Yabkowitz R, Dixit VM (1992) The A20 zinc finger protein protects cells from tumor necrosis factor cytotoxicity. J Biol Chem 267:12424-12427

[51] Ott I, Fischer E, Miyagi Y, Mueller B, Ruf W (1998) A role for tissue factor in cell adhesion and migration mediated by interaction with actin-binding protein 280. J Cell Biol 140:1241-1253

[52] Parry GC, Mackman N (1994) A set of inducible genes expressed by activated human monocytic and EC contain kappa B-like sites that specifically bind c-Rel-p65 heterodimers. J Biol Chem 269:20823-20825

[53] Parry GC, Mackman N (1995) Transcriptional regulation of tissue factor expression in human EC. Arterioscler Thromb Vasc Biol 15:612-621

[54] Pober JS, Cotran RS (1990a) Cytokines and endothelial cell biology. Physiol Rev 70:427-451

[55] Pober JS, Cotran RS (1990b) The role of EC in inflammation. Transplantation 50:537-544

[56] Read MA, Whitley MZ, Gupta S, Pierce JW, Best J, Davis RJ, Collins T (1997) Tumor necrosis factor alpha-induced E-selectin expression is activated by the nuclear factor-kappaB and c-JUN N-terminal kinase/p38 mitogen-activated protein kinase pathways. J Biol Chem 272:2753-2761

[57] Regnier CH, Song HY, Gao X, Goeddel DV, Cao Z, Rothe M (1997) Identification and Characterization of an IkB kinase. Cell 90:373-383

[58] Risau W (1997) Mechanisms of angiogenesis. Nature 386:671-674

[59] Rothe M, Pan MG, Henzel WJ, Ayres TM, Goeddel DV (1995) The TNFR2-TRAF signaling complex contains two novel proteins related to baculoviral inhibitor of apoptosis proteins. Cell 83:1243-1252

[60] Rottingen JA, Enden T, Camerer E, Iversen JG, Prydz H (1995) Binding of human factor VIIa to tissue factor induces cytosolic Ca(2+) signals in J82 cells, transfected COS-1 cells, Madin-Darby canine kidney cells and in human EC induced to synthesize tissue factor. J Biol Chem 270:4650-4660

[61] Roy N, Deveraux QL, Takahashi R, Salvesen GS, Reed JC (1997) The c-IAP-1 and c-IAP-2 proteins are direct inhibitors of specific caspases. EMBO J 16:6914-6925

[62] Salvesen GS, Dixit VM (1997) Caspases: intracellular signaling by proteolysis. Cell 91:443-446

[63] Schouten GJ, Vertegaal AC, Whiteside ST, Israel A, Toebes M, Dorsman JC, van der Eb AJ, Zantema A (1997) IkappaB alpha is a target for the mitogen-activated 90 kDa ribosomal S6 kinase. EMBO J 16:3133-3144

[64] Shu HB, Takeuchi M, Goeddel DV (1996) The tumor necrosis factor receptor 2 signal transducers TRAF2 and c-IAP1 are components of the tumor necrosis factor receptor 1 signaling complex. Proc Natl Acad Sci USA 93:13973-13978

[65] Stehlik C, de Martin R, Binder BR, Lipp J (1998a) Cytokine induced expression of porcine inhibitor of apoptosis protein (iap) family member is regulated by NF-kappa B. Biochem Biophys Res Commun 243:827-832

[66] Stehlik C, de Martin R, Kumabashiri I, Schmid JA, Binder BR, Lipp J (1998b) Nuclear factor (NF)-kappaB-regulated X-chromosome-linked iap gene expression protects EC from tumor necrosis factor alpha-induced apoptosis. J Exp Med 188:211-216

[67] van Antwerp DJ, Martin SJ, Kafri T, Green D, Verma IM (1996) Suppression of TNF-alpha induced apoptosis by NF-kappaB. Science 274:787-789

[68] van Hinsbergh VW, Vermeer M, Koolwijk P, Grimbergen J, Kooistra T (1994) Genistein reduces tumor necrosis factor alpha-induced plasminogen activator inhibitor-1 transcription but not urokinase expression in human EC. Blood 84:2984-2991

[69] Wallach D (1997) Cell death induction by TNF: a matter of self control. Trends Biochem Sci 22(4):107-109

[70] Wang CY, Mayo MW, Baldwin AS, Jr. (1996) TNF- and cancer therapy-induced apoptosis: potentiation by inhibition of NF-kappaB. Science 274:784-787

[71] Waters C, Hancock D, Evan G (1990) Identification and characterisation of the egr-1 gene product as an inducible, short-lived, nuclear phosphoprotein. Oncogene 5:669-74

[72] Wertheimer SJ, Myers CL, Wallace RW, Parks TP (1992) Intercellular adhesion molecule-1 gene expression in human EC. Differential regulation by tumor necrosis factor-alpha and phorbol myristate acetate. J Biol Chem 267:12030-12035

[73] Whitley MZ, Thanos D, Read MA, Maniatis T, Collins T (1994) A striking similarity in the organization of the E-selectin and beta interferon gene promoters. Mol Cell Biol 14:6464-6475

[74] Wong GH, Elwell JH, Oberley LW, Goeddel DV (1989) Manganous superoxide dismutase is essential for cellular resistance to cytotoxicity of tumor necrosis factor. Cell 58:923-931

[75] Woronicz JD, Gao X, Cao Z, Rothe M, Goeddel DV (1997) IκB kinase-ß: NF-κB activation and complex formation with IκB kinase-α and NIK. Science 278:866-869

[76] Wrighton C, Hofer-Warbinek, R., Moll, T., Eytner, R., Bach, F.H. and de Martin, R. (1996) Inhibition of endothelial cell activation by adenovirus-mediated expression of IκBα, an inhibitor of the transcription factor NF-κB. J Exp Med 183:1013-1022

[77]   Yamaoka S, Courtois G, Bessia C, Whiteside ST, Weil R, Agou F, Kirk HE, Kay RJ, Israel A (1998) Complementation cloning of NEMO, a component of the IκB kinase complex essential for NF-κB activation. Cell 93:1231-1240

[78]   Yin M-Y, Christeron LB, Yamamoto Y, Kwak Y-T, Xu S, Mercurio F, Barbosa M, Cobb MH, Gaynor R (1988) HTLV-I Tax protein binds to MEKK1 to stimulate IκB kinase activity and NF-κB activation. Cell 93:875-884

[79]   Yu K, Morioka H, Fritze LM, Beeler DL, Jackman RW, Rosenberg RD (1992) Transcriptional regulation of the thrombomodulin gene. J Biol Chem 267:23237-23247

[80]   Yuan J (1997) Transducing signals of life and death. Curr Opin Cell Biol 9:247-251

[81]   Zandi E, Rothwarf DM, Delhase M, Hayakawa M, Karin M (1997) The IκB kinase complex (IKK) contains two kinase subunits, IKKα and IKKß, necessary for IκB phosphorylation and NF-κB activation. Cell 91:243-252

[82]   Zhang Y, Deng Y, Luther T, Muller M, Ziegler R, Waldherr R, Stern DM, Nawroth PP (1994) Tissue factor controls the balance of angiogenic and antiangiogenic properties of tumor cells in mice. J Clin Invest 94:1320-1327

[83]   Zhong H, SuYang H, Erdjument Bromage H, Tempst P, Ghosh S (1997) The transcriptional activity of NF-kappaB is regulated by the IkappaB-associated PKAc subunit through a cyclic AMP-independent mechanism. Cell 89:413-424

Vascular Endothelium: Mechanisms of Cell Signaling
J.D. Catravas et al. (Eds.)
IOS Press, 1999

CELLULAR AND MOLECULAR REGULATION OF TYPE II NITRIC OXIDE SYNTHASE EXPRESSION IN VASCULAR SMOOTH MUSCLE CELLS

Hanfang Zhang, Leslie Fuchs, Nandor Marczin, and John D. Catravas
Vascular Biology Center, Medical College of Georgia
Augusta, Georgia 30912-2500, USA

Abstract

The induction of Type II nitric oxide synthase (NOS) may play important roles in many pathologic events. High output of nitric oxide has been observed in the serum of septic patients and in animal models of sepsis, and may be responsible for the reduced in vascular reactivity to inotropes and hypotension observed in septic shock and as side-effects of cytokine therapy. Pretreatment with antisense oligonucleotide specific to Type II NOS significantly inhibits the lipopolysaccharide (LPS)-induced Type II NOS protein expression and activity in rat, as well as the LPS-induced vascular hyporeactivity to norepinephrine and congestion in the small mesenteric arteries of the small intestine. The induction of Type II NOS in rat vascular smooth muscle cells is significantly reduced by microtubule depolymerizing reagents, but not by microflament depolymerizing reagents. The regulation of Type II NOS induction by protein synthesis inhibitor is biphasic. At lower concentrations, cyclohexmide super-induces type II NOS expression by LPS, but at higher concentrations, it inhibits. The mechanisms of induction of Type II NOS are species-dependent. In marked contrast to mouse macrophage Type II NOS promoter, the downstream NF-κB site in rat vascular smooth muscle cells is not a crucial regulator of induction by cytokines and LPS. Instead, it requires the coexistence of at least two NF-κB sites and other elements in the 5'-flanking region of the gene.

1. Introduction

Nitric oxide (NO) plays important roles in the physiology and pathophysiology of nearly every organ system. NO is synthesized by one of three isozymes of nitric oxide synthase (NOS), each a product of a different gene. Type I and III NOS (or nNOS and eNOS, respectively) are constitutively expressed in neuronal and endothelial cells, respectively, and their activity is regulated by changes in intracellular calcium concentration [1, 2]. However, Type II NOS (or iNOS) is induced by immunomodulators, such as interleukin-1β (IL-1β), or bacterial lipopolysaccharide (LPS), and its activity is calcium independent

[3]. Type II NOS induction is implicated in many pathologic events, such as host defense against infections and tumors, inflammation, and autoimmune diseases. The up-regulation of Type II NOS in vascular smooth muscle cells by the immunomodulators results in high output of NO, and may be responsible for the cardiovascular collapse seen in septic shock [4-11] and in the side effects of anti-tumor therapy with cytokines [12-14]. Understanding the cellular and molecular mechanisms of Type II NOS induction will allow to propose and test pharmacological interventions aimed at preventing or reversing NO dysfunctions. Recent evidence suggests that the induction of Type II NOS may be species- and cell type-dependent. Exposure of rats to LPS has served as a useful model of septic shock, and the high output of NO by rat vascular smooth muscle cells may be important in the pathophysiology of septic shock. Herein, we will summarize evidence that Type II NOS induction is involved in the pathogenesis of septic shock, and review the cellular and molecular regulation of rat Type II NOS induction in rat vascular smooth muscle cells.

2. Septic Shock and Type II NOS Induction

Numerous studies have indicated that the induction of Type II NOS may participate in the pathogenesis of septic shock. Since Type II NOS lacks calcium regulation, it will produce NO continuously for the lifetime of the enzyme once it is induced in the vasculature [15, 16]. This results in overproduction of NO and persistent stimulation of soluble guanylate cyclase (sGC) causing prolonged smooth muscle relaxation. Increased serum levels of nitrite/nitrate, the stable products of NO, is found in animals [5, 17-19] and patients with septic shock [20-22], and Type II NOS mRNA is increased in aorta, pulmonary artery, and heart of animals injected with LPS [4, 23]. LPS and cytokines, IL-1β and TNF-α, inhibit vasoconstrictor-induced contractions of isolated vascular preparations in an endothelium-independent manner [6, 10, 24-29]. This impairment of contractility is associated with activation of sGC and increased production of cGMP [6, 24, 26-28]. The maximal force of contraction of carotid arterial rings in response to vasoconstrictors is reduced in LPS-treated wild-type mice, but not in LPS-treated Type II NOS-knockout mice. Further, the Type II NOS inhibitors improve contractile responses in LPS-treated wild-type mice. These data suggest that induction of Type II NOS mediates the impairment of vascular contraction after LPS treatment [29]. A number of studies have reported that NOS inhibitors inhibit LPS- or cytokine-induced hypotension in animal models of sepsis [5, 8, 30-35], and increase systemic vascular resistance and blood pressure in patients with septic shock [36-39]. While Laubach et al. reported that Type II NOS-knockout mice were not resistant to LPS-induced death [40], Wie et al. reported that Type II NOS-knockout mice were resistant to lipopolysaccharide-induced mortality [41]. MacMicking et al. further observed decreased early death and prevention of the fall in blood pressure in anesthetized Type II NOS-knockout mice, but not in conscious Type II NOS-knockout mice. The existence of both Type II NOS-dependent and Type II NOS-independent routes to LPS induced death was suggested [42].

In order to demonstrate Type II NOS induction in the pathogenesis of septic shock and to eliminate the non-specific inhibition of Type I and III NOS, we recently reported the effects of antisense oligonucleotide to Type II NOS on hemodynamic and vascular changes induced by LPS in rats [43]. Three groups received LPS (5 mg/kg iv) after one of the following pretreatments: 1) antisense (AS) oligonucleotide to Type II NOS; 2) mismatch (MM) oligonucleotide; and 3) saline, 12 and 24 hr before LPS. The fourth group received saline only as control. Type II NOS induction was determined by conversion of ^{3}H-L-arginine to ^{3}H-L-citrulline and by Western blot analysis. Figure 1

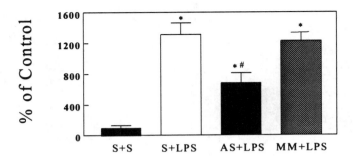

Figure 1. Conversion of ^{3}H-L-arginine to ^{3}H-L-citrulline illustrated as percentage of control (S+S) in lung homogenates from rats receiving S, LPS, AS, or MM oligonucleotides. Values represent means ± SE; n=6 rats per group. *p < 0.05 vs. S+S; #p < 0.05 vs. S+LPS.

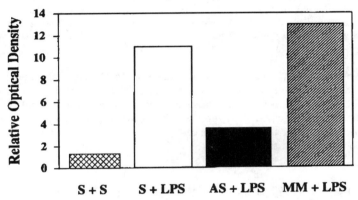

Figure 2. Expression of Type II NOS protein in aorta of rats receiving S, LPS, AS, or MM oligonucleotides. Type II NOS protein was quantitated by immunoblotting and densitometry. Values represent average optical density of Type II NOS obtained from 2 rats aorta per group.

shows that in lung homogenates, the control (Saline+Saline) group only generated 14.6±1.1 pmol of citulline /mg protein per 40 min of citulline (100%). A significant enhancement in the conversion of ^{3}H-L-arginine to ^{3}H-L- citrulline was observed in the LPS (Saline+LPS) group, compared to control. Pretreatment with antisence oligonucleotide to Type II NOS, but not mismatch oligonucleotide, inhibited the LPS-induced increase in ^{3}H-L-arginine to ^{3}H-L-citrulline conversion (Fig. 1). The expression of Type II NOS protein in aorta is shown in Figure 2. LPS increased Type II NOS protein expression, and the antisense oligonucleotide largely reduced Type II NOS protein expression in LPS-treated rats. After LPS injection, small mesentary arteries were isolated, and the vascular reactivity was studied in endothelium-denuded vessels. Figure 3 shows the effect of antisense and mismatch oligonucleotides on LPS-induced vascular hyporeactivity to norepinephrine (NE). The dose-response curve to NE was significantly shifted to the right, and the maximal contractile response was decreased compared with the saline+saline control group. Pretreatment with antisense oligonucleotide completely prevented the LPS-induced rightward shift and the decrease in the maximal contraction to NE. However, pretreatment with mismatch oligonucleotide did not prevent the LPS-

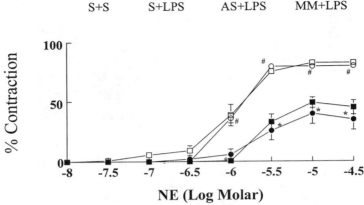

NE (Log Molar)

Figure 3. Dose-response curves to norepinephrine (NE) in small mesentric arteries from rats receiving S, LPS, AS, or MM oligonuleotides. Intraluminal diameter (in µm) in isolated vessels at 40 mmHg intraluminal pressure was 262 ± 24 in LPS group, 254 ± 16 in AS group, and 250 ± 10 in MM group. Values represent means $\pm$ SE; n=6 rats per group. *p < 0.05 vs. S+S; #p < 0.05 vs. S+LPS.

induced hyporeactivity to NE. Further, LPS caused significant congestion in the small mesenteric arteries of the small intestine in rats. The congestion was prevented by pretreatment with antisense but not mismatch oligonucleotide (data not shown) [43]. These studies strongly support the hypothesis that activation of the Type II NOS pathway is a major factor responsible for reduced contractile responsiveness of vessels and hypotension associated with septic shock.

3. Cytoskeletal Regulation of Type II NOS Induction in Vascular Smooth Muscle Cells

Two major components of the cytoskeleton system, microtubules and microfilaments, may play a pivotal role in the regulation of cell shape, intracellular transportation, secretion, and signal transduction [44]. Alterations in the microfilament structure stimulate the expression of certain proteolytic enzymes in fibroblasrs and LLC-PKI cells [45, 46]. Disassembly of microtubules increases the mitogenic activity of growth factors [47-50] and prevents gene expression of positive acute phase proteins in hepatocytes [51]. Depolymerization of microtubules is associated with activation of several genes, including urokinase type plasminogen activator [46, 52] and IL-1β [53, 54]. Moreover, microtubules may be involved in the release of TNF-α and in the regulation of TNF-α receptor in macrophages [55, 56].

In light of the relationship between the organization of the cytoskeletal apparatus of the cytoplasm and the activation of certain genes, we have investigated the role of microtubules and microfilaments in the regulation of Type II NOS induction in rat aortic smooth muscle cells (RASMC). Figure 4a shows that in vehicle-treated control cells, microtubules are abundant and frequently form bundles. Cells treated with the microtubule depolymerizing reagent, colchicine, however, are largely depleted from microtubules (Fig. 4c). Taxol, a plant-derived drug that enhances microtubule assembly, promotes the formation of dense bundles of microtubules (Fig. 4e) and prevents microtubule depolymerization induced by colchicine (Fig. 4g).

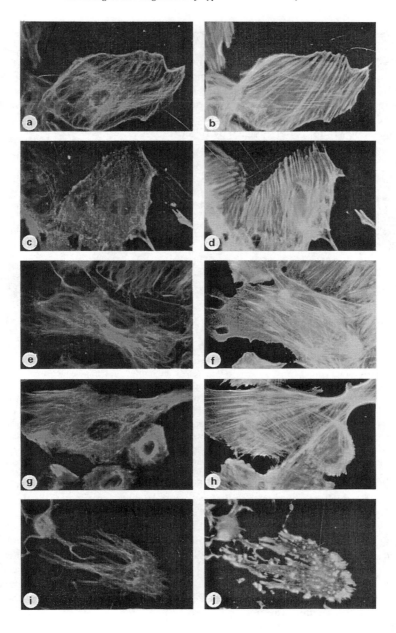

Figure 4. Modulation of microtubule and microfilament assembly in rat aortic smooth muscl cells. Shown are indirect anti-tubulin immunofluorescence images for β-tubulin (a, c, e, g, i and fluorescein phalloidin fluorescence images for actin filaments (b, d, f, h, j) of contro RASMC (a, b), or cells treated with colchicine (5 μM, c, d), taxol (10 μM, e, f) taxol+colchicine (g, h), and cytochalasin D (I, j).

Next, the effect of microtubule depolymerizing agents on the type II NOS induction was studied in RASMC. Neither nocodazole nor colchicine has an effect on basal cGMP levels. However, they significantly prevent the enhancement of cGMP induced by LPS (Fig. 5A), whereas they have virtually no effect on the cGMP increase elicited by the NO donor, sodium nitroprusside, suggesting that the effect of nocodazole and colchicine is not related to a direct action on sGC activity. Taxol, stabilizing the microtubule assembly, significantly prevents the inhibitory effects of nocodazole and colchicine on cGMP formation induced by LPS (Fig. 5A).

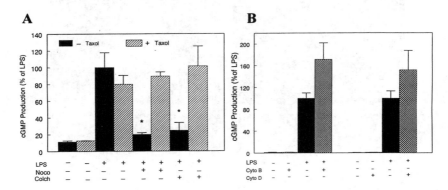

Figure 5. Panel A, effects of microtubule disassembly and stabilization on production o cGMP in rat aortic smooth muscle cells. Cells were chilled to 4°C, and incubated in th presence of vehicle, nocodazole (Noco, 1 μM) or colchicine (Colch, 10 μM) for 90 min Cells were then warmed to 37°C and incubated for additional 30 min prior to addition o LPS (1 μg) for 3 hr (solid columns). The effects of nocodazole or colchcine on the cGM production was reversed by microtubule stabilization reagent, taxol (10 μM) (hatche columns). **Panel B,** effects of microfilamen disassembly on the production of GMP i RASMC. Cells were incubated with vehicle or cytochalasin B or D (10 μM) for 60 mi prior to addition of LPS for 3 hr. *p< 0.05 from corresponding vehicle value.

Further, we investigate the effect of depolymerization of microfilaments on the Type II NOS induction. As shown in Figure 4i and 4j, the microfilament depolymerizing reagent, cytochalasin D changes the cell shape dramatically, and produces significant alterations in actin staining, by completely eliminating stress-fibre like structures. Despite the change in cell morphology, cytochalasin B and cytochalasin D do not inhibit the enhanced cGMP production induced by LPS (Fig. 5B). Moreover, neither microtubule depolymerizing reagents nor microfilament depolymerizing reagents affect Type III NOS activity in endothelial cells [57], suggesting a further difference between the inducible vs. the constitutive NO pathway. The differential regulation of the inducible and constitutive pathways by the dynamic assembly of microtubules might represent a basis for novel therapeutic treatment in septic shock. In contrast to our results, Fernandes et al. reported that in mouse macrophages depolymerizing microfilaments prevented the induction of Type II NOS, whereas microtubule depolymerizing reagent had a much smaller effect [58]. The discrepancy between our results in RASMC and that in macrophages may suggest that elements of cytoskeleton mediating the Type II NOS induction may vary in different cell types, or species.

A   **B**

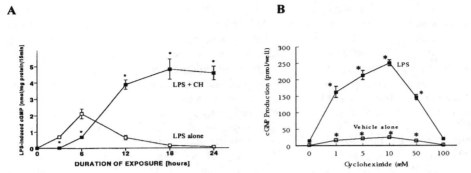

Figure 6. Panel A, Time-dependent effects of cycloheximide (CH) on LPS-induced cGMP production in rat aortic smooth muscle cells. Cells were incubated with LPS alone or LPS in combination with CH (10 μM). At the indicated time point, the production of cGMP was analyzed. *p< 0.05 compared to corresponding LPS value. **Panel B,** Concentration-dependent effects of CH on LPS-induced cGMP production in RASMC. Different concentrations of CH were incubated with or without LPS for 24 hr, and then the production of cGMP was analyzed. *p< 0.05 compared to control values in the absence of CH.

4. Protein Synthesis Inhibition and Type II Nos Induction in Vascular Smooth Muscle Cells

Cultured vascular smooth muscle cells do not express type II NOS protein at rest, and it is suggested that cytokine-induced expression of Type II NOS requires new protein synthesis, since inhibition of protein synthesis by cyclohexmide (CH) prevents the release of NO and formation of cGMP [6, 24, 27]. While investigating the induction of Type II NOS in vascular smooth muscle cells, we observed increased cGMP levels after CH exposure [59] (Fig. 6A). In response to LPS alone, cGMP accumulation peak after 6 hr and steadily declines over the next 18 hr. When LPS is combined with CH, the short-term LPS-induced Type II NOS activity is inhibited. Further, Type II NOS activity increases beyond the peak reached by LPS stimulation alone and remains elevated for 24 hr (Fig. 6A). Figure 6B show that the regulation by CH of Type II NOS induction is biphasic. At lower concentrations, CH super-induces Type II NOS expression by LPS, but at higher concentrations, it inhibits the induction by LPS. We hypothesize that at low concentration, CH may interfere with a negatively regulating repressor mechanism that is normally responsible for offsetting LPS- or cytokine-induced NO synthesis in vascular smooth muscle cells, and this mechanism is more sensitive to CH inhibition than Type II NOS protein synthesis. The mechanism by which CH super-induces Type II NOS induction by LPS may be at the transcriptional level since low concentrations of protein synthesis inhibitor enhance Type II NOS promoter activity in the macrophage cell line, RAW 264.7 [60] and super-induce NF-κB binding activity in the pre-B cell line, epithelial cell line, and hepatocytes stimulated by LPS or cytokines [61-63].

5. Induction of the Rat Type Ii Nos Promoter in Vascular Smooth Muscle Cells

One of the required transcription factors responsible for cytokine-, and LPS-induced Type II NOS induction appears to be NF-κB [16, 64], and the activation of NF-κB in sepsis has been reported in human [65] and animals [19]. In most cells, NF-κB is present in a non-

DNA binding form in the cytoplasm. This complex is composed of two DNA binding proteins and a third inhibitory subunit, IκB [66-68]. The latter inhibits DNA binding of NF-κB and appears to be responsible for the cytoplasmic localization of the complex [69]. Covalent modification through phosphorylation and subsequent degradation of IκB appears to trigger the release of NF-κB with DNA binding activity [70, 71].

The molecular mechanisms and the potential importance of NF-κB in Type II NOS induction have been studied by cloning the mouse Type II NOS promoter and expressing of the promoter-reporter gene constructs in a cultured mouse macrophage cell line, RAW 264.7 [64, 72-75]. The fully functional promoter of the mouse Type II NOS is 1.0 kb size with Region I (-48 to -209) as the core promoter and Region II (-913 to -1029) as the enhancer, since Region II is orientation and distance independent [76]. It has been demonstrated, by progressive deletion from the 5'-end of the promoter, that the construct up to -85bp, containing a downstream NF-κB binding site confers the inducibility of the Type II NOS promoter by LPS in a dose-dependent manner [74]. The region -890 to -1002bp, containing the upstream NF-κB site was also important for the full Type II NOS promoter activity [64, 77]. Moreover, site-directed mutagenesis and deletion experiments showed that either NF-κB site has significant inducibility in response to LPS and cytokines, and that two NF-κB sites in those two regions confer the full promoter activity. Interferon regulatory factor-1 (IRF-1) binding sites in the upstream region are responsible for the synergistic effect of IFN-γ with LPS [78, 79]. It has also been reported that pyrrolidine dithiocarbamate (PDTC), an inhibitor of NF-κB, diminishes the ability of macrophages to produce NO in response to LPS and cytokines [80].

Unlike the mouse Type II NOS gene promoter, construct up to -1.09 [75], or -3.8 [81] of the 5'-flanking region of the human Type II NOS gene, containing a functional NF-κB binding site, do not respond well to LPS or cytokines. Recently, promoter analysis of the human Type II NOS showed that the first -3.8 kb upstream of the gene resulted in only basal promoter activity and demonstrated at most a slight response to cytokines. A three to five-fold induction was found in promoter segments containing up to -5.8 and -7.0 kb, and a ten-fold activation was observed in a construct containing -16 kb of the promoter [81]. The same group recently reported that a NF-κB site at -5.8 kb, with a cluster of additional four NF-κB sites located at -3.8 to -7.2 kb, may be important in the induction of human Type II NOS. However, the inducibility of the mutant at this -5.8 kb NF-κB site was decreased by only 37% [82], indicating that other elements in the promoter may be required together with NF-κB for full promoter induction. The remarkable difference between human and mouse in the promoter structure suggests species-dependent differences in Type II NOS induction.

The 5'-regions of the rat Type II NOS gene were recently published [83, 84]. The -1.7 kb rat Type II NOS promoter was transfected into Swiss 3T3 fibroblasts, and induced by IL-1β. Only a three-fold induction was observed which is very low for Type II NOS. Subsequently, the same group showed that -526 bp from the transcription starting site conferred the same inducibility to IL-1β as the -1.7 kb, with about three fold induction in mesangial cells [85], indicating that the down stream NF-κB site may be crucial.

We recently cloned the -3.2 kb and -5.1 kb of the 5'-region of the rat Type II NOS gene [84]. The DNA fragments were linked to a luciferase-containing vector (PGL3-Basic). We have employed a homologous system (rat type II NOS promoter in rat aortic smooth muscle cells) to eliminate possible species differences in the regulation of the gene. To study the transcriptional regulation of the rat Type II NOS gene promoter, constructs containing different lengths of the 5'-flanking region of Type II NOS were prepared and transfected into RASMC. Promoter activities were studied after 6 hr. of exposure to cytokine mix (IL-1β + TNF-α) or LPS. The PGL3-Basic DNA construct (without any promoter and enhancer) exhibited 38±9 light units of luciferase activity, and all five Type II NOS promoter-reporter constructs (Fig. 7) exhibited similar basal activities (41 to 59 light units). The basal activities of PGL3-basic and the five promoter-reporter constructs were not statistically different from each other (p = 0.45 by ANOVA). The

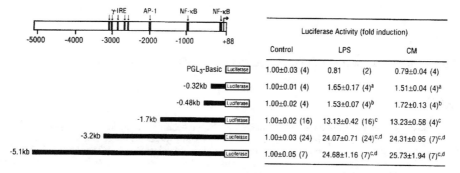

	Luciferase Activity (fold induction)		
	Control	LPS	CM
PGL₃-Basic [Luciferase]	1.00±0.03 (4)	0.81 (2)	0.79±0.04 (4)
-0.32kb ▬[Luciferase]	1.00±0.01 (4)	1.65±0.17 (4)ᵃ	1.51±0.04 (4)ᵃ
-0.48kb ▬▬[Luciferase]	1.00±0.02 (4)	1.53±0.07 (4)ᵇ	1.72±0.13 (4)ᵇ
-1.7kb ▬▬▬▬[Luciferase]	1.00±0.02 (16)	13.13±0.42 (16)ᶜ	13.23±0.58 (4)ᶜ
-3.2kb ▬▬▬▬▬[Luciferase]	1.00±0.03 (24)	24.07±0.71 (24)ᶜ,ᵈ	24.31±0.95 (7)ᶜ,ᵈ
-5.1kb ▬▬▬▬▬▬[Luciferase]	1.00±0.05 (7)	24.68±1.16 (7)ᶜ,ᵈ	25.73±1.94 (7)ᶜ,ᵈ

Figure 7. Inducibility of different length rat Type II NOS promoter constructs in response to LPS or CM in rat aortic smooth muscle cells. The constructs containing different lengths of the 5'-flanking region of Type II NOS gene are shown on the left with certain restriction sites and transcription factor binding sites identified. Each construct DNA was transfected into RASMC. Luciferase activity was determined in RASMC incubated with LPS (5 μg/ml) or a cytokine mixture (CM) for 6 hr. following the transfection of the constructs. Data are expressed as fold induction from the respective unstimulated controls. Means ± S.E (number of determinations). a, p < 0.0002 vs controls; b, p < 0.01 vs controls; c, p< 0.0002 vs control; and d, p < 0.0004 vs the -1.7 kb construct.

PGL3-Basic DNA construct did not respond to stimulation by cytokine mix or LPS, and the -316 bp and -484 bp constructs, containing a single NF-κB site, with sequence identical to the corresponding regions of the -3.2 kb construct, responded only slightly to either cytokine mix or LPS (Fig. 7). However, the -1.7 kb construct exhibited a 13-fold increase in luciferase activity in response to LPS or cytokine mix (CM), whereas both the -3.2 kb and -5.1 kb constructs produced a 24- fold induction in luciferase activity in response to CM or LPS (Fig. 7), indicating that the 1.9 kb upstream of -3.2 kb may not be important in rat Type II NOS regulation. Our data differ from those of Eberhardt et al. in which the -1.7 kb rat iNOS promoter shows only three-fold induction in response to IL-1 [83, 85]. The most likely reason for this difference may lie in the Swiss 3T3 fibroblasts and mesangial cells used by Eberhardt et al. to study the induction of the rat iNOS promoter construct. These two cell types may exhibit different mechanisms of inducibility from those of RASMC and may not be suitable for studying Type II NOS induction.

6. Conclusion

The induction of Type II NOS and subsequent high output of NO may play important roles in many pathologic events. The up-regulation of Type II NOS in vascular smooth muscle cells by LPS and cytokines may be responsible for the cardiovascular collapse observed in septic shock and in the side effects of anti-tumor therapy with cytokines. The regulation of Type II NOS induction is complex, and it may be species and cell type dependent. In rat vascular smooth muscle cells, the regulation of Type II NOS induction may involve in the microtubule system, and a labile protein which is very sensitive to the low concentrations of protein synthesis inhibitors. In contrast to mouse Type II NOS promoter, the co-existence of two NF-κB sites in the rat promoter are necessary for the full induction of the gene. Understanding the cellular and molecular mechanisms of Type II NOS induction will allow to propose and test pharmacological interventions aimed at preventing or reversing NO dysfunctions.

Acknowledgements

This work was supported by grant HL52958 from the NHLBI of the NIH.

References

[1] Mayer B, Schmidt K, Humbert P and Bohme E, Biosynthesis of endothelium-derived relaxing factor: a cytosolic enzyme in porcine aortic endothelial cells Ca^{2+}-dependently converts L-arginine into an activator of soluble guanylyl cyclase. *Biochem. Biophys. Res. Commun.* **164**(2): 678-85, 1989.

[2] Busse R and Mulsch A, Calcium-dependent nitric oxide synthesis in endothelial cytosol is mediated by calmodulin. *FEBS. Lett.* **265**(1-2): 133-6, 1990.

[3] Nathan C and Xie QW, Nitric oxide synthases: roles, tolls, and controls. *Cell* **78**(6): 915-8, 1994.

[4] Weigert AL, Higa EM, Niederberger M, McMurtry IF, Raynolds M and Schrier RW, Expression and preferential inhibition of inducible nitric oxide synthase in aortas of endotoxemic rats. *J. Am. Soc. Nephrol.* **5**(12): 2067-72, 1995.

[5] Kilbourn RG, Jubran A, Gross SS, Griffith OW, Levi R, Adams J and Lodato RF, Reversal of endotoxin-mediated shock by NG-methyl-L-arginine, an inhibitor of nitric oxide synthesis. *Biochem. Biophys. Res. Commun.* **172**(3): 1132-8, 1990.

[6] Beasley D, Schwartz JH and Brenner BM, Interleukin 1 induces prolonged L-arginine-dependent cyclic guanosine monophosphate and nitrite production in rat vascular smooth muscle cells. *J. Clin. Invest.* **87**(2): 602-8, 1991.

[7] Beasley D, Cohen RA and Levinsky NG, Endotoxin inhibits contraction of vascular smooth muscle in vitro. *Am. J. Physiol.* **258**(4 Pt 2): H1187-92, 1990.

[8] Szabo C, Southan GJ and Thiemermann C, Beneficial effects and improved survival in rodent models of septic shock with S-methylisothiourea sulfate, a potent and selective inhibitor of inducible nitric oxide synthase. *Proc. Natl. Acad. Sci. USA* **91**(26): 12472-6, 1994.

[9] Szabo C, Mitchell JA, Thiemermann C and Vane JR, Nitric oxide-mediated hyporeactivity to noradrenaline precedes the induction of nitric oxide synthase in endotoxin shock. *Brit. J. Pharmacol.* **108**(3): 786-92, 1993.

[10] Umans JG, Wylam ME, Samsel RW, Edwards J and Schumacker PT, Effects of endotoxin in vivo on endothelial and smooth-muscle function in rabbit and rat aorta. *Am. Rev. Respir. Dis.* **148**(6 Pt 1): 1638-45, 1993.

[11] McKenna TM, Prolonged exposure of rat aorta to low levels of endotoxin in vitro results in impaired contractility. Association with vascular cytokine release. *J. Clin. Invest.* **86**(1): 160-8, 1990.

[12] Shahidi H and Kilbourn RG, The role of nitric oxide in interleukin-2 therapy induced hypotension. *Cancer Metast. Rev.* **17**(1): 119-26, 1998.

[13] Hibbs JB, Jr., Westenfelder C, Taintor R, Vavrin Z, Kablitz C, Baranowski RL, Ward JH, Menlove RL, McMurry MP, Kushner JP and et al., Evidence for cytokine-inducible nitric oxide synthesis from L-arginine in patients receiving interleukin-2 therapy. *J. Clin. Invest.* **89**(3): 867-77, 1992.

[14] Ochoa JB, Curti B, Peitzman AB, Simmons RL, Billiar TR, Hoffman R, Rault R, Longo DL, Urba WJ and Ochoa AC, Increased circulating nitrogen oxides after human tumor immunotherapy: correlation with toxic hemodynamic changes. *J. Natl. Cancer Inst.* **84**(11): 864-7, 1992.

[15] Knowles RG and Moncada S, Nitric oxide as a signal in blood vessels. *Trends Biochem. Sci.* **17**(10): 399-402, 1992.

[16] Xie Q and Nathan C, The high-output nitric oxide pathway: role and regulation. *J. Leukoc. Biol.* **56**(5): 576-82, 1994.

[17] Cunha FQ, Assreuy J, Moss DW, Rees D, Leal LM, Moncada S, Carrier M, CA OD and Liew FY, Differential induction of nitric oxide synthase in various organs of the mouse during endotoxaemia: role of TNF-alpha and IL-1-beta. *Immunology* **81**(2): 211-5, 1994.

[18] Lai CS and Komarov AM, Spin trapping of nitric oxide produced in vivo in septic-shock mice. *FEBS. Lett.* **345**(2-3): 120-4, 1994.

[19] Liu SF, Ye X and Malik AB, In vivo inhibition of nuclear factor-kappa B activation prevents inducible nitric oxide synthase expression and systemic hypotension in a rat model of septic shock. *J. Immunol.* **159**(8): 3976-83, 1997.

[20] Ochoa JB, Udekwu AO, Billiar TR, Curran RD, Cerra FB, Simmons RL and Peitzman AB, Nitrogen oxide levels in patients after trauma and during sepsis. *Ann. Surg.* **214**(5): 621-6, 1991.

[21] Goode HF, Howdle PD, Walker BE and Webster NR, Nitric oxide synthase activity is increased in patients with sepsis syndrome. *Clin. Sci.* **88**(2): 131-3, 1995.

[22] Wong HR, Carcillo JA, Burckart G, Shah N and Janosky JE, Increased serum nitrite and nitrate concentrations in children with the sepsis syndrome. *Crit. Care Med.* **23**(5): 835-42, 1995.

[23] Liu SF, Barnes PJ and Evans TW, Time course and cellular localization of lipopolysaccharide-induced inducible nitric oxide synthase messenger RNA expression in the rat in vivo. *Crit. Care Med.* **25**(3): 512-8, 1997.

[24] Beasley D, Cohen RA and Levinsky NG, Interleukin 1 inhibits contraction of vascular smooth muscle. *J. Clin. Invest.* **83**(1): 331-5, 1989.

[25] Fleming I, Gray GA, Julou-Schaeffer G, Parratt JR and Stoclet JC, Incubation with endotoxin activates the L-arginine pathway in vascular tissue. *Biochem. Biophys. Res. Commun.* **171**(2): 562-8, 1990.

[26] Beasley D, Interleukin 1 and endotoxin activate soluble guanylate cyclase in vascular smooth muscle. *Am. J. Physiol.* **259**(1 Pt 2): R38-44, 1990.

[27] Busse R and Mulsch A, Induction of nitric oxide synthase by cytokines in vascular smooth muscle cells. *FEBS. Lett.* **275**(1-2): 87-90, 1990.

[28] Schini VB, Junquero DC, Scott-Burden T and Vanhoutte PM, Interleukin-1 beta induces the production of an L-arginine-derived relaxing factor from cultured smooth muscle cells from rat aorta. *Biochem. Biophys. Res. Commun.* **176**(1): 114-21, 1991.

[29] Gunnett CA, Chu Y, Heistad DD, Loihl A and Faraci FM, Vascular effects of LPS in mice deficient in expression of the gene for inducible nitric oxide synthase. *Am. J. Physiol.* **275**(2 Pt 2): H416-21, 1998.

[30] Kilbourn RG, Gross SS, Jubran A, Adams J, Griffith OW, Levi R and Lodato RF, NG-methyl-L-arginine inhibits tumor necrosis factor-induced hypotension: implications for the involvement of nitric oxide. *Proc. Natl. Acad. Sci. USA* **87**(9): 3629-32, 1990.

[31] Thiemermann C and Vane J, Inhibition of nitric oxide synthesis reduces the hypotension induced by bacterial lipopolysaccharides in the rat in vivo. *Eur. J. Pharmacol.* **182**(3): 591-5, 1990.

[32] Hollenberg SM, Cunnion RE and Zimmerberg J, Nitric oxide synthase inhibition reverses arteriolar hyporesponsiveness to catecholamines in septic rats. *Am. J. Physiol.* **264**(2 Pt 2): H660-3, 1993.

[33] Tracey WR, Nakane M, Basha F and Carter G, In vivo pharmacological evaluation of two novel type II (inducible) nitric oxide synthase inhibitors. *Can. J. Physiol. Pharm.* **73**(5): 665-9, 1995.

[34] Perrella MA, Hsieh CM, Lee WS, Shieh S, Tsai JC, Patterson C, Lowenstein CJ, Long NC, Haber E, Shore S and Lee ME, Arrest of endotoxin-induced hypotension by transforming growth factor beta1. *Proc. Natl. Acad. Sci. USA* **93**(5): 2054-9, 1996.

[35] Liaudet L, Feihl F, Rosselet A, Markert M, Hurni JM and Perret C, Beneficial effects of L-canavanine, a selective inhibitor of inducible nitric oxide synthase, during rodent endotoxaemia. *Clin. Sci.* **90**(5): 369-77, 1996.

[36] Petros A, Bennett D and Vallance P, Effect of nitric oxide synthase inhibitors on hypotension in patients with septic shock. *Lancet* **338**(8782-8783): 1557-8, 1991.

[37] Schilling J, Cakmakci M, Battig U and Geroulanos S, A new approach in the treatment of hypotension in human septic shock by NG-monomethyl-L-arginine, an inhibitor of the nitric oxide synthetase. *Intens. Care Med.* **19**(4): 227-31, 1993.

[38] Petros A, Lamb G, Leone A, Moncada S, Bennett D and Vallance P, Effects of a nitric oxide synthase inhibitor in humans with septic shock. *Cardiovasc. Res.* **28**(1): 34-9, 1994.

[39] Ketteler M, Cetto C, Kirdorf M, Jeschke GS, Schafer JH and Distler A, Nitric oxide in sepsis-syndrome: potential treatment of septic shock by nitric oxide synthase antagonists. *Kidney Int.- Suppl.* **64**: S27-30, 1998.

[40] Laubach VE, Shesely EG, Smithies O and Sherman PA, Mice lacking inducible nitric oxide synthase are not resistant to lipopolysaccharide-induced death. *Proc. Natl. Acad. Sci. USA* **92**(23): 10688-92, 1995.

[41] Wei XQ, Charles IG, Smith A, Ure J, Feng GJ, Huang FP, Xu D, Muller W, Moncada S and Liew FY, Altered immune responses in mice lacking inducible nitric oxide synthase. *Nature* **375**(6530): 408-11, 1995.

[42] MacMicking JD, Nathan C, Hom G, Chartrain N, Fletcher DS, Trumbauer M, Stevens K, Xie QW, Sokol K, Hutchinson N and et al., Altered responses to bacterial infection and endotoxic shock in mice lacking inducible nitric oxide synthase. *Cell* **81**(4): 641-50, 1995.

[43] Hoque AM, Papapetropoulos A, Venema RC, Catravas JD and Fuchs LC, Effects of antisense oligonucleotide to iNOS on hemodynamic and vascular changes induced by LPS. *Am. J. Physiol.* **275**(3 Pt 2): H1078-83, 1998.

[44] Bershadaky AD and Vasiliev JM, Cytoskeleton and internal organization of the cell. In: *cytoskeleton* (Eds. Bershadaky AD and Vasiliev JM), pp. 167-201. Plenum Press, New York, 1989.

[45] Unemori EN and Werb Z, Reorganization of polymerized actin: a possible trigger for induction of procollagenase in fibroblasts cultured in and on collagen gels. *J. Cell Biol.* **103**(3): 1021-31, 1986.

[46] Botteri FM, Ballmer-Hofer K, Rajput B and Nagamine Y, Disruption of cytoskeletal structures results in the induction of the urokinase-type plasminogen activator gene expression. *J. Biol. Chem.* **265**(22): 13327-34, 1990.

[47] Crossin KL and Carney DH, Evidence that microtubule depolymerization early in the cell cycle is sufficient to initiate DNA synthesis. *Cell* **23**(1): 61-71, 1981.

[48] Crossin KL and Carney DH, Microtubule stabilization by taxol inhibits initiation of DNA synthesis by thrombin and by epidermal growth factor. *Cell* **27**(2 Pt 1): 341-50, 1981.

[49] Otto AM, Microtubules and the regulation of DNA synthesis in fibroblastic cells. (A minireview). *Cell Biol. Int.* **6**(1): 1-18, 1982.

[50] Otto AM and Jimenez de Asua L, Microtubule-disrupting agents can independently affect the prereplicative period and the entry into S phase stimulated by prostaglandin F2 alpha and fibroblastic growth factor. *J. Cell. Physiol.* **115**(1): 15-22, 1983.

[51] Carter KC, Cooper R, Papaconstantinou J and Ritchie DG, Microtubule depolymerization inhibits the regulation of alpha 1-acid glycoprotein mRNA by hepatocyte stimulating factor. *J. Biol. Chem.* **264**(1): 515-9, 1989.

[52] Lee JS, von der Ahe D, Kiefer B and Nagamine Y, Cytoskeletal reorganization and TPA differently modify AP-1 to induce the urokinase-type plasminogen activator gene in LLC-PK1 cells. *Nucleic Acids Res.* **21**(15): 3365-72, 1993.

[53] Manie S, Schmid-Alliana A, Kubar J, Ferrua B and Rossi B, Disruption of microtubule network in human monocytes induces expression of interleukin-1 but not that of interleukin-6 nor tumor necrosis factor-alpha. Involvement of protein kinase A stimulation. *J. Biol. Chem.* **268**(18): 13675-81, 1993.

[54] Ferrua B, Manie S, Doglio A, Shaw A, Sonthonnax S, Limouse M and Schaffar L, Stimulation of human interleukin 1 production and specific mRNA expression by microtubule-disrupting drugs. *Cell. Immunol.* **131**(2): 391-7, 1990.

[55] Ding AH, Porteu F, Sanchez E and Nathan CF, Downregulation of tumor necrosis factor receptors on macrophages and endothelial cells by microtubule depolymerizing agents. *J. Exp. Med.* **171**(3): 715-27, 1990.

[56] Ding AH, Porteu F, Sanchez E and Nathan CF, Shared actions of endotoxin and taxol on TNF receptors and TNF release. *Science* **248**(4953): 370-2, 1990.

[57] Marczin N, Jilling T, Papapetropoulos A, Go C and Catravas JD, Cytoskeleton-dependent activation of the inducible nitric oxide synthase in cultured aortic smooth muscle cells. *Brit. J. Pharmacol.* **118**(5): 1085-94, 1996.

[58] Fernandes PD, Araujo HM, Riveros-Moreno V and Assreuy J, Depolymerization of macrophage microfilaments prevents induction and inhibits activity of nitric oxide synthase. *Eur. J. Cell Biol.* **71**(4): 356-62, 1996.

[59] Marczin N, Go CY, Papapetropoulos A and Catravas JD, Induction of nitric oxide synthase by protein synthesis inhibition in aortic smooth muscle cells. *Br J Pharmacol* **123**(5): 1000-8, 1998.

[60] Oguchi S, Weisz A and Esumi H, Enhancement of inducible-type NO synthase gene transcription by protein synthesis inhibitors. Activation of an intracellular signal transduction pathway by low concentrations of cycloheximide. *FEBS. Lett.* **338**(3): 326-30, 1994.

[61] Sen R and Baltimore D, Inducibility of kappa immunoglobulin enhancer-binding protein NF-kappa B by a posttranslational mechanism. *Cell* **47**(6): 921-8, 1986.

[62] Menegazzi M, Guerriero C, Carcereri de Prati A, Cardinale C, Suzuki H and Armato U, TPA and cycloheximide modulate the activation of NF-kappa B and the induction and stability of nitric oxide synthase transcript in primary neonatal rat hepatocytes. *FEBS. Lett.* **379**(3): 279-85, 1996.

[63] Newton R, Adcock IM and Barnes PJ, Superinduction of NF-kappa B by actinomycin D and cycloheximide in epithelial cells. *Biochem. Biophys. Res. Commun.* **218**(2): 518-23, 1996.

[64] Spink J, Cohen J and Evans TJ, The cytokine responsive vascular smooth muscle cell enhancer of inducible nitric oxide synthase. Activation by nuclear factor-kappa B. *J. Biol. Chem.* **270**(49): 29541-7, 1995.

[65]   Bohrer H, Qiu F, Zimmermann T, Zhang Y, Jllmer T, Mannel D, Bottiger BW, Stern DM, Waldherr R, Saeger HD, Ziegler R, Bierhaus A, Martin E and Nawroth PP, Role of NFkappaB in the mortality of sepsis. *J. Clin. Invest.* **100**(5): 972-85, 1997.

[66]   Urban MB, Schreck R and Baeuerle PA, NF-kappa B contacts DNA by a heterodimer of the p50 and p65 subunit. *EMBO J.* **10**(7): 1817-25, 1991.

[67]   Siebenlist U, Franzoso G and Brown K, Structure, regulation and function of NF-kappa B. *Annu. Rev. Cell Biol.* **10**: 405-55, 1994.

[68]   Baeuerle PA and Baltimore D, I kappa B: a specific inhibitor of the NF-kappa B transcription factor. *Science* **242**(4878): 540-6, 1988.

[69]   Baeuerle PA and Baltimore D, Activation of DNA-binding activity in an apparently cytoplasmic precursor of the NF-kappa B transcription factor. *Cell* **53**(2): 211-7, 1988.

[70]   Ghosh S and Baltimore D, Activation in vitro of NF-kappa B by phosphorylation of its inhibitor I kappa B. *Nature* **344**(6267): 678-82, 1990.

[71]   Brown K, Park S, Kanno T, Franzoso G and Siebenlist U, Mutual regulation of the transcriptional activator NF-kappa B and its inhibitor, I kappa B-alpha. *Proc. Natl. Acad. Sci. USA* **90**(6): 2532-6, 1993.

[72]   Lowenstein CJ, Alley EW, Raval P, Snowman AM, Snyder SH, Russell SW and Murphy WJ, Macrophage nitric oxide synthase gene: two upstream regions mediate induction by interferon gamma and lipopolysaccharide. *Proc. Natl. Acad. Sci. USA* **90**(20): 9730-4, 1993.

[73]   Xie QW, Whisnant R and Nathan C, Promoter of the mouse gene encoding calcium-independent nitric oxide synthase confers inducibility by interferon gamma and bacterial lipopolysaccharide. *J. Exp. Med.* **177**(6): 1779-84, 1993.

[74]   Xie QW, Kashiwabara Y and Nathan C, Role of transcription factor NF-kappa B/Rel in induction of nitric oxide synthase. *J. Biol. Chem.* **269**(7): 4705-8, 1994.

[75]   Kleinert H, Euchenhofer C, Ihrig-Biedert I and Forstermann U, Glucocorticoids inhibit the induction of nitric oxide synthase II by down-regulating cytokine-induced activity of transcription factor nuclear factor-kappa B. *Mol. Pharmacol.* **49**(1): 15-21, 1996.

[76]   Alley EW, Murphy WJ and Russell SW, A classical enhancer element responsive to both lipopolysaccharide and interferon-gamma augments induction of the iNOS gene in mouse macrophages. *Gene* **158**(2): 247-51, 1995.

[77]   Kim YM, Lee BS, Yi KY and Paik SG, Upstream NF-kappaB site is required for the maximal expression of mouse inducible nitric oxide synthase gene in interferon-gamma plus lipopolysaccharide-induced RAW 264.7 macrophages. *Biochem. Biophys. Res. Commun.* **236**(3): 655-60, 1997.

[78]   Martin E, Nathan C and Xie QW, Role of interferon regulatory factor 1 in induction of nitric oxide synthase. *J. Exp. Med.* **180**(3): 977-84, 1994.

[79]   Spink J and Evans T, Binding of the transcription factor interferon regulatory factor-1 to the inducible nitric-oxide synthase promoter. *J. Biol. Chem.* **272**(39): 24417-25, 1997.

[80]   Schreck R, Meier B, Mannel DN, Droge W and Baeuerle PA, Dithiocarbamates as potent inhibitors of nuclear factor kappa B activation in intact cells. *J. Exp. Med.* **175**(5): 1181-94, 1992.

[81]   De Vera ME, Shapiro RA, Nussler AK, Mudgett JS, Simmons RL, Morris SM, Jr., Billiar TR and Geller DA, Transcriptional regulation of human inducible nitric oxide synthase (NOS2) gene by cytokines: initial analysis of the human NOS2 promoter. *Proc. Natl. Acad. Sci. USA* **93**(3): 1054-9, 1996.

[82]   Taylor BS, de Vera ME, Ganster RW, Wang Q, Shapiro RA, Morris SM, Jr., Billiar TR and Geller DA, Multiple NF-kappaB enhancer elements regulate cytokine induction of the human inducible nitric oxide synthase gene. *J. Biol. Chem.* **273**(24): 15148-56, 1998.

[83]   Eberhardt W, Kunz D, Hummel R and Pfeilschifter J, Molecular cloning of the rat inducible nitric oxide synthase gene promoter. *Biochem. Biophys. Res. Commun.* **223**(3): 752-6, 1996.

[84]   Zhang H, Chen X, Teng X, Snead C and Catravas JD, Molecular cloning and analysis of the rat inducible nitric oxide sythase gene promoter in aortic smooth muscle cells. *Biochem. Pharmacol.* **55**: 1873-1880, 1998.

[85]   Eberhartt W, Pluss C, Hummel R and Pfeilschifter J, Molecular mechanisms of inducible nitric oxide synthase gene expression by IL-1 and cAMP in rat mesangial cells. *J. Immunol.* **160**: 4961-4969, 1998.

Vascular Endothelium: Mechanisms of Cell Signaling
J.D. Catravas et al. (Eds.)
IOS Press, 1999

ALLOGENEIC AND XENOGENEIC INTERACTIONS BETWEEN ENDOTHELIAL CELLS AND HUMAN T CELLS DURING TRANSPLANT REJECTION

Marlene L. Rose

Department of Cardiac Surgery, National Heart and Lung Institute, Imperial College School of Medicine, Heart Science Centre, Harefield Hospital, Harefield, Middlesex, UB9 6JH, UK

Abstract

Human and porcine endothelial cells express on their cell surfaces many of the molecules, which can cause activation of T cells. Of particular importance is expression of Major Class II Histocompatibilty (HLA- DR, DP and DQ) molecules which are essential for activation of CD4 + T cells and subsequent maturation of the various effector mechanisms leading to allograft rejection. Cells which cause activation of resting CD4+ T cells are called Antigen Presenting Cells (APCs); the essential pre-requisite for APCs are expression of MHC class II molecules and accessory molecules which interact with T ligands. It is established that dendritic cells, monocytes and B cells are APC but in humans many parenchymal cells such as fibroblasts, smooth muscle cells and epithelial cells can be induced to express MHC class II antigens by IFNγ. Data is presented which shows that both human and porcine endothelial cells, but not other parenchymal cells, act as APC and stimulate resting CD4+ T cells, however they utilise different second signals. Human and endothelial cells use LFA/3 whereas porcine endothelial cells present CD86 to human T cells. Porcine CD86 and porcine MHC class II molecules are recognised by human T cells and results in vigorous T cell activation and production of Interleukin-2. There is some compatibility between human cytokines and porcine endothelial cells; thus IFNγ is species specific but human TNFα induces MHC class II, VCAM-1, and CD86 on porcine endothelial cells. It is highly likely that human and porcine endothelial cells will directly interact and activate recipient T cells after allogeneic or xenogeneic implantation.

Approximately 36,000 allogeneic transplants are performed throughout the world each year, of which the majority are kidney transplants. About 5,000 hearts, 6,500 livers and 1,200 lung transplant are performed. Solid organ transplantation has become so successful that the number of available human donors cannot meet the demand. One solution to this problem is to use donors from another species (i.e. xenogeneic donors). Pigs are the species of choice, being physiologically similar to humans and ethically more acceptable than primates. The existence of naturally occurring human IgM antibodies to glycosylated residues on pig endothelial cells, mediating hyperacute rejection of pig organs perfused with human blood, was the initial barrier to using pigs as organ donors for human beings. However, use of transgenic pigs and other strategies to reduce antibody-mediated rejection are likely to overcome this particular barrier [1]. There is thus considerable interest in role human T cells will have in mediating acute rejection of porcine xenografts.   Endothelial cells forming the interface between donor and recipient are the first donor cells to be recognised by the host's immune system, this fact plus the observation that they express numerous molecules able to activate lymphocytes has stimulated much research into their precise role in transplant rejection.   It is our view that endothelial cells are pivotal in rejection, both in controlling the egress of inflammatory cells into the allografted organ but also by acting as specific antigen presenting cells, i.e. presenting foreign molecules to the immune system (Fig 1).

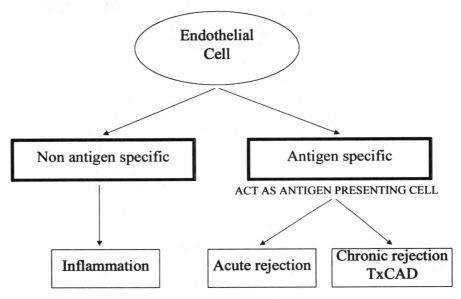

Fig 1. Role of endothelial cells in transplant rejection
(TxCAD = transplant associated coronary artery disease)

Rejection is mediated by both cell mediated and humoral mechanisms but the relative importance of these pathways differs in acute and chronic rejection.   Currently, interactions between human and pig can only be summised from *in vitro* experiments.

There follows a brief description of the basic mechanisms of transplant rejection, as it applies to allotransplantation. This Chapter will then describe the role of endothelial cells in this process and go on to consider interactions between pig endothelial cells and human T cells.

1. Basic mechanism of rejection

The major stimulus for rejection of allografted organs is recognition of foreign antigens coded by the Major Histocompatibilty Complex (MHC). Class I (HLA-ABC) and Class II (HLA-DR, DP, DQ) antigens are highly polymorphic glycoproteins encoded by the MHC locus found on chromosome 6 in humans. The frequency of circulating T cells which recognise foreign MHC molecules is very large (estimated at an astounding 0.1-1% of circulating T cells) - a fact which almost certainly accounts for the vigour of the anti-allograft response.

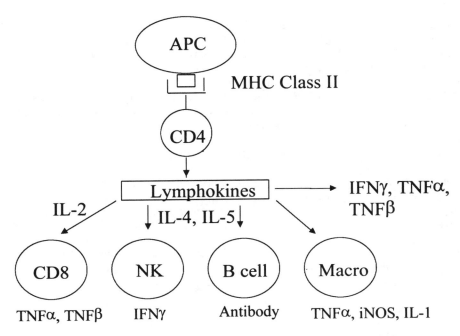

Fig 2. Diagrammatic representation of T cell activation illustrating pivotal role of MHC class II antigens presented by APC. Activated CD4+ T cells produce a cascade of lymphokines resulting in maturation of CD8 T cells, NK cells,, B cells and macrophages, which themselves produce further cytokines. It is likely that IFNg, iNOS and TNF are directly damaging to the graft.

Rejection is initiated by the CD4+ T cell subset recognising MHC class II antigens on antigen presenting cells (APC) within the graft (Fig 2). Recognition of foreign MHC molecules results in CD4+ T cell activation and release of cytokines (IL-2, IL-4, IL-5, IL-6, IFNγ, TNFα, TNFβ) which allow maturation of the effector mechanisms of rejection, namely maturation of CD8 + cytotoxic T cells, infiltration of macrophages, maturation of NK cells and lymphokine activated killer cells (LAK) and antibody formation (Fig 2). These effector mechanisms have been listed for the sake of completeness; there is little evidence that NK or LAK cells are important in allograft rejection. Indeed, the precise effector mechanisms which cause graft dysfunction are unknown; although CD8+ cytotoxic T cells are invariably found in allografts experimental studies have shown that CD8 + T cells are not essential for rejection [2]. It is quite possible that a direct effect of cytokines, in particular TNFα and IFNγ may are toxic to allografted cells. For example, TNFα has a negative ionotropic effect on cardiac myocytes [3] and elevated levels of TNFα have been reported in the serum of patients in heart failure [4]. Similarly, induction of inducible nitric oxide synthase by activated macrophages and possibly endothelial cells may be an important effector mechanism, and has been associated with contractile dysfunction after cardiac transplantation [5].

Activation of CD4+ T cells is thus pivotal in initiating acute rejection (Fig 2). In view of the fact that CD4+ T cells are activated by foreign MHC class II molecules, understanding the quantitative and qualitative distribution of these molecules on the allografted organ is of considerable importance. The advent of monoclonal antibodies, use of frozen sections and advances in immunocytochemical techniques have revolutionised knowledge about the normal distribution of MHC molecules in different tissues. Class II (HLA-DR and DP) antigens, originally thought to be restricted to macrophages, dendritic cells, monocytes and activated T cells have now been described on human endothelial cells and epithelial cells [6,7]. The expression of class II on human endothelial cells has been described in every organ [6,8] and it is particular striking on the microvessels i.e. capillaries, arterioles and venules. The large vessel endothelium (such as aorta, pulmonary artery, saphenous vein) are negative for MHC class II expression [8].

1.1. Pathways of antigen presentation and Antigen Presenting Cells

The term Antigen Presenting Cell (APC) has a specific meaning to immunologists: it means the cell is able to present antigen to resting T cells i.e. is able to cause activation of resting T cells. Only specialised cells (traditionally recognised as B cells, dendritic cells and monocytes) can perform this task. T cells recognise nominal antigen as processed peptides presented by self-MHC molecules. An important step in the understanding of alloreactivity came with the discovery that T cells can engage and respond to allogeneic MHC molecules directly (Fig 3).

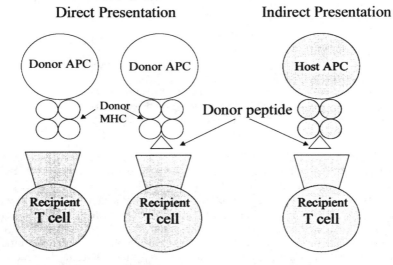

Fig 3. Recipient T cells recognise donor MHC determinants on donor APC (direct presentation)
or they recognise donor MHC peptides which have been processed and presented by host APC
(indirect presentation

This form of antigen recognition, termed direct presentation or the direct pathway is responsible for the strong proliferative response to alloantigens seen *in vitro* and quite possibly the early acute rejection seen in non-immunosuppressed animals after transplantation of MHC mismatched organs. However, T cells can also recognise allogeneic peptides that have been processed and presented within self-MHC molecules by recipient APC in the same manner that T cells recognise nominal antigen (Fig 3). This pathway is termed the indirect route or indirect pathway of T cell activation. Alloantigens shed from the graft are likely to be treated as exogenous antigen by recipient APC and will therefore be presented within MHC class II molecules to activate recipient CD4+ T cells.

A number of experimental studies have exemplified this phenomenon [9-11]. The direct and indirect pathway of T cell recognition will equally apply to T cell recognition of xenoantigens expressed by porcine endothelial cells; the questions being wither human T cells recognise porcine Swine Leukocyte Antigens (SLA) directly or via processing by human APC.

Any graft cell expressing class II antigens will be able to activate the indirect pathway - is likely that damaged endothelial cells are an important source of graft derived MHC class II antigens - since these are the only parenchymal cells expressing class II in the heart. The contribution indirect recognition of endothelial MHC class II makes to cellular rejection is currently not known. However, the question which has received much attention in recent years is whether endothelial cells can cause direct allostimulation of resting T lymphocytes (see below and 12 for review). There are two reasons for this: first is that direct recognition of allo-MHC molecules results in a 'strong' response, the number of T cells recognising MHC molecules directly is 10-100 higher than those recognising nominal antigen, resulting in a strong *in vitro* proliferative response. Second is that it is known that expression of MHC class II is not sufficient to cause T cell activation.

One of the important concepts to emerge in recent years is the knowledge that T cells require two signal to become activated [13], one is occupancy of the T cell receptor the second is activation of one of the many 'accessory molecules' present on T cells (Fig 4). Much attention has focused on the B7 (CD80, CD86) family of receptors [14] known to be essential as second signals on APC of bone -marrow origin (e.g., monocytes, B cells and dendritic cells); B7 receptors interact with CD28 molecules on the surface of resting T cells and blockade of this pathway inhibits dendritic cell stimulated mixed lymphocyte responses *in vitro* [15]. It is thought that interaction of resting T cell receptor with antigen in the absence of costimulation results in T cells being rendered anergic [16] or depleted by apoptosis [17] on APC. Another T cell surface antigen CTLA4 binds CD80 and CD86 with 10-20 times greater affinity than CD28 [18]. Thus CTLA4-Ig acts as a strong competitive inhibitor of CD28 mediated T cell activation. Injection of this fusion protein into rodents results in long term survival of MHC mismatched cardiac allografts [19,20,21] and human islet xenografts [22].

2. Acute rejection

The consequences of T cell activation described above leads to infiltration of the graft with inflammatory cells (T cells and monocytes) - a process termed acute rejection. The majority of patients have one or two acute rejection episodes in the first 6 months following transplantation. Acute rejection may be suspected clinically but it is always confirmed by histological assessment of biopsies. In particular, endomyocardial biopsy is an essential part of the management of patients following cardiac transplantation. Acute rejection invariably responds to anti-T cell depletion therapy, steroids and Cyclosporine.

3. Chronic rejection

Chronic rejection, presenting as a rapidly progressing obliterative vascular disease occurring in the transplanted heart, is the major cause of late death and repeat transplantation after cardiac transplantation. This disease is variously termed cardiac allograft vasculopathy or transplant associated coronary artery disease (TxCAD). This

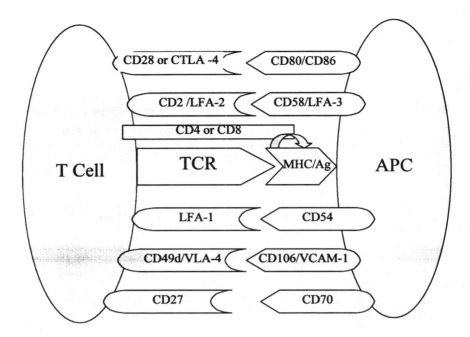

Fig 4. Diagrammatic representation of possible interactions
between receptors on T cells and their appropriate ligands on APC.

same phenomenon is also present in renal, lung and liver allografts and has been designated chronic rejection, obliterative bronchiolitis and vanishing bile duct syndrome respectively. Chronic rejection does not respond to currently used immunosuppressive drugs (cytolytic anti-T cell agents, steroids and Cyclosporine) - which primarily inhibit T cell mediated immune responses. The reported incidence of TxCAD, detected by routine angiography varies greatly between cardiac transplant centres. Incidences of 18% at one year progressing to 44% at three years have been reported [23]. Use of more accurate and sensitive methods of detecting intimal hyperplasia, such as intracoronary ultrasound [24], is likely to increase the reported incidence of the disease.

3.1. Histology of TxCAD

There are a number of reviews which describe the histological differences between TxCAD and spontaneous CAD and the various risk factors, both immunological and non-immunological have been described [25]. Importantly the lesions are limited to the allograft and involve both arterial and venous structures - demonstrating the role of the alloimmune response in the aetiology. It is interesting that TxCAD is a much more diffuse disease than spontaneous CAD, affecting the entire length of the epicardial vessels; the intimal proliferation is concentric as opposed to the eccentric plaque found in spontaneous CAD. These differences suggest the whole endothelium is the target of damage in TxCAD. Because the epicardial branches, including the intramyocardial branches are affected by TxCAD, coronary artery bypass surgery for revascularisation is usually precluded.

4. Properties of Endothelial cells

The phenotypic properties of endothelial cells and their response to cytokines gives them pivotal role in initiating acute and chronic allograft rejection in three distinct ways:
1. They allow extravasation of inflammatory cells into the graft
2. They act as antigen presenting cells
3. They are the target of the alloimmune response.

In principal, porcine endothelial cells will perform the same functions in a xenograft environment as human EC perform in an allograft environment. There will however be differences in terms of compatibility between human cytokines and porcine EC receptors, and human T cell recognition of SLA. The following information is described first for allogeneic interactions and second for xenogeneic interactions.

5. Allogeneic Interactions

5.1. Adhesion molecules and lymphocyte migration

There is currently extensive research on the role of endothelial adhesion molecules in controlling lymphocyte recirculation and extravasation of inflammatory cells. There are many excellent reviews of this subject [26], which is not within the remit of this article. However, a number of immunocytochemical studies have investigated the role of these molecules in acute and chronic rejection [8, 27, 28, 29]. Immunocytochemistry of frozen sections of human heart, coronary artery, aorta, pulmonary artery and endocardium have revealed differences with regard to basal expression of these molecules (Table 1).

Table 1. Distribution of adhesion molecules, MHC molecules and vWf in endothelial cells derived from microvessels and large vessels of the human cardiovascular system. *

	myocardial biopsies			large vessels		
	capillaries	arterioles	venules	coronary	PA	aorta
CD31	++	++	++	++	++	++
ICAM-1	++	+	+	++	+	+
VCAM-1	neg	+/-	+/-	+	neg	neg
E-selectin	neg	neg	+/-	+	+/-	+/-
VWf	+/-	++	++	++	++	++
Class I	++	+	+	++	+	+
Class II	++	+/-	+/-	++	neg	neg

*Summarised from references 7 and 8. ++ strong, even expression, + strong but patchy expression, +/- weak and patchy expression

PECAM (CD31), generally acknowledged to be a marker of endothelial cells was strongly expressed on all endothelium. In contrast, von Willebrands factor , also used as a marker of endothelial cells was strongly expressed on the larger vessels but was very weak on capillaries. ICAM -1 (CD54) was constitutivley expressed on endothelial cells from all vessels but was particularly strong on capillaries and EC lining the coronary artery. The coronary arteries were rather surprising, as they were found to basely express VCAM-1 (CD106) as well as ICAM-1 (8). VCAM-1 was not found to be expressed on any of the other large vessels. All coronary arteries investigated at this centre have expressed an 'activated phenotype'. Indeed an investigation of the cell phenotypes expressed in normal coronary artery and coronary artery with TxCAD [29] has not found any significant differences.   Possible explanations for this phenomenon are discussed below. Immunocytochemistry of frozen sections of normal endomyocardial biopsies show weak expression of E-selectin (CD62E) and VCAM-1: the capillaries being negative for these markers and venules showing patchy expression of E-selectin and VCAM-1. However, during acute (cell mediated) rejection, there is upregulation of VCAM-1 on capillary endothelial cells in close apposition to infiltrating T cells, this is not surprising since interaction between endothelial VCAM-1 with the T cell $\beta1$ integrins ($\alpha4\beta1$) is a requirement for T cell migration across endothelial cells.   Experimental studies confirm the importance of these adhesion molecules in acute rejection; thus antibodies against VCAM-1 [30] or ICAM-1 [31] produce allograft survival.

5.2. Expression of MHC class II molecules on human endothelial cells

Since MHC class II antigens initiate allograft rejection, it is of interest to describe the distribution of these molecules on endothelial cells of different origins (Table 1).   All endothelial cells constitutively express MHC class I molecules and many endothelial cells constitutively express MHC class II molecules.   However, there is an interesting heterogeneity with regard to constitutive expression of class II antigens; the large vessels (aorta, pulmonary artery, endocardium, umbilical vein, umbilical artery) are negative but the capillaries within all organs examined are strongly positive (Table 1).   Arterioles and venules within the heart show weak or patchy basal expression of MHC class II antigens. It was surprising to find that all pieces of coronary artery we examined expressed MHC class II molecules, as well as VCAM-1 and ICAM-1 [8].   The coronaries were either obtained from heart donors deemed unsuitable for transplantation, or they were removed from the explanted heart of patients requiring transplantation (for diseases not involving

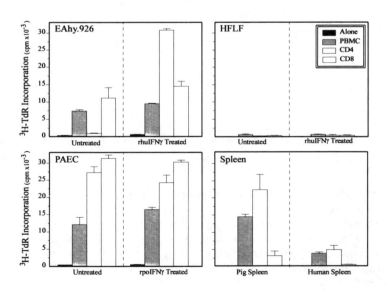

Fig 5.   Proliferative response of human CD4[+] or CD8[+] T cells to the human endothelial cell line (EAHY926), human foetal lung fibroblasts (HFLF), porcine aortic endothelial cells, porcine spleen or human spleen measured 6 days after co-culture. (Reproduced courtesy of Dr C Bravery).

the coronary artery). These molecules may therefore have been upregulated during procedures prior to harvest. The most common endothelial cells used in cell culture are those derived from umbilical vein endothelial cells, these do not express MHC class II antigens *in situ* and it is therefore not surprising that they are also negative *in vitro*. However, interestingly, cardiac microvascular endothelial cells, which are positive *in situ*, lose their class II after two weeks in culture [32]. This observation raises the interesting possibility that factors in normal serum act to maintain class II expression *in vivo*. The most likely candidate being IFNγ since this is the only cytokine which is able to induce MHC class II on human endothelial cells [33].

5.3. Endothelial cells as Antigen Presenting Cells – Human Studies

The fact that human endothelial cells constitutively express MHC class II molecules has stimulated a number of workers to ask whether endothelial cells directly cause allostimulation of resting T cells. We and others [34, 35] have cultured stringently purified CD4 + T cells with pure passaged human umbilical vein endothelial cells and looked for T cell proliferation (measured by uptake of 3H-thymidine) at day 6. The endothelial cells are treated with mitomycin C to stop them proliferating, any proliferation which is detected is thus due to responding T cells (Fig 5).

The results in Fig 5 show the response of CD4+ T cell to human endothelial cells (Eahy.926), porcine aortic endothelial cells (PAEC) and fetal lung fibroblasts. It can be seen that provided IFN γ is used to upregulate MHC class II, there is a strong proliferative response to human EC, but not to fibroblasts. There is also a strong response to PAEC, which is independent of IFNγ treatment. The reason for this is that PAEC class II expression persists in culture. That the response was direct and not indirect was proven by the findings that responder T cells were free of contaminating APC [34]. The majority of studies use endothelial cells of foetal origin (from the umbilical vein); we have confirmed this finding using endothelial cells from adult aorta, coronary artery and microvascular and in addition have shown that smooth muscle cells derived from the same vessel fail to stimulate allogeneic T cells [36].

When restimulated, T cells responded to endothelial cells giving kinetics similar to that seen in the primary response [37], there is no evidence for anergy induction.

It must be concluded therefore that donor endothelial cells can present alloantigen to recipient T cells. There is an important species difference between rodents and humans; rodents do not constitutively express MHC class II antigens on their endothelial cells. This may explain why it is easier to suppress transplant rejection in rodents than it is in humans. Thus in rodents the only MHC class II positive cells of donor origin in the graft are cells (dendritic cells and macrophages) of bone-marrow origin. These cells have a finite life span and in addition they migrate from the graft to lodge in other organs. Thus after about two weeks the rodent allografted organ is bereft of donor MHC class II presenting cells. In contrast, in humans, endothelial expression of donor MHC class II antigens ensures persistence of donor class II for long periods (if no indefinitely) after transplantation [38]. It follows, that understanding the signals that allow human endothelial cells to stimulate T cells may lead to new strategies of preventing rejection. We have questioned whether endothelial cells utilise the B7 pathway to stimulate T cells, and [39, 12] demonstrated that endothelial cells do not express B7 receptors and stimulate T cells via another accessory molecule, LFA-3. The possibility that second signals other than B7 could be important in allograft rejection is supported by the evidence of skin allograft rejection in CD28 deficient mice [40], blocking the receptor for LFA3 prolongs cardiac allograft survival in primates [41] and use of antibodies against ICAM-1 induces tolerance in a murine model of allograft rejection [31]. The fact that it has been shown that 'adhesion molecules' such as VCAM-1, ICAM-1 and ICAM-2 can act a costimulatory signals inducing T cell proliferation *in vitro* [42, 43] suggests they could act as costimulatory molecules on endothelial cells. In addition the possibility that extracellular matrix molecules (fibronectin, collagen, lamenin) via interaction with β1 integrin receptors on lymphocytes can act as second signals should also be considered [44].

6. Xenogeneic Interactions

6.1. Recognition of PAEC by human T cells

Like humans, pig endothelial cells constitutively express MHC class I and MHC class II antigens [45, 46]. Thus staining frozen sections of pig heart, kidney and aorta all show class II to be present on the capillaries and large vessel endothelial cells. Most of the in vitro studies have been done using cultured porcine aortic endothelial cells. Interestingly these cells continue to express class MHC class II antigens in culture [45]. Culturing purified CD4+ T cells with PEAC produces a strong T cell proliferative response, accompanied by considerable Interleukin-2 production [45, 47]. It is not necessary to use IFNγ to upregulate MHC antigens to produce this response and it is inhibited by mabs to Class II [45]. CD8+ T cells also proliferate in response to untreated PAEC, presumably in response to swine MHC class I antigens, although this has not been formally proven using blocking mabs [45]. As with the human studies above, this is direct recognition since the T cells are free of contaminating monocytes (they cannot proliferate to PHA). It is interesting that unlike human EC, PEAC bind CTLA-4-Ig demonstrating the existence of B7 molecules [45, 47], which were later shown to be CD86 [48, 49]. Thus CD86 is found constitiutively on PAEC and is also upregulated after treatment with species specific IFNγ [49]. Porcine CD86 is recognised by human T cells, thus transient transfection of human EC with porcine CD86 results in enhanced proliferation of human T cells [48] equivalent to that produced by PAEC. The expression of CD86 explains the greater proliferation and IL-2 production by T cells activated by porcine EC (45 and Fig 6) as it is known that stimulation of human T cells through CD28 stabilises and enhances IL-2 transcription [50]. It also explains the element of Cyclosporine resistance found when culturing PEAC with human T cells [49]. It is not surprising that human T cells recognise porcine SLA class II antigens as there are large areas of conservation of class II (HLA-DR) molecules across species.

6.2. Molecular compatibilties between human cytokines and PAEC

After allograft transplantation, it is known that amplification of the cellular response (i.e. maturation of effector cells and their migration into the graft) depends on local release of inflammatory cytokines (see Fig 2) and their effect on the local endothelium. In order to test the compatibility between human cytokines and PEAC we tested the effect of human TNFα, IL-1β, IL-4 and IFNγ on the expression of MHC molecules and adhesion molecules expressed by PAEC [51]. IFNγ was species specific, thus only porcine IFNγ induced swine DR and DQ and upregulated CD86 on PAEC [51]. In contrast, human TNFα was found to cross-react on PAEC producing upregulation of VCAM-1, MHC class II and CD86 on PAEC. This is not surprising, comparison of nucleotide sequences of the human and porcine TNFα gene have shown 85% sequence homology [52] and porcine VCAM-1 shows large homology with human VCAM-1 [53]. It has also been shown that porcine VCAM-1 mediates binding of human T cells to activated PEAC [54]. Our own studies have demonstrated that human T cells migrate across PEAC, although to a lesser extent than human EC (Liddington and Rose in preparation).

7. Role of endothelial cells in chronic rejection

It may well be that initial damage to coronary endothelium is mediated by CD4+ T cell recognition of foreign HLA molecules, but the paradox is that whereas T cell damage to the myocardium is limited and controlled by immunosuppressive drugs, initial damage to the coronary endothelium, in some patients, progresses to TxCAD. It must be remembered that the mainstay immunosuppressive drug, Cyclosporine, acts by inhibiting *early* events in T cell activation, namely transcription of IL-2 [55]. T cell activation leads to maturation of a number of different effector pathways (Fig 2) depending on the release of different cytokines. Thus production of cytokines IL-4 and IL-5 will lead to antibody production. Some studies report that production of these cytokines are less sensitive to Cyclosporine than IL-2 production [56] and proliferating B cells are known to be less sensitive to Cyclosporine than T cells [57]. It is therefore not surprising that despite the heavy immunosuppression received by patients after solid organ transplantation, the majority make a vigorous antibody response against the allografted organ (reviewed in 58).

It is our hypothesis that a sustained antibody response against HLA and non-HLA antigens on donor endothelial cells leads to TxCAD. The most common way of detecting antibodies formed after transplantation is a complement dependent cytotoxicity test against a panel of HLA typed leukocytes (termed Panel Reactive Antibodies or PRA test) or donor cells (termed a donor specific response). Clinical studies have reported an association between antibody producers and development of chronic rejection [59] after cardiac transplantation. Thus Suciu- Foca et al reported a 90% 4-year actuarial survival in patients who had not made antibody following cardiac transplantation versus 38% 4-year survival in the antibody producer's [60]. These authors looked for anti-HLA antibodies, but our own studies have shown a correlation between anti-endothelial antibodies and chronic rejection [61]. Using gel electrophoreses to separate endothelial peptides according to molecular weight followed by probing blots with patients'sera, we found that the majority of patients who had TxCAD had antibodies against endothelial peptides of 56/58kDa. A similar association between anti-endothelial antibodies, detected by flow cytometry and chronic rejection has been reported after renal transplantation [62]. Since the western blot test (61) detected antibodies against unrelated HUVEC, it is clear that donor specific HLA antigens could not be involved. Use of SDS gel electrophoresis and amino acid sequencing revealed that the most immunogeneic endothelial peptide (at 56/58kDa) was the intermediate filament vimentin and other immunoreactive peptides were identified as triose phosphate isomerase and glucose regulating protein - in all 40 different proteins were identified which reacted with patients IgM [63]. Vimentin is the intermediate filament characteristic but not restricted to endothelial cells and fibroblasts. Whereas smooth muscle cells predominantly express desmin as their intermediate filament they co-express desmin and vimentin when migrating or proliferating. Vimentin is diffusely expressed in the intima and media of normal and diseased coronary arteries. Our working hypothesis is that antibodies to vimentin reflect disease activity in the coronary arteries - but the outstanding questions are how vimentin, a cytosolic protein is exposed to the immune system and whether and how the antibodies are damaging.

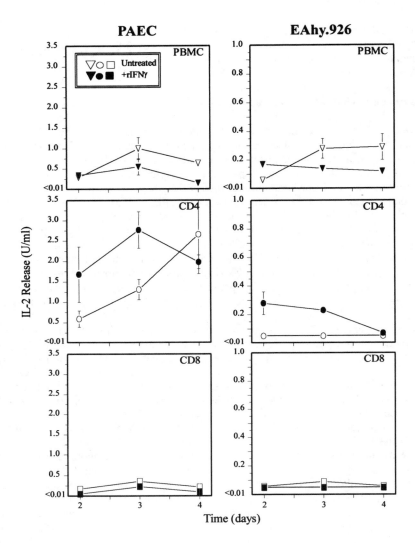

Fig 6. Interleukin 2 production by CD4⁺, CD8⁺ T cells and PBMC responding to porcine aortic endothelial cells (PAEC) or human endothelial cells (Eahy.926) after 2, 3 and 4 days of co-culture. (Reproduced by courtesy of Dr C Bravery).

The serum derived from our patients does not exhibit complement dependent cytotoxicity against endothelial cells derived from HUVEC or aorta, nor does it exhibit antibody dependent cellular cytotoxicity. This is not surprising with the exception of serum from patients with Kawasaki disease, where IgM antibodies are directly cytotoxic to endothelial cells in the presence of complement [64] anti-endothelial antibodies have not been found to mediate complement mediated damage to endothelial cells. However, complement mediated lysis is a severe and acute form of damage, usually associated with hyperacute rejection. It is more important to investigate whether anti-endothelial antibodies can mediate more subtle forms of damage. Recently a number of reports have demonstrated that antibodies from patients with autoimmune disease [65] or anti-HLA antibodies [66] can activate endothelial cells. We believe the information that antibodies can activate endothelial cells is very promising and should be explored as a mechanism whereby antibodies could damage endothelial cells in both autoimmune disease and chronic rejection after solid organ transplantation.

References

[1] Bach FH, Ferran C., Hechenleitner P et al. Accomodation of vascularised xenografts: Expression of "protective genes" by donor endothelial cells in a host Th2 cytokine environment. Nature Medicine 1997:3: 196-204.

[2] Steinmuller D. Which T cells mediate allograft rejection ? Transplantation 1985: **40**: 229-233.

[3] Ungureanu-Longrois D, Balligand JL, Simmons WW et al. Induction of nitric oxide synthase activity by cytokines in ventricular myocytes is necessary but not sufficient to decrease contractile responses to beta-adrenergic agonists. Circulation Research 1995: **77**: 494-502.

[4] Matsumori A, Yamada T, Suzuki H, Matoba Y, Sasayama S. Increased circulating cytokines in patients with myocarditis and cardiomyopathy. British Heart J. 1994: **72**: 561-566.

[5] Lewis N.P., Tsao PS, Rickenbacher PR et al. Induction of nitric oxide synthase in the human cardiac allograft is associated with contractile dysfunction of the left ventricle. Circulation 1996: **93**: 720-729.

[6] Daar AS, Fuggle SV, Fabre JW, Morris PJ. The detailed distribution of MHC class II antigens in normal human organs. Transplantation 1984: **38**: 292-297.

[7] Rose ML, Coles MI, Griffin RJ, Pomerance A, Yacoub MH. Expression of class I and class II major histocompatibilty antigens in normal and transplanted human heart. Transplantation 1986: **41**: 776-780.

[8] Page CS, Rose ML, Piggott R, Yacoub MH. Heterogeneity of vascular endothelial cells. Am J Pathology 1992: **141**: 673-683.

[9] Parker KE, Dalchau R, Fowler VJ, Priestly CA, Carter CA, Fabre JW. Stimulation of CD4+ T lymphocytes by allogeneic MHC peptides presented on autologous antigen presenting cells. Transplantation 1992: 53: 918-24.

[10] Terness P, Dufter C, Otto G, Opelz G. Allograft survival following immunisation with membrane bound or soluble peptide MHC class I donor antigens: factors relevant for the induction of rejection by indirect recognition. Transplant International 1996: 9: 2-8.

[11] Liu Z, Colovai AI, Tugulea S et al. Indirect recognition of donor HLA-DR peptides in organ allograft rejection. J Clin Invest. 1996: 98: 1150-1157.

[12] Pober JS, Orosz CG, Rose ML, Savage COS. Can graft endothelial cells initiate a host anti-graft immune response? Transplantation 1996: 61: 343-349.

[13] Janeway CAJ, Bottomly K. Signals and signs for lymphocyte responses. Cell 1994: 57: 275-

[14] June CH, Blustone JA, Nadler LM, Thompson CB. The B7 and CD28 receptor families. Immunology Today 1994: 15: 321-331.

[15] Tan P, Anasetti C, Hansen JA et al. Induction of alloantigen specific hyporesponsiveness in human T lymphocytes by blocking interaction of CD28 with its natural ligand B7/BB1. J Exp Med 1993: 177: 165-

[16] Schwartz RH. A cell culture model for T lymphocyte clonal anergy. Science 1990: **248**: 1349

[17] Liu Y, Jabeway CAJ. Interferon γ plays a criticial role in induced cell death of effector T cells: a possible third mechanism of self-tolerance. J Exp. Med 1990; 172: 1735.

[18] Linsley PS, Brady W, Urnes M, Grosmire LS, Damle NK, Ledbetter JA.

[19] CTLA-4 is a second receptor for the B cell activation antigen B7. J Exp Med. 1991: **147**: 561-569.

[20] Turka LA, Linsley PS, Lin H et al. T cell activation by the CD28 ligand B7 is required for cardiac allograft rejection in vivo. Proc. Natl. Acad Sci USA 1992: **89**: 11102-

[21] Lin H, Bolling SF, Linsley PS et al. Long term acceptance of major histocompatibilty complex mismatched cardiac allografts induced by CTLA4-Ig plus donor specific transfusions. J Exp Med 1993: 178: 1801-

[22] Pearson TC, Alexandre DZ, Winn KJ, Linsley PS, Lowry RP, Larsen CP. Transplantation tolerance induced by CTLA4-Ig. Transplantation 1994: 57: 1701.

[23] Lenschow D, Zeng Y, Thistlethwaite J et al. Long term survival of xenogeneic pancreatic islet grafts induced by CTLA4-Ig. Science 1992: 257; 789-

[24] Gao SJ, Schroeder JS, Alderman EL, Hunt SA, Valantine HA, Weiederhold V. Prevalence of accelerated coronary artery disease in heart transplant survivors. Comparison of cyclosporine and axathiprine regimens. Circulation 1989: 8: III100-105.

[25] Johnson JA, Kobashigawa JA. Quantitative analysis of transplant coronary artery disease with use of intracoronary ultrasound. J Heart & Lung Transplantation 1995: 14: S198-202.

[26] Hosenpud JD, Shipley GD, Wagner CR. Cardiac allograft vasculopathy: current concepts, recent developments, and future directions. J Heart & Lung Transplantation 1992: 11: 9-23.

[27] Springer TA. Traffic signals for lymphocyte recirculation and leukocyte emigration; The mutistep paradigm. Cell 1994: 76: 301-314.

[28] Briscoe DM, Schoen FJ, Rice GE, Bevilacqua MP, Ganz P, Pober JS. Induced expression of endothelial-leukocyte adhesion molecules in human cardiac allografts. Transplantation 1991: 51: 537-539.

[29] Taylor PM, Rose ML, Yacoub MH and Piggott R. Induction of vascular adhesion molecules during rejection of human cardiac allografts. Transplantation 1992: 54: 451-457.

[30] Taylor PM, Rose ML, Yacoub MH. Coronary artery immunogenecity: a comparison between explanted recipient or donor hearts and transplanted hearts. Transplant Immunology 1993: 1: 294-301.

[31] Orosz CG, Ohye RG, Pelletier RP et al. Treatment with anti-vascular cell adhesion molecules 1 monoclonal antibody induces long-term murine cardiac allograft acceptance. Transplantation 1993: 56: 453-460.

[32] Isobe M, Yagita H, Okumura K, Ihara A. Specific acceptance of cardiac allograft after treatment with antibodies to ICAM-1 and LFA-1. Science 1992: 255: 1125-

[33] McDouall RM, Yacoub MH, Rose ML. Isolation, culture and characterisation of MHC class II positive microvascular endothelial cells from the human heart. Microvascular Research 1996: 51: 137-152.

[34] Pober JS, and Cotran RS. The role of endothelial cells in inflammation. Transplantation 1990: 50: 537-544.

[35] Page CS, Holloway N, Smith H, Yacoub MH, Rose ML. Alloproliferative responses of purified CD4+ and CD8+ T cell subsets to human vascular endothelial cells in the absence of contaminating accessory cells. Transplantation 1994: 57: 1628-

[36] Savage C O S, Hughes CCW, McIntyre BW, Piracy JK, Pober J.S. Human CD4+ T cells proliferate to HLA-DR + allogeneic vascular endothelium: identification of accessory interactions. Transplantation 1993: 56, 128-

[37] McDouall RM, Page CS, Hafizi H, Yacoub MH, Rose ML. Alloproliferation of purified CD4+ T cells to adult human heart endothelial cells and study of second signal requirements. Immunology, 1996: *in press.*

[38] Savage COS, Brooks CJ. Human vascular endothelial cells do not induce anergy in allogeneic CD4+ T cells unless costimulation is prevented. Transplantation 1995: 60: 734-740.

[39] Rose ML, Navarette C, Yacoub MH, Festenstein H. Persistence of donor specific class II antigens in allografted human heart two years after transplantation. Human Immunol. 1988: 23: 179-182.

[40] Page C S, Thompson C, Yacoub M H. and Rose M L. Human endothelial cell stimulation of allogeneic T cells via a CTLA-4 independent pathway. Transplant Immunology 1994: 2: 342-347.

[41] Kawai K, Shahinian A, Mak TW, Ohashi PS. Skin allograft rejection in CD28-deficient mice. Transplantation 1996: 61: 352-355.

[42] Kaplon AG, Hochman PS, Michler RE et al. Short course single agent therapy with an LFA-3-IgG1 fusion protein prolongs primate cardiac allograft survival. Transplantation 1996: 61: 356-363.

[43] VanSeventer GA, Shimizy Y, Horgan KJ, Shaw S. The LFA-1 ligand ICAM-1 provides a costimulatory signal for T cell receptor mediated activation of resting T cells. J Immunol 1990: 144: 4579-

[44] Damle N, Aruffo A. Vascular cell adhesion molecule induces T cell antigen receptor dependent activation by CD4+ T lymphocytes. Proc. Natl. Acad Sci 1991: 88: 6403-

[45] Yamada A, Nikaido T, Nojima Y, Schlossman S, Morimoto C. Activation of human CD4+ T lymphocytes. Interaction of fibronectin with VLA-5 receptor on CD4 cells induces the AP-1 transcription factor. J Immunology 1991: 146: 53-56.

[46] Bravery C, Batten P, Yacoub M, Rose ML. Direct recognition of SLA and HLA like class II molecules on porcine endothelium by human T cells results in t cell activation and release of Interleukin-2. Transplantation 1995; 60: 1024-1033.

[47] Choo JK, Seebach JD, Nickeleit V, Shimizu A, Lei H, Sachs D, Madsen JC. Species differences in the expression of major histocompatibility complex antigens on coronary artery endothelium: implications for cell mediated xenoreactivity. Transplantation 1997; 64: 1315-1322.

[48] Murray AG, Khodadquist MM, Pober JS, Bothwell ALM. Porcine aortic endothelial cells activte human t cells: direct presentation of MHC antigens and costimulation by ligands for human CD2 and CD28. Immunity 1994: 1: 57-63

[49] Maher SE, Karmann K, Min W, Hughes CCW, Pober JS, Bothwell ALM. Porcine endothelial CD86 is a major costimulator of xenogeneic human T cells. Cloning, Sequencing, and functional expression in human endothelial cells. J Immunol. 1996: 157: 3838-3844.

[50] Davis TA, Craighead N, Williams AJ, Scadron A, June CH, Lee KP. Primary porcine endothelial cells express membrane bound B7-2 (CD86) and a soluble factor that co-stimulate cyclosporine resistnet CD28 dependent human Tcell proliferation. Int. Immunol. 1996, 8: 1099-1111.

[51] Ward, S.G. CD28: a signalling perspective. J Biochem 1996, 318: 361-377.

[52] Batten P, Yacoub MH, Rose ML. Effect of human cytokines (IFNγ, TNFα, IL-1β, Il-4) on porcine endothelial cells: induction of MHC and adhesion molecules and functional significance of these changes. Immunology, 1996: 87: 127-133.

[53] Pauli U, Beutler B, Peterhans E. Porcine tumor necrosis factor alpha; cloning with the polymerase chain reaction and determination of the nucleotide sequence. Gene, 1989: 185-192.

[54] Tsang YTM, Haskard DO, Robinson MK. Cloning and expression kinetics of porcine vascular cell adhesion molecule. Biochem. Biophys. Res. Comm. 1994: 201: 805-812.

[55] Mueller JP, Evans MJ, Cofielli R, Rother RP, Matis LA, Elliott EA. Porcine vascular cell adhesion molecule (VCAM) mediates endothelial cell adhesion to human T cells. Transplantation 1995, 60: 1299-1306.

[56] Clipstone NA, Crabtree GR. Identification of calcineurin as a key signalling enzyme in T lymphocyte activation. Nature 1992: 357: 695-697.

[57] Han CW, Imamura M, Hashino S et al. Differential effects of the immunosuppressants cyclosporin A, FK506, and KM2210 on cytokine expression. Bone Marrow Transplantation 1995: 15: 733-739.

[58] Morris RE. Rapamycin: FK506's fraternal twin or distant cousin? Immunology Today 1991: 12: 137-140.

[59] Rose M L. Antibody mediated rejection following cardiac transplantation. Transplantation Reviews 1993: 7: 140-152.

[60] Rose EA, Smith CR, Petrossian GA, Barr ML, Reemtsma K. Humoral immune responses after cardiac transplantation: correlation with fatal rejection and graft atheroscleosis. Surgery 1989: 106: 203-8.

[61] Suciu-Foca N., Reed E, Marboe C et al. The role of anti-HLA antibodies in heart transplantation. Transplantation 1991: 51: 716-724.

[62] Dunn M J, Crisp S J, Rose ML, Taylor PM, Yacoub MH. Antiendothelial antibodies and coronary artery disease after cardiac transplantation. Lancet 1992: 339: 1566-70.

[63] Al Hussein KA, Talbot D, Proud D, Taylor RMR, Shenton BK. The clinical significance of post transplantation non-HLA antibodies in renal transplantation. Transplant International 1995: 8: 214-220.

[64] Wheeler C H, Collins A., Dunn M J, Crisp S J, Yacoub MH, Rose ML. Characterisation of endothelial antigens associated with transplant associated coronary artery disease. J Heart & Lung Transplantation 1995: 14: S188-97.

[65] Leung DY, Collins MT, Lapierre LA, Geha RS, Pober JS. Immunoglobulin M antibodies present in the acute phase of Kawasaki syndrome lyse cultured vascular endothelial cells stimulated by gamma interferon. J Clin. Investig. 1986, 77: 1428-1435

[66] Carvalho D., Savage C OS, Black C M and Pearson JD. IgG antiendothelial cell autoantibodies from scleroderma patients induce leukocyte adhesion to human vascular endothelial cells in vitro. J Clin. Investigation 1996: 97: 1-9.

[67] Harris PE, Bian H, Reed EF. Induction of high affinity growth factor receptor expression and proliferation in human endothelial cells by anti-HLA antibodies: A possible mechanism for transplant atherosclerosis. J Immunol. 1997, 159: 5697-5704.

Part II

Inflammation / Immunology

Vascular Endothelium: Mechanisms of Cell Signaling
J.D. Catravas et al. (Eds.)
IOS Press, 1999

CYTOKINE ACTIVATION OF ENDOTHELIAL CELLS: AN OLD PARADIGM WITH NEW ELEMENTS

Marta Muzio, Andrea Doni, Giuseppe Peri, Barbara Bottazzi, Marco Metra[t], Livio Dei Cas[t], Alberto Mantovani[§]

Istituto di Ricerche Farmacologiche "Mario Negri", via Eritrea 62 - 20157 Milan, Italy; [t]Division of Cardiology, Spedali Riuniti di Brescia, Italy; [§]also at Dept. Biotechnology, Section of General Pathology, University of Brescia, Italy

Abstract

Endothelial cells have long been viewed as a passive lining of blood vessels. It is now evident that upon exposure to environmental signals, cytokines in particular, vascular cells undergo profound changes in gene expression and function that allow these cells to participate actively in inflammatory reactions, immunity, and thrombosis. Different mediators (e.g., IL-1, IL-6 and TNF) activate relatively distinct sets of functions. The molecular basis of these same activation programs will be discussed.

1. Introduction

In the last years the concept that endothelial cells, rather than being a passive barrier between blood elements and tissues, represent a metabolically active organ has been consolidated. More in particular emphasis has been given to the role played by endothelial cells in the determination and maintenance of inflammatory reactions which take place in tissues [1-4]. All the crucial aspects which characterise inflammation, from the release of chemoattractants for different leukocyte populations to the expression and functional activation of adhesion molecules of different classes, from the induction of a pro-thrombotic activity on the luminal surface to the transmigration and functional activation of the motile elements, are mainly determined by the early metabolic response of the endothelial cells to the inflammatory signals [1-4].

In order to rationalise a vast amount of information, several years ago we have defined such complex series of molecular events which take place in endothelial cells (EC) upon exposure to the classical pro-inflammatory cytokines (such as Interleukin-1 (IL-1) and Tumor Necrosis Factor (TNF)) as the induction of the "protrombotic-proinflammatory" programme [1,4,5]. In this review we will concentrate only on selected recent aspects of the molecular events which take place in EC. We will not recapitulate the list of the many known genes or activities which have been found "induced" upon activation, but rather concentrate on what has been learned recently about the mechanisms by which some of these genes or activities are induced. We will also emphasize the production and action of relatively novel mediators.

2. Cytokine regulation of EC function

2.1. Primary proinflamamtory cytokines

As previously described in detail, interleukin 1 (IL-1) and tumor necrosis factor (TNF) induce the expression of a functional program related to thrombosis and inflammation. Briefly, these cytokines facilitate thrombus formation by inducing procoagulant activity, inhibiting the thrombomodulin/protein C anticoagulation pathway and blocking fibrin dissolution via stimulation of the type I inhibitor of plasminogen activator.

These cytokines induce production of autacoids in EC, including prostanoids (PGI2 in particular), platelet activating factor (PAF) and nitric oxide (NO). NO produced by EC also has an autocrine function. Experiments suggest that NO inhibits cytokine-induced expression of adhesion molecules and cytokine production by EC [6-8]. The effects are mediated by inhibition of NF-kB through the induction and stabilization of NF-kB inhibitor [6,9]. Thus, constitutively produced NO may tonically inhibit the expression of NF-kB-dependent pro-inflammatory genes and attenuate the pro-inflammatory response of EC.

Inflammatory cytokines promote leukocyte extravasation by altering the rheology of microcirculation via NO and prostaglandins and by inducing adhesion molecules and chemotactic cytokines [4]. The regulated expression of adhesion molecules in the multistep process of recruitment has been the object of recent extensive reviews and chemokine production is discussed below.

The membrane attack complex of complement (C) augments TNF-induced expression of adhesion molecules [10] and induces tissues factor (TF) by inducing IL-1α [11]. Interestingly, in turn, IL-1 augments production of C3 and factor B by EC. The first long pentraxin PTX3, also known as TSG14, is one of the many genes identified in cytokine-activated EC [12,13]. It is a secreted molecule consisting of a C-terminal domain, encoded by the 3rd exon, with sequence and structural similarity to classical pentraxins (e.g. CRP), coupled with an unrelated N-terminal portion. PTX3 is produced by various cell types in vitro, prominently by EC and mononuclear phagocytes. Intriguingly, after LPS administration to mice, PTX3 is expressed predominantly by heart and skeletal muscle EC [13]. Recent results suggest that PTX3 binds C1q and activates C and thus may represent a mechanism of amplification of innate immunity [14]. Moreover, elevated levels of PTX3 have been detected in patients with acute myocardial infarction (unpublished).

IL-1 and TNF induce production of various cytokines in EC, including various chemokines, colony stimulating factors (CSF), IL-6 and IL-1 itself [2,4]. *In vitro* culture of EC results in spontaneous expression of IL-1α and refraction of the response to exogeneous IL-1 [4]. Endogeneous IL-1 may represent a mediator that limits the lifespan of EC in culture, possibly by acting in the nucleus [15]. IL-1 receptor antagonist (IL-1ra) is not produced by EC, but these cells may represent a major target for the therapeutic activity of IL-1ra *in vivo* [4]. The hematopoietic growth factors GM-CSF, G-CSF, IL-3 and erythropoietin have been shown to affect EC [4,16]. By and large, these factors are relatively weak agonists, which affect migration and proliferation and amplify EC responsiveness to other signals [16]. In the same studies M-CSF was generally inactive. Analysis of receptor expression revealed that EC express c-kit; the β chain common to the GM-CSF, IL-3 and IL-5 receptors; the α IL-3 and αGM chains, but not αIL-5 nor c-fms. TNF and IFNγ augment expression of IL-3Rα chain [17]; accordingly IL-3 and TNF

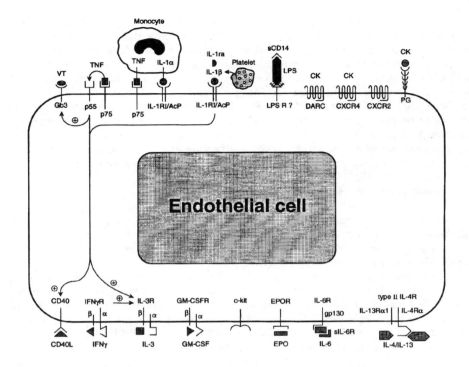

Fig. 1 - Cytokine receptors in endothelial cells. The location of the receptor does not imply a differential distribution on the luminal versus abluminal surface of the EC. Abbreviations: CK, chemokine; DARC, Duffy antigen receptor for chemokines; Gb3 globotriaosylceramide; L, ligand; LPS, lipopolysaccharide; PG, proteoglycan; R, receptor; VT, verotoxin.

synergize in terms of induction of IL-8 and adhesion molecules and the same occurs with IFNγ in terms of class II MHC. It has been speculated that the ability of various hemopoietic cytokines to affect EC is a reflection of the common ontogenetic origin of hematopoietic and endothelial elements in blood islands [16].

EC express both the p55 and the p75 TNF receptor (TNFR), the latter being the most abundant on the cell membrane [18] (Fig. 1). The p55R is expressed at much lower levels on the membrane itself but is more abundant overall, and is detectable mainly in the Golgi apparatus and in cytoplasmic vacuoles [18]. TNF activates EC predominantly via p55 [19,20]. The contribution of p75 is best observed at low TNF concentrations, consistently with the 'ligand passing' model of function of this molecule. The transmembrane form of TNF is the prime ligand of p75 and it may play an important role in juxtacrine interactions between EC and monocytes [21-23].

EC express only the type I IL-1R. Under resting conditions or upon activation EC do not express the type II decoy receptor, a molecule without a demonstrable role in signalling, capable of blocking IL-1 [24]. The mRNA coding for the IL-1R accessory protein is detectable at low levels in EC [Saccani S. unpublished].

Various stimuli induce production not of IL-11 [4] but of copious amounts of IL-6 and leukemia inhibitory factor (LIF) [25] in EC [4]. IL-6 production is elicited by IL-1, TNF, IL-4, IL-13, oncostatin M, IL-17 [26], infectious agents and their products, and hypoxia [27]. NFIL-6 is involved in the latter response [27]. Original studies on IL-6 production by human umbelical vein EC (HUVEC) concluded that this cytokine did not affect several EC functions [28], a conclusion repeatedly confirmed, despite indications of involvement of this molecule in angiogenesis and vascular tumor formation. Observations in IL-6-deficient knockout mice prompted a reexamination of the interaction of IL-6 with EC. HUVEC express the signal transducing gp130 chain but not the IL-6R chain (Fig. 1). Soluble IL-6R and IL-6 alone did not affect EC function, but the two together induced chemokine production in EC, with no other measurable response. IL-6/IL-6R complexes activated STAT3 in EC [29]. Hence, recent *in vitro* and *in vivo* data suggest that IL-6 plays an unsuspected role as a pathway of amplification of leukocyte recruitment and that, in concert with its soluble receptor, it activates a unique functional program in EC.

2.2. Hematopoietic growth factors

EC are an important source of CSFs. Hematopoietic growth factors produced by EC include stem cell factor, G-CSF, GM-CSF, and M-CSF. CSF production is induced or augmented by a variety of stimuli including LPS, IL-1 and TNF and minimally modified low-density lipoproteins (MM-LDL) [4,16].

The hematopoietic growth factors GM-CSF, G-CSF, IL-3 and erythropoietin have been shown to affect EC [4,16]. By and large, these factors are relatively weak agonists, which affect migration and proliferation and amplify EC responsiveness to other signals (16). In the same studies M-CSF was generally inactive. Analysis of receptor expression revealed that EC express c-kit; the § chain common to the GM-CSF, IL-3 and IL-5 receptors; the αGM chains but not αIL-5 nor c-fms. TNF and IFNγ augment expression of IL-3Rα chain [17]; accordingly IL-3 and TNF synergize in terms of induction of IL-8 and adhesion molecules and the same occurs with IFNγ in terms of class II MHC. It has been speculated that the ability of various hemopoietic cytokines to affect EC is a reflection of the common ontogenetic origin of hematopoietic and endothelial elements in blood islands [16].

2.3. Antiinflammatory cytokines

Information on the interaction of IL-10 with vascular endothelium is scanty and fragmentary. This cytokine was a weak stimulus for expression of chemokines and IL-6 in mouse Polyoma middle T (PmT) immortalized EC lines and amplified the action of IL-1 and TNF [30]. This effect was associated with prolongation of mRNA half life. Stimulation of HUVEC was variable and not reproducible. The effect of IL-10 on IL-8 production has been the object of conflicting reports [31,32]. IL-10 was reported to inhibit antigen presentation by human dermal microvascular EC [33], induction of tetrahydrobiopterine in HUVEC [34], amplification by LPS of irradiation-induced apoptosis [35] and IL-1γ induction of adhesion molecules [36].

IL-4 has growth factor activity and induces uPA in micro but not in macrovascular EC (for review [4,37]). It is intriguing that IL-4 and IL-13, but not IL-10, inhibited induction of RANTES expression in EC stimulated by IFNγ and TNF [38]. IL-4 selectively induces VCAM-1 and inhibits ICAM-1 and E-selectin expression. IL-4 is a weak inducer of IL-6 and MCP-1 in EC and amplifies production of these mediators in concert with other stimuli (for review [4]). Recently it was shown that IL-13 has similar activities on EC [39]. Sharing of receptor components may underlie the similarity of action of IL-4 and IL-13 in EC [40]. EC do not express the common γ chain [40]. It is intriguing that these cytokines have divergent effects on monocytes (where they inhibit), and EC (where they amplify production of certain cytokines). Stimulation of certain EC function may be important in the induction and local expression of TH2 type responses, by, for instance, inducing recruitment of eosinophils and basophils and favouring the transition to the late phase reaction.

2.4. Chemokines

Chemokines are a key element in the multistep process of leukocyte recruitment and are produced by EC in response to molecules involved in inflammatory reactions, immunity and thrombosis. The chemokine repertoire of EC includes members of both the CXC (IL-8, IP10, ENA78 and groα) and CC (MCP-1, MCP-3, RANTES) family of chemokines, with most studies focused on the prototypic molecules IL-8 and MCP-1.One interesting pathway of chemokine induction is represented by monocytes [21-23] and platelets [41], which can activate local EC via juxtacrine pathways involving adhesion molecules, IL-1 and TNF.

Given the different spectrum of action of chemokines, one would expect MCP-1 and IL-8 to be independently regulated. However there are few examples of selective regulation. It was found that IFNγ selectively induces MCP-1 in microvascular EC [42] as found also in monocytes, where this molecule stimulates MCP-1 and inhibits IL-8.

Recently, Schall et al. reported the identification of a unique chemokine, fractalkine, representative of a new class: it is a transmembrane molecule consisting of a mucin and a chemokine domain. It is induced by IL-1 in EC and is recognized by mononuclear cells [43].

In general, the spectrum of action of chemokines is restricted to leukocytes, but recent evidence suggests that some members of this superfamily of inflammatory mediators may affect EC function. IL-8, groα and other CXC chemokines were reported to induce EC migration and proliferation in vitro and to be angiogenic *in vivo* [44]. The expression of high affinity receptors and responsiveness to IL-8 of EC has however been the object of conflicting results [45,46].

In common with platelet factor 4, IP10 was shown to have angiostatic properties *in vivo* and represent the ultimate mediator of the anti-angiogenic activity of IL-12 (47), though conflicting results have been obtained as to its capacity to inhibit bFGF-induced proliferation of HUVEC *in vitro* [48,49]. A three amino acid motif (ELR), is conserved in members of the CXC family which activate neutrophils. Recent results, including the action of molecules with or without the ELR motif and the activity of IL-8 muteins, suggest that the presence or absence of an ELR motif dictates whether CXC chemokines induce or inhibit angiogenesis [50]. However, the observation that groβ inhibits angiogenesis is not consistent with this model of function [51].

Three types of chemokine binding sites have been identified. The presence and type of signalling chemokine receptors on EC is controversial [44-46]. The promiscuous chemokine receptor identical to the Duffy blood group antigen (DARC) is expressed by EC at post-capillary venules *in vivo*, but not by endothelial cells *in vitro* [52]. Finally, heparin and heparin-like proteoglycans on endothelial cells present at least some chemokines to leukocytes in the multistep process of recruitment [53].

In conclusion, EC cells, strategically located at the tissue/blood interface, produce and present at least some chemokines to circulating leukocytes. Chemokines, when produced in massive amounts, as in cancer or chronic inflammation, could contribute to systemic anti-inflammation [54], by inducing for instance in concert with PAF rapid release of the TNF p75R and of the IL-1 typeII decoy receptor [55]. Recent evidence also suggests that at least certain chemokines act on EC exerting pro- or anti-angiogenic activity. It will be important to define unequivocally the structural basis and receptors involved in the divergent action of chemokines on EC.

2.5. Interferons and IL-12

IFNγ was the first molecularly identified cytokine shown to affect EC [2]. IFNγ induces EC expression of MHC class II antigens and of the invariant chain, augments expression of MHC class I and CD40 [56-58], amplifies responses to TNF, slowly stimulates ICAM-1 expression and augments LPS-induced production of IL-1. Engagement of CD40 amplifies induction of adhesion molecules [58]. Thus, reciprocal mutual stimulation may occur when CD40L expressing cells interact with EC.

IL-12 is a heterodimeric cytokine active on T cells and NK cells with antitumor activity. Recently IL-12 was shown to have potent in vivo anti-angiogenic activity [47]. Circumstantial evidence suggests that IL-12 does not act per se on EC, but rather via induction of IFNγ [47]. IFNs are known to have antiangiogenic activity and IFNγ is used in the treatment of human hemangiomas. IFNγ, in turn, may act on EC via induction of the CXC chemokine IP-10 (see below). Thus, IL-12 may set in motion a cytokine cascade involving IFNγ and IP10, which eventually results in inhibition of angiogenesis.

3. Molecular basis of EC activation by IL-1

IL-1 is a prototypic endothelial cell activator. Substantial progress has been recently made in defining the signaling pathway of IL-1 receptor.

Two transmembrane receptors for IL-1 have been cloned and characterized, IL-1 receptor type I (IL-1RI) and IL-1 receptor type II (IL-1RII) [59,60] with the type II receptor acting as a negative regulator or decoy target [24,59-61]. Recently a third surface molecule designated IL-1RAcP has been identified and unlike IL-1RI and IL-1RII, IL-1RAcP itself does not bind IL-1, but augments the affinity of IL-1 for IL-1RI [62]. Both I_-1RI and IL-1RAcP mediate IL-1 activities [61-64]. To note EC express detectable levels of IL-1RI and IL-1RAcP but do not express the decoy IL-1RII. As expected EC are fully responsive to the activation induced by IL-1 treatment [65].

Since the cytoplasmic domains of the IL-1RI and IL-1RAcP have no similarity to other characterized mammalian transmembrane receptors and no resemblance to any enzymatic activity it has been speculated that they will use a novel pathway of signal transduction.

Following IL-1 treatment, several IL-1-mediated intracellular events have been observed, including an increase in diacylglicerol (DAG) [66], ceramide [67] and Ser-Thr protein phosphorylation [68]. IL-1 also activates a novel protein kinase cascade which eventually results in the phosphorylation of hsp27 [69]. Notably a very early event occurring in a number of cell types after treatment with IL-1 is the activation of distinct transcription factors (including c-Jun, NF-kB and Elk) which subsequently drive the transcriptional regulation of different cytokine genes (see [70,71] for a review). A prototypic example of this is represented by the induction of NF-kB after IL-1 treatment of the cells; the biochemical cascade occurring from the IL-1R signalling complex to NF-kB activation has been very recently defined (see Fig. 2 for a schematic representation).

A biochemical approach has led to the identification of a novel protein kinase called IRAK, for IL-1R Associated Kinase, which associates with the IL-1R signalling complex [72]. It is a novel Ser-Thr kinase which, together with the Drosophila protein Pelle, belongs to a novel subfamily of protein kinases. It is important to note that genetic studies examining the formation of dorsoventral polarity of the *Drosophila* embryo have shed light on the intracellular signalling pathway of IL-1 induced NF-kB activation [73]. The protein Dorsal, a homologue of NF-kB, is activated during embryogenesis. Like NF-kB, Dorsal activity is suppressed by an I-kB-like molecule designated Cactus. Activation of Dorsal is initiated by the interaction of an extracellular ligand with the membrane-bound receptor designated Toll. A potential connection between the IL-1 receptors and Toll signalling pathways was found on the basis of the sequence similarity shared by the intracellular domains of IL-1RI, IL-1RAcP and Toll [74]. Two other genetically identified molecules, the adapter protein Tube and the Ser/Thr kinase Pelle, function downstream of Toll to activate Dorsal [75,76]. Therefore it is not surprising, that IRAK shows significant homology to Pelle indicating a further level of similarity between this two pathways of signal transduction.

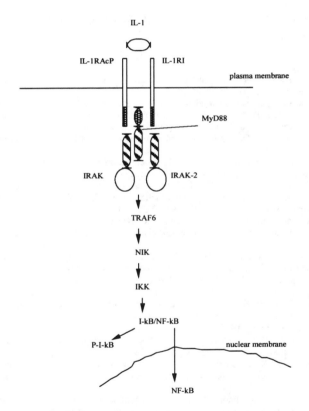

Fig. 2 - An overview of IL-1-induced NF-kB activation signaling cascade.
IRAK indicates IL-1 receptor associated kinase, NIK indicates NF-kB inducing kinase, IKK indicates I-kB kinase, TRAF6 belongs to the TRAF family of signal transducing proteins that are characterized by a conserved carboxy-terminal TRAF-C domain and an alpha helical TRAF-N domain. TRAF originally indicated TNFR associating factor.

Searching EST databases for additional proximal mediators of IL-1 signaling a novel member of the Pelle/IRAK family was identified and molecularly cloned (IRAK-2).

IRAK-2 [77]. Both IRAK and IRAK-2 are recruited to the IL-1R signaling complex by the adapter moleule MyD88 that bridges the cytoplasmic tails of the receptors (IL-1RI and IL-1RAcP) to the N-terminal domain of either IRAK or IRAK-2 (IRAKs for clarity) [77,78].

Downstream to the IL-1 receptor signaling complex, IRAKs bind the adapter molecule TRAF6 that biochemically links them to the downstream protein kinase NIK (for NF-kB inducing kinase) [79,80].

Finally NIK phosphorylates and subsequently activates the I-kB kinase complex or IKK (including the kinases IKKα and IKKβ and additional unknown components) that is now directly responsible for the Ik-B phosphorylation and consequent NF-kB activation [81-85].

Acknowledgements

This work was supported by Centro per lo Studio dello Scompenso Cardiaco.

References

[1]   Mantovani A. and Dejana E.Cytokines as communication signals between leukocytes and endothelial cells. *Immunol.Today.* 1989;10:370-375
[2]   Pober J. and Cotran R.S.Cytokines and endothelial cell biology. *Physiol.Rev.* 1990;70:427-451
[3]   Libby P. and Hansson G.K.Biology of disease. Involvement of the immune system in human atherogenesis: current knowledge and unanswered questions. *Lab.Invest.* 1991;64:5-15
[4]   Mantovani A., Bussolino F. and Dejana E. Cytokine regulation of endothelial cell function. *FASEB.J.* (1992); 6:2591-2599
[5]   Mantovani A., Bussolino F. and Introna M. Cytokine regulation of endothelial cell function: from molecular level to the bed side. *Immunol.Today.* (1997); 18:231-239
[6]   De Caterina R., Libby P., Peng H.B., et al Nitric oxide decreases cytokine-induced endothelial activation. Nitric oxide selectively reduces endothelial expression of adhesion molecules and proinflammatory cytokines. *J.Clin.Invest.* (1995); 96:60-68
[7]   Peng H.B., Rajavashisth T.B., Libby P. and Liao J.K. Nitric oxide inhibits macrophage-colony stimulating factor gene transcription in vascular endothelial cells. *J.Biol.Chem.* (1995); 270:17050-17055
[8]   Zeiher A.M., Fisslthaler B., Schray Utz B. and Busse R. Nitric oxide modulates the expression of monocyte chemoattractant protein 1 in cultured human endothelial cells. *Circ.Res.* (1995); 76:980-986
[9]   Peng H.B., Libby P. and Liao J.K. Induction and stabilization of I kappa B alpha by nitric oxide mediates inhibition of NF-kappa B. *J.Biol.Chem.* (1995); 270:14214-14219
[10]   Kilgore K.S., Shen J.P., Miller B.F., Ward P.A. and Warren J.S. Enhancement by the complement membrane attack complex of tumor necrosis factor-alpha-induced endothelial cell expression of E-selectin and ICAM-1. *J.Immunol.* (1995); 155:1434-1441
[11]   Saadi S., Holzknecht R.A., Patte C., Stern D.M. and Platt J.L. Complement-mediated regulation of tissue factor activity in endothelium . *J.Exp.Med.* (1995); 182:1807-1814
[12]   Breviario F., d'Aniello E.M., Golay J., et al Interleukin-1-inducible genes in endothelial cells. Cloning of a new gene related to C-reactive protein and serum amyloid P component. *J.Biol.Chem.* (1992); 267:22190-22197
[13]   Introna M., Vidal Alles V., Castellano M., et al Cloning of mouse PTX3, a new member of the pentraxin gene family expressed at extrahepatic sites. *Blood* (1996); 87:1862-1872
[14]   Bottazzi B., Vouret-Craviari V., Bastone A., et al Multimer formation and ligand recognition by the long pentraxin PTX3: similarities and differences with the short pentraxins C reactive proteins and serum amyloid P component. *J.Biol.Chem.* (1997); 272:32817-32829
[15]   Maier J.A., Statuto M. and Ragnotti G. Endogenous interleukin 1 alpha must be transported to the nucleus to exert its activity in human endothelial cells. *Mol.Cell Biol.* (1994); 14:1845-1851
[16]   Bussolino F., Bocchietto E., Silvagno F., Soldi R., Arese M. and Mantovani A. Actions of molecules which regulate hemopoiesis on endothelial cells: memoirs of common ancestors? *Pathol.Res.Pract.* (1994); 190:834-839

[17] Korpelainen E.I., Gamble J.R., Smith W.B., Dottore M., Vadas M.A. and Lopez A.F. Interferon-gamma upregulates interleukin-3 (IL-3) receptor expression in human endothelial cells and synergizes with IL-3 in stimulating major histocompatibility complex class II expression and cytokine production. *Blood.* (1995); 86:176-182

[18] Bradley J.R., Thiru S. and Pober J.S. Disparate localization of 55-kd and 75-kd tumor necrosis factor receptors in human endothelial cells. *Am.J.Pathol.* (1995); 146:27-32

[19] Mackay F., Loetscher H., Stueber D., Gehr G. and Lesslauer W. Tumor necrosis factor alpha (TNF-alpha)-induced cell adhesion to human endothelial cells is under dominant control of one TNF receptor type, TNF-R55. *J.Exp.Med.* (1993); 177:1277-1286

[20] Paleolog E.M., Delasalle S.A., Buurman W.A. and Feldmann M. Functional activities of receptors for tumor necrosis factor-alpha on human vascular endothelial cells. *Blood* (1994); 84:2578-2590

[21] Grell M., Douni E., Wajant H., et al The transmembrane form of tumor necrosis factor is the prime activating ligand of the 80 kDa tumor necrosis factor receptor. *Cell* (1995); 83:793-802

[22] Schmid E.F., Binder K., Grell M., Scheurich P. and Pfizenmaier K. Both tumor necrosis factor receptors, TNFR60 and TNFR80, are involved in signaling endothelial tissue factor expression by juxtacrine tumor necrosis factor alpha. *Blood.* (1995); 86:1836-1841

[23] Lukacs N.W., Strieter R.M., Elner V., Evanoff H.L., Burdick M.D. and Kunkel S.L. Production of chemokines, interleukin-8 and monocyte chemoattractant protein-1, during monocyte endothelial cell interactions. *Blood.* (1995); 86:2767-2773

[24] Colotta F., Dower S.K., Sims J.E. and Mantovani A. The type II 'decoy' receptor: novel regulatory pathway for interleukin-1. *Immunol.Today.* (1994); 15:562-566

[25] Grosset C., Jazwiec B., Taupin J.L., et al In vitro biosynthesis of leukemia inhibitory factor/human interleukin for DA cells by human endothelial cells: differential regulation by interleukin-1 alpha and glucocorticoids. *Blood.* (1995); 86:3763-3770

[26] Fossiez F., Djossou O., Chomarat P., et al T- cell IL-17 induces stromal cells to produce proinflammatory and hematopoietic cytokines . *J.Exp.Med.* (1996); 183:2593-2603

[27] Yan S.F., Tritto I., Pinsky D., et al Induction of interleukin 6 (IL-6) by hypoxia in vascular cells. Central role of the binding site for nuclear factor-IL-6. *J.Biol.Chem.* (1995); 270:11463-11471

[28] Sironi M., Breviario F., Proserpio P., et al IL-1 stimulates IL-6 production in endothelial cells. *J.Immunol.* (1989); 142:549-553

[29] Romano M., Sironi M., Toniatti C., et al Role of IL-6 and its soluble receptor in induction of chemokines and leukocyte recruitment. *Immunity.* (1997); 6:315-325

[30] Sironi M., Munoz C., Pollicino T., et al Divergent effects of interleukin-10 on cytokine production by mononuclear phagocytes and endothelial cells. *Eur.J.Immunol.* (1993); 23:2692-2695

[31] Chen C.C. and Manning A.M. TGF-beta1, IL-10 and IL-4 differentially modulate the cytokine-induced expression of the IL-6 and IL-8 in human endothelial cells. *Cytokine* (1996); 8:58-65

[32] Debeaux A.C., Maingay J.P., Ross J.A., Fearon K.C.H. and Carter D.C. Interleukin-4 and interleukin-10 increase endotoxin- stimulated human umbilical vein endothelial cell interleukin-8 release. *J.Interferon.Cytokine Res.* (1995); 15:441-445

[33] Vora M., Yssel H., de Vries J.E. and Karasek M.A. Antigen presentation by human dermal microvascular endothelial cells. Immunoregulatory effect of IFN-gamma and IL-10. *J.Immunol.* (1994); 152:5734-5741

[34] Schoedon G., Schneemann M., Blau N., Edgell C.J. and Schaffner A. Modulation of human endothelial cell tetrahydrobiopterin synthesis by activating and deactivating cytokines: new perspectives on endothelium-derived relaxing factor. *Biochem.Biophys.Res.Commun.* (1993); 196:1343-1348

[35] Eissner G., Kohlhuber F., Grell M., et al Critical involvement of transmembrane tumor necrosis factor-alpha in endothelial programmed cell death mediated by ionizing radiation and bacterial endoxin. *Blood* (1995); 86:4184-4193

[36] Krakauer T. IL-10 inhibits the adhesion of leukocytic cells to IL-1-activated human endothelial cells. *Immunol.Lett.* (1995); 45:61-65

[37] Wojta J., Gallicchio M., Zoellner H., Filonzi E.L., Hamilton J.A. and Mcgrath K. Interleukin-4 stimulates expression of urokinase-type-plasminogen activator in cultured human foreskin microvascular endothelial cells. *Blood* (1993); 81:3285-3292

[38] Marfaingkoka A., Devergne O., Gorgone G., et al Regulation of the production of the RANTES chemokine by endothelial cells - Synergistic induction by IFN-gamma plus TNF-alpha and inhibition by IL-4 and IL-13. *J.Immunol.* (1995); 154:1870-1878

[39] Sironi M., Sciacca F.L., Matteucci C., et al Regulation of endothelial and mesothelial cell function by interleukin-13: selective induction of vascular cell adhesion molecule-1 and amplification of interleukin-6 production. *Blood* (1994); 84:1913-1921

[40] Garcia de Frutos P., Hardig Y. and Dahlback B. Serum amyloid P component binding to C4b-binding protein. *J.Biol.Chem.* (1995); 270:26950-26955

[41] Kaplanski G., Farnarier C., Kaplanski S., et al Interleukin-1 induces interleukin-8 secretion from endothelial cells by a juxtacrine mechanism. *Blood* (1994); 84:4242-4248

[42] Brown Z., Gerritsen M.E., Carley W.W., Strieter R.M., Kunkel S.L. and Westwick J. Chemokine gene expression and secretion by cytokine- activated human microvascular endothelial cells - Differential regulation of monocyte chemoattractant protein-1 and interleukin-8 in response to interferon- gamma. *Am.J.Pathol.* (1994); 145:913-921

[43] Bazan J.F., Bacon K.B., Hardiman G., et al A new class of membrane-bound chemokine with a CX3C motif. *Nature* (1997); 385:640-644

[44] Koch A.E., Polverini P.J., Kunkel S.L., et al Interleukin-8 as a macrophage-derived mediator of angiogenesis. *Science* (1992); 258:1798-1801

[45] Schonbeck U., Brandt E., Petersen F., Flad H.D. and Loppnow H. IL-8 specifically binds to endothelial but not to smooth muscle cells. *J.Immunol.* (1995); 154:2375-2383

[46] Petzelbauer P., Watson C.A., Pfau S.E. and Pober J.S. IL-8 and angiogenesis: Evidence that human endothelial cells lack receptors and do not respond to IL-8 in vitro. *Cytokine* (1995); 7:267-272

[47] Voest E.E., Kenyon B.M., O'Reilly M.S., Truitt G., D'Amato R.J. and Folkman J. Inhibition of angiogenesis in vivo by interleukin-12. *J.Natl.Cancer Inst.* (1995); 87:581-586

[48] Luster A.D., Greenberg S.M. and Leder P. The IP-10 chemokine binds to a specific cell surface heparan sulfate site shared with platelet factor 4 and inhibits endothelial cell proliferation. *J.Exp.Med.* (1995); 182:219-231

[49] Angiolillo A.L., Sgadari C., Taub D.D., et al Human interferon-inducible protein 10 is a potent inhibitor of angiogenesis in vivo. *J.Exp.Med.* (1995); 182:155-162

[50] Strieter R.M., Polverini P.J., Kunkel S.L., et al The functional role of the ELR motif in CXC chemokine-mediated angiogenesis . *J.Biol.Chem.* (1995); 270:27348-27357

[51] Cao Y.H., Chen C., Weatherbee J.A., Tsang M. and Folkman J. gro-beta, a -C-X-C- chemokine, is an angiogenesis inhibitor that suppresses the growth of Lewis lung carcinoma in mice. *J.Exp.Med.* (1995); 182:2069-2077

[52] Peiper S.C., Wang Z.X., Neote K., et al The Duffy antigen receptor for chemokines (DARC) is expressed in endothelial cells of Duffy negative individuals who lack the erythrocyte receptor. *J.Exp.Med.* (1995); 181:1311-1317

[53] Rot A. Endothelial cell binding of NAP-1/IL-8: role in neutrophil emigration. *Immunol.Today.* (1992); 13:291-294

[54] Ley K., Baker J.B., Cybulsky M.I., Gimbrone M.A. and Luscinskas F.W. Intravenous interleukin-8 inhibits granulocyte emigration from rabbit mesenteric venules without altering L-selectin expression or leukocyte rolling. *J.Immunol.* (1993); 151:6347-6357

[55] Colotta F., Orlando S., Fadlon E.J., Sozzani S., Matteucci C. and Mantovani A. Chemoattractants induce rapid release of the interleukin 1 type II decoy receptor in human polymorphonuclear cells. *J.Exp.Med.* (1995); 181:2181-2188

[56] Hollenbaugh D., Mischel Petty N., Edwards C.P., et al Expression of functional CD40 by vascular endothelial cells. *J.Exp.Med.* (1995); 182:33-40

[57] Yellin M.J., Brett J., Baum D., et al Functional interactions of T cells with endothelial cells: the role of CD40L-CD40-mediated signals. *J.Exp.Med.* (1995); 182:1857-1864

[58] Karmann K., Hughes C.C., Schechner J., Fanslow W.C. and Pober J.S. CD40 on human endothelial cells: inducibility by cytokines and functional regulation of adhesion molecule expression. *Proc.Natl.Acad.Sci.U.S.A.* (1995); 92:4342-4346

[59] McMahan C.J., Slack J.L., Mosley B., et al A novel IL-1 receptor, cloned from B cells by mammalian expression, is expressed in many cell types. *EMBO J.* (1991); 10:2821-2832

[60] Sims J.E., March C.J., Cosman D., et al cDNA espression cloning of the IL-1 receptor, a member of the immunoglobulin superfamily. *Science* (1988); 241:585-589

[61] Colotta F., Re F., Muzio M., et al Interleukin-1 type II receptor: a decoy target for IL-1 that is regulated by IL-4. *Science* (1993); 261:472-475

[62] Greenfeder S.A., Nunes P., Kwee L., Labow M., Chizzonite R. and Ju G. Molecular cloning and characterization of a second subunit of the interleukin 1 receptor complex. *J.Biol.Chem.* (1995); 270:13757-13765

[63] Korherr C., Hofmeister R., Wesche H. and Falk W. A critical role for interleukin-1 receptor accessory protein in interleukin-1 signaling. *Eur.J.Immunol.* (1997); 27:262-267

[64]　Wesche H., Korherr C., Kracht M., Falk W., Resch K. and Martin M.U. The interleukin-1 receptor accessory protein (IL-1RAcP) is essential for IL-1-induced activation of interleukin-1 receptor-associated kinase (IRAK) and stress-activated protein kinases (SAP kinases). *J.Biol.Chem.* (1997); 272:7727-7731

[65]　Colotta F., Sironi M., Borre A., et al Type II interleukin-1 receptor is not expressed in cultured endothelial cells and is not involved in endothelial cell activation. *Blood* (1993); 81:1347-1351

[66]　Rosoff P.M., Savage N. and Dinarello C.A. Interleukin-1 stimulates diacylglycerol production in T lymphocytes by a novel mechanism. *Cell* (1988); 54:73-81

[67]　Mathias S., Younes A., Kan C.C., Orlow I., Joseph C. and Kolesnick R.N. Activation of the sphingomyelin signaling pathway in intact EL4 cells and in a cell-free system by IL-1 beta. *Science* (1993); 259:519-522

[68]　Guesdon F. and Saklatvala J. Identification of a cytoplasmic protein kinase regulated by IL-1 that phosphorylates the small heat shock protein, hsp27. *J.Immunol.* (1991); 147:3402-3407

[69]　Freshney N.W., Rawlinson L., Guesdon F., et al Interleukin-1 actives a novel protein kinase cascade that results in phosphorylation of Hsp27. *Cell* (1994); 78:1039-1049

[70]　Dinarello C.A. Interleukin-1 and interleukin-1 antagonism. *Blood* (1991); 77:1627-1652

[71]　Dinarello C.A. Biological basis for IL-1 in disease. *Blood* (1996); 87:2095-2147

[72]　Cao Z., Henzel W.J. and Gao X. IRAK: a kinase associated with the interleukin-1 receptor. *Science* (1996); 271:1128-1131

[73]　Lemaitre B., Nicolas E., Michaut L., Reichhart J.M. and HoffmannJA. The dorsoventral regulatory gene cassette spatzle/Toll/cactus controls the potent antifungal response in Drosophila adults. *Cell* (1996); 86:973-983

[74]　Gay N.J. and Keith F.J. Drosophila Toll and IL-1 receptor. *Nature* (1991); 351:355-356

[75]　Galindo R.L., Edwards D.N., Gillespie S.K. and Wasserman S.A. Interaction of the pelle kinase with the membrane-associated protein tube is required for transduction of the dorsoventral signal in Drosophila embryos. *Development* (1995); 121:2209-2218

[76]　Norris J.L. and Manley J.L. Functional interactions between the pelle kinase, Toll receptor, and tube suggest a mechanism for activation of dorsal. *Gene.Develop.* (1996); 10:862-872

[77]　Muzio M., Ni J., Feng P. and Dixit V.M. IRAK (Pelle) family member IRAK-2 and MyD88 as proximal mediators of IL-1 signaling. *Science* (1997); 278:1612-1615

[78]　Wesche H., Henzel W.J., Shillinglaw W., Li S. and Cao Z. MyD88: an adapter that recruits IRAK to the IL-1 receptor complex. *Immunity* (1997); 7:837-847

[79]　Cao Z., Xiong J., Takeuchi M., Kurama T. and Goeddel D.V. TRAF6 is a signal transducer for interleukin-1. *Nature* (1996); 383:443-446

[80]　Malinin N.L., Boldin M.P., Kovalenko A.V. and Wallach D. MAP3K-related kinase involved in NF-kappaB induction by TNF, CD95 and IL-1. *Nature* (1997); 385:540-544

[81]　Regnier C.H., Song H.Y., Gao X., Goeddel D.V., Cao Z. and Rothe M. Identification and characterization of an IkappaB kinase. *Cell* (1997); 90:373-383

[82]　DiDonato J.A., Hayakawa M., Rothwarf D.M., Zandi E. and Karin M. A cytokine-responsive IkappaB kinase that activates the transcription factor NF-kappaB. *Nature* (1997); 388:548-554

[83]　Mercurio F., Zhu H., Murray B.W., et al IKK-1 and IKK-2: cytokine-activated IkappaB kinases essential for NF-kappaB activation. *Science* (1997); 278:860-866

[84]　Woronicz J.D., Gao X., Cao Z., Rothe M. and Goeddel D.V. IkappaB kinase-beta: NF-kappaB activation and complex formation with IkappaB kinase-alpha and NIK. *Science* (1997); 278:866-869

[85]　Zandi E., Rothwarf D.M., Delhase M., Hayakawa M. and Karin M. The IkappaB kinase complex (IKK) contains two kinase subunits, IKKalpha and IKKbeta, necessary for IkappaB phosphorylation and NF-kappaB activation. *Cell* (1997); 91:243-252

Vascular Endothelium: Mechanisms of Cell Signaling
J.D. Catravas et al. (Eds.)
IOS Press, 1999

SHEAR STRESS-MEDIATED REGULATION OF ERK1/2 IN ENDOTHELIAL CELLS: SIGNAL TRANSDUCTION PATHWAYS

Bradford C. Berk and Oren Traub
University of Rochester Medical Center, Cardiology Unit
Box 679, Rochester, NY 14646, USA
email: Bradford_Berk@urmc.rochester.edu

Abstract

Mechanical forces are important modulators of cellular function in various tissues and are particularly important in the cardiovascular system. The endothelial cell layer, by virtue of its unique location in the vessel wall, is exposed to fluid forces of much greater magnitude than those experienced by other mammalian tissues and thus has developed mechanically-related responses to fluid shear stress. While the effects of shear on endothelial cell function have been well studied, the mechanisms by which endothelial cells sense mechanical stimuli and convert them to biochemical signals are not well characterized. In this review, we discuss the role of MAP kinases as mediators of fluid shear stress-dependent signal transduction. In addition, we show that PKC is involved in the fluid shear stress-mediated ERK1/2 activation as well as characterize PKC-ε as the necessary isoform for this signaling pathway. Based on results for ERK1/2 we propose four potential mechanosensing mechanisms in endothelial cells. Characterization of endothelial cell signaling mechanisms will provide insight into how hemodynamic forces modulate endothelial cell function. This knowledge is important not only to our understanding of the pathogenesis of atherosclerosis but also to a wide variety of biological processes that are modulated by physical forces such as bone growth, muscle hypertrophy, and hair cell sound transduction.

1. Introduction

Numerous studies suggest that normal functioning of the endothelium is critical in limiting the development of atherosclerosis as illustrated by the correlation between risk factors for atherosclerosis (smoking, high cholesterol, high homocysteine, decreased estrogen, increasing age, and hypertension) and endothelial dysfunction [1]. A major role of the endothelial cells is to detect changes in hemmodynamic state and maintain vascular homeostasis. In particular, endothelial cells are ideally situated to respond to changes in physical forces. The frictional force that blood exerts on the endothelium is termed fluid shear stress. The nature of fluid shear stress experienced by endothelial cells is a function of blood flow patterns throughout the vasculature generated by the cardiac cycle. In "linear" areas of the vasculature, blood flows in ordered laminar patterns in a pulsatile fashion dependent on the cardiac cycle and endothelial cells experience pulsatile fluid shear stress with fluctuations in magnitude that yield a mean positive shear stress. This flow pattern should be distinguished from the steady flow pattern which is often used in experimental preparations which generates a *steady* positive shear stress, being temporally and spatially uniform. While steady fluid shear stress generally stimulates many of the same endothelial cell responses as pulsatile stress, there are some qualitative and quantitative differences [2-4]. At areas of abrupt curvatures in the vasculature, as in the carotid bifurcation, the laminar flow of blood is disrupted and separated flow patterns result. Specifically, the medial wall of the carotid bulb experiences higher fluid shear stress while the lateral wall experiences recirculation vortices which vary with the cardiac cycle resulting in flow reversal [5]. Thus, the lateral area of the carotid bulb experiences *oscillatory* shear stress (periodic flow reversal with time-average shear stress approaching zero) and low mean shear stress. The significance of these flow patterns is demonstrated by studies that correlate development of atherosclerotic lesions (fatty streaks and small plaques) with areas of the carotid that experience these flow reversals with low time-averaged shear stress [5, 6]. Regions of the carotid bifurcation that experience pulsatile and mean positive shear stress as the result of laminar blood flow patterns, however, are relatively protected from atherosclerosis. Other investigators have confirmed these observations throughout the vasculature [7]. The mechanisms by which the physical force generated by fluid shear stress is transduced into biological signals remain undefined.

NO appears to be a key mediator of the atheroprotective effects of fluid shear stress on the blood vessel wall. NO has been reported to play a role in platelet aggregation and leukocyte binding to the endothelium, in inhibition of vascular smooth muscle tone and growth, and in alteration of lipoprotein metabolism [8]. The ability of fluid shear stress to regulate some of these processes is abrogated by inhibitors of NO production suggesting that fluid shear stress may exert its effects through the release of NO. Further, it has been postulated that the beneficial effects of regular aerobic training, including its anti-atherogenic properties, may be mediated through fluid shear stress-induced increases in NO secretion [9]. NO is produced by a unique enzyme present in the endothelium, termed endothelial nitric oxide synthase (eNOS) [10-12]. Fluid shear stress is the most potent physiologic stimulus for NO production in endothelial cells. Rapid increases in NO production are due to post-translational activation of eNOS while chronic alterations in eNOS expression are due to changes in gene expression.

Experiments by our laboratory and others [13, 14] indicate that two distinct signaling pathways (a Ca^{2+}-dependent and a Ca^{2+}-independent pathway) are involved in shear-mediated increases in NO production [15]. We compared NO production in response to the Ca^{2+}-ionophore A23187 with fluid shear stress. While A23187 increased NO production by 3 to 6-fold, fluid shear stress stimulated NO production by 10- to 30-fold above static levels. The initial rapid increase in NO required Ca^{2+}, while the sustained increase in NO production was independent of changes in intracellular Ca^{2+} [16]. Further experiments by our laboratory have demonstrated that eNOS was phosphorylated in response to fluid shear stress [16]. Although the relationship between eNOS phosphorylation and NO production is unclear, phosphorylation may regulate the activity of eNOS. To better understand how fluid shear stress influences eNOS activity and expression, it will be necessary to identify upstream mediators of eNOS function which are activated by fluid shear stress, such as protein kinases.

2. Mitogen-Activated Protein Kinases: Likely Signaling Molecules in the Transduction of Fluid Shear Stress

Several features of the endothelial cell response to fluid shear stress are analogous to receptor-mediated signaling: dependence on G proteins, increase in intracellular calcium, and changes in gene expression (Table 1). The family of kinases termed mitogen-activated protein (MAP) kinases are potential candidates to mediate some of the effects of fluid shear stress on endothelial cells. MAP kinases are ubiquitously expressed serine/threonine protein kinases that are activated in response to a variety of extracellular stimuli involved in cell growth, transformation, and differentiation. The extracellular signal regulated

Table 1: Endothelial cell responses to fluid shear stress: temporal classification.

Initiation of Signaling (< 1 minute)

- K+ channel activation
- IP$_3$ and DAG elevation
- cGMP increase
- Calcium increase
- Acute end responses (NO, PGI$_2$ release)

Signaling cascades; Transcription factor activation; Gene regulation (1 minute to 1 hour)

- G protein activation
- MAP kinase signaling
- NFkB activation
- SSRE-dependent gene regulation: (PDGF-B, c-jun)
- bFGF upregulation
- Pinocytosis stimulated

Adaptive responses to new hemodynamic conditions (1-6 hours)

- Reorganization of luminal surface
- Cell alignment
- Completion of cytoskeletal rearrangement
- Increased mechanical stiffness
- Decreased fibronectin synthesis
- Changes of TM expression
- Stimulation of histidine decarboxylase
- Enhanced LDL metabolism
- Induced MHC antigen expression

Gene regulation and protein synthesis; Cell-wide adaptive responses (> 6 hours)

- SSRE-dependent gene regulation: (eNOS, tPA, TGF-β, ICAM-1, c-fos, MCP-1)
- Stimulation of HSP-70
- Downregulation of ET-1
- Cytoskeletal rearrangement
- Focal adhesion rearrangement
- Transient rearrangement of Golgi

kinases (ERK1/2), members of the MAP kinase family have many potential substrates, including other protein kinases (p90rsk, MAPKAP, Raf-1, MEK), transcription factors (c-myc, c-jun, c-fos, p62TCF), enzymes (cPLA2) and cell surface proteins (EGF receptor), and thus have many effects on cellular physiology and gene expression [15] (Figure 1).

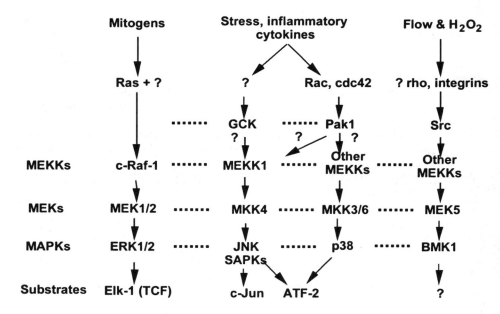

Figure 1. MAP kinase activation pathways. A common theme in the stimulation of MAP kinase family members is activation by an immediate upstream MAP kinase kinase (MEK) which is, in turn, activated by an immediate upstream MAP kinase kinase (MEKK). Different stimuli activate different signaling pathways leading to individual MAP kinase activation.

The pathway for ERK1/2 activation in response to growth factors has been well characterized and serves as a model for fluid shear stress-mediated signal transduction (Figure 2). The MAP and ERK kinase (MEK-1) is a dual specificity kinase that phosphorylates ERK1/2 on T-E-Y. MEK-1 is itself regulated by a MAP kinase kinase kinase, one of which has been identified as Raf-1. Raf-1 is activated by translocation to the membrane and association with the small GTP-binding protein, ras. The GTPase activity of ras is regulated by a complex involving Grb2 and mSOS which are recruited and activated by a tyrosine kinase receptor [17]. We have recently reported that ERK1/2 is activated by fluid shear stress in endothelial cells in a time- and force-dependent manner [18]. These data, combined with observations that eNOS contains multiple consensus sites for phosphorylation by a variety of kinases including ERK1/2 [15], make this pathway a likely candidate to participate in the stimulation of sustained NO production in response to fluid shear stress. Additionally, several fluid shear stress-responsive genes contain elements (e.g., AP-1) [19, 20] that may be influenced by ERK1/2-mediated phosphorylation of transcription factors [15] such as c-fos, c-jun, and c-myc. Importantly this pathway appears to be conserved in mammalian cells as shown by the ability of fluid shear stress to stimulate ERK1/2 in fibroblasts (Figure 3).

    Another member of the MAP kinase family shown to be regulated by fluid shear stress is the stress-activated protein kinase (JNK/SAPK). Two laboratories have shown increases in JNK activity by fluid shear stress, although with varying kinetics [21, 22]. Preliminary results in our laboratory show that fluid shear stress inhibits TNF-stimulated JNK activity in endothelial cells (unpublished observations), a finding consistent with the recently reported ability of fluid shear stress to inhibit endothelial cell apoptosis [23, 24]. Additional experiments by our laboratory indicate that other members of the MAP kinase

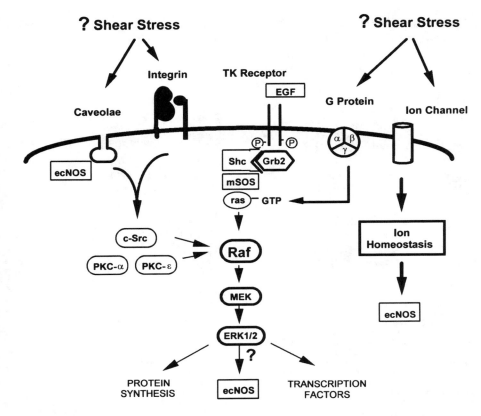

Figure 2. Proposed model of fluid shear stress-mediated mechanotransduction in endothelial cells. Primary mechanosensors (e.g. integrins, caveolae, G proteins, ion channels) transduce physical stimuli into biochemical signals. Several stimuli serve to activate Raf-1, including tyrosine phosphorylation by c-Src or c-Src-like kinases, serine and threonine phosphorylation by PKC, and GTP-bound ras. Raf-1 activates MEK which in turn activates ERK1/2. Sustained generation of NO may result from the effects of ERK1/2 or through direct effects of mechanosensors (e.g. caveolae) themselves.

family, p38 and BMK-1 (ERK5), are also activated by fluid shear stress in endothelial cells [25].

3. Fluid Shear Stress Leads to Phosphorylation and Activation of ERK1/2 in a Force- and Time-Dependent Manner

Published results from our laboratory demonstrate that ERK1/2 is phosphorylated in response to fluid shear stress in a force-dependent manner and that phosphorylation correlates with ERK1/2 kinase activity (Figure 4). Compared with static conditions, fluid shear stress at 12 dynes/cm^2 activated ERK1/2 with a peak at 10 min and return to baseline by 60 min . These data show activation kinetics similar to those previously reported by our laboratory using other techniques [18, 26]. Western blotting with an antibody for ERK1/2 that detects both the phosphorylated and unphosphorylated form of the kinases showed that cellular ERK1/2 levels remained constant throughout the fluid shear stress time-course. These results demonstrate that ERK1/2 is phosphorylated in

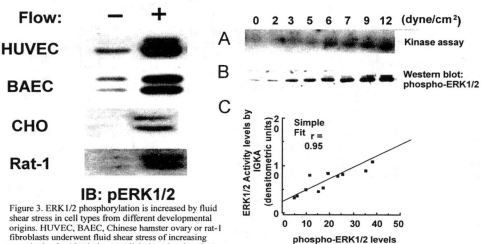

IB: pERK1/2

Figure 3. ERK1/2 phosphorylation is increased by fluid shear stress in cell types from different developmental origins. HUVEC, BAEC, Chinese hamster ovary or rat-1 fibroblasts underwent fluid shear stress of increasing magnitudes for 10 min in a parallel plate chamber. Lysates were separated by SDS-PAGE and Western blotting with anti-phosphospecific-ERK1/2 antibody performed. Fluid shear stress increased ERK1/2 phosphorylation in all cells tested, with the response in endothelial cells being significantly more robust.

Figure 4. ERK1/2 phosphorylation is directly proportional to ERK1/2 activity and increases with shear stress. HUVEC underwent fluid shear stress of increasing magnitudes for 10 minutes. (A) Lysates were run on SDS-PAGE containing myelin basic protein. Protein was renatured and incubated with 32P-ATP for 1 hour. The gel was dried and autoradiography was performed to measure kinase activity. (B) Lysates were separated by SDS-PAGE and Western blotting with anti-phosphospecific-ERK1/2 antibody performed. (C) Densitometry was performed on the gels in A and B. ERK1/2 activity and phosphorylation were directly correlated with r = 0.95.

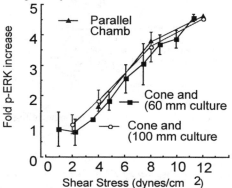

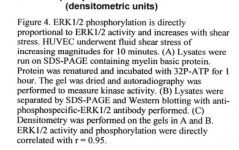

Figure 5. ERK1/2 phosphorylation and activation is increased by fluid shear stress. HUVEC underwent fluid shear stress of increasing magnitudes for 10 minutes in either a parallel plate chamber or a cone and plate viscometer. Lysates were separated by SDS-PAGE and Western blotting with anti-phosphospecific-ERK1/2 antibody performed. Fluid shear stress increased ERK1/2 phosphorylation in a force-dependent manner with no significant difference between the two apparatus tested.

response to fluid shear stress with time-course similar to receptor agonists, such as thrombin and EGF [18].

Time course kinetics for ERK1/2 phosphorylation using a cone and plate viscometer were compared to results obtained on the parallel plate chamber (Figure 5). While the kinetics of activation were similar for early time points (< 30 min), levels of pERK1/2 were significantly higher at time points >30 min when compared with results using the parallel plate chamber. One likely explanation for this persistent elevation is that vasoactive mediators released by the endothelium in response to fluid shear stress become concentrated in the relatively low volume (1-4 mL) of medium used in the cone and plate viscometer. Many vasoactive mediators are released by endothelial cells in response to fluid shear stress [27] and may affect ERK1/2 phosphorylation. These results indicate that the use of the cone and plate viscometer yields results similar to those obtained with the parallel plate chamber for early time points, but not for longer time points.

In summary, ERK1/2 is an excellent biological marker to use for analysis of fluid shear stress signal transduction based on the following properties: (1) ERK1/2 responds to shear stress in a force- and time-dependent manner; (2) shear mediated ERK1/2 activation is conserved across several cell lines from different developmental origins; (3) measurement of ERK1/2 phosphorylation and/or activity is quick, simple, relatively inexpensive, and does not necessarily require radioactivity; and (4) ERK1/2 demonstrates a response to fluid shear stress that is relatively rapid, thus short periods of stimulation are often sufficient for studies characterizing fluid shear stress responsivity.

4. Fluid Shear Stress Activation of ERK1/2 Is Protein Kinase C-Dependent

Fluid shear stress has been shown to activate phospholipase C [28], resulting in the cleavage of PIP_2 into inositol 1,4,5-trisphosphate, a calcium-mobilizing second messenger, and diacylglycerol, an activator of protein kinase C (PKC). Indeed, recent studies have implicated PKC in cellular responses to fluid shear stress, such as endothelin-1 production [29], PDGF expression [30] and cytoskeletal reorganization [31]. Previous studies by our laboratory have suggested that PKC is also required for the fluid shear stress-mediated activation of ERK1/2 [18]. We investigated the role of PKC in fluid shear stress-mediated signaling and show that PKC-ε, but not PKC-α or PKC-ζ, is required for ERK1/2 activation by fluid shear stress.

4.1. ERK1/2 Activation by Shear Stress is PKC-Dependent and Calcium-Independent

Several investigators have reported that PKC is activated in response to various mechanical stimuli such as stretch, pressure and shear [32]. To determine the role of PKC in ERK1/2 activation by fluid shear stress, cells were exposed to 1 µM phorbol 12, 13 dibutyrate (PDBu) for 24 hr prior to fluid shear stress to downregulate PKC. ERK1/2 activation by fluid shear stress was significantly inhibited by PDBu pretreatment, (28±3% of control) as shown by immunoblotting with the ERK1/2 phosphospecific antibody [33]. Pretreatment with the protein kinase inhibitor, staurosporine (2 nM, 30 min), reduced ERK1/2 activation to 10±6% of control levels. Levels of phosphorylated ERK1/2 in cells maintained in static culture were not changed by either treatment (data not shown). These data suggest that PKC is necessary for the fluid shear stress-mediated activation of ERK1/2.

Mechanical stimuli cause a rapid increase in intracellular calcium concentration [34], and our laboratory has previously reported that fluid shear stress at 12 dynes/cm^2 for 10 min increases intracellular calcium [35]. To determine if the fluid shear stress-mediated increase in intracellular calcium was necessary for ERK1/2 activation, cells were treated with the Ca^{2+}-chelator BAPTA-AM (75 µM, 30 min), and the fluid shear stress stimulus was performed in a Ca^{2+}-free balanced salt solution supplemented with EDTA (10 mM) in order to inhibit the fluid shear stress-mediated increase in intracellular calcium. Basal levels of ERK1/2 activation (data not shown) and ERK1/2 activation by fluid shear stress were unaffected by pretreatment with BAPTA [33], suggesting that a rise in intracellular calcium is not necessary for ERK1/2 activation by fluid shear stress. These results demonstrate that the fluid shear stress-mediated activation of ERK1/2 is PKC-dependent and calcium-independent.

4.2. Endothelial Cells Express Several Different PKC Isoforms

At least eleven PKC isoforms have been described, each possessing unique characteristics and perhaps playing different roles in cell signaling. A classification system for the PKC family has emerged that separates the different isoforms into four distinct classes [36] (Table 2).

Table 2. Protein Kinase C Isoform Classification

Group	Isoform	Phorbol-responsive?	Translocation?
Classical	α, β, γ	Yes	Yes
Novel	$\delta, \varepsilon, \theta, \eta$	Yes	Yes/No
Atypical	$\lambda/\iota, \zeta$	No	No
Eccentric	μ	No	??

The "classical" PKC isoforms, which include α, βI, βII, and γ, are described as calcium-independent and phorbol ester-responsive enzymes. The second and third class are the "novel" PKC isoforms (including δ, ε, θ, η) and the "atypical" PKC isoforms (including ζ, λ/ι). The novel isoforms lack the calcium-binding domains that are present on the classical isoforms, yet still retain the phorbol ester-binding domains. Hence, the novel isoforms are described as calcium-independent and phorbol ester-responsive PKC isoforms. In contrast, the atypical isoforms lack both the calcium-binding sites as well as the phorbol ester-binding domains and are described as calcium-independent and phorbol ester-unresponsive. The final group, termed "eccentric," contains the recently discovered and little studied PKC-μ isoform. Because ERK1/2 activation by fluid shear stress is phorbol ester-responsive but calcium independent; our results suggest that some member(s) of the novel class (δ, ε, θ, η) are involved in the signaling pathway that leads to activation of ERK1/2. To determine which PKC isoforms were expressed in endothelial cells, we performed Western blotting with isoform-specific antibodies on endothelial cell lysates. Endothelial cells express primarily three PKC isoforms: PKC-α, PKC-ε, and PKC-ζ while no significant immunoreactivity was detected for PKC-β, $-\gamma$, $-\delta$, $-\theta$, $-\eta$, and $-\lambda/\iota$. Thus, the only member of the novel class present in endothelial cells is PKC-ε.

4.3. Effect of PDBu treatment on PKC Isoform Expression

Because fluid shear stress-mediated activation of PKC was significantly attenuated by 24 hr pretreatment with PDBu, we determined the time-dependent change in PKC isoform levels. While brief stimulation with PMA (200 nM, 10 min) had no effect on PKC levels, prolonged exposure of cells to PDBu caused downregulation of PKC-α (100% by 24 hr) and PKC-ε (100% by 12 hr). PKC-ζ levels were unaffected. PDBu treatment had no effect on either cellular ERK1/2 levels or on EGF-mediated ERK1/2 activation. These results are consistent with the characteristics of the different PKC-isoforms described above and suggest that PKC–ζ is not involved in ERK1/2 activation by fluid shear stress as it was unaffected by PDBu treatment.

4.4. Measurement of PKC Activity by Translocation Assay

To determine whether the PKC isoforms expressed in endothelial cells translocate upon cell stimulation, the intracellular localization of the PKC isoforms was determined by centrifugal fractionation, SDS-PAGE separation, and Western blotting (Figure 6). Western analysis showed that in the unstimulated state, both PKC–α and PKC–ζ were evenly distributed in the cytosolic and membrane fractions while PKC–ε was localized solely to the membrane fraction. After stimulation with PMA (200 nM, 10 min), PKC–α translocated to the membrane fraction but little difference was observed in the distribution of PKC–ε and PKC–ζ. Since PKC–ε was already localized to the membrane fraction (though whether nuclear or membrane is unknown) and because there was little difference in cellular localization of PKC–ζ in response to PMA, this method of measuring PKC activity

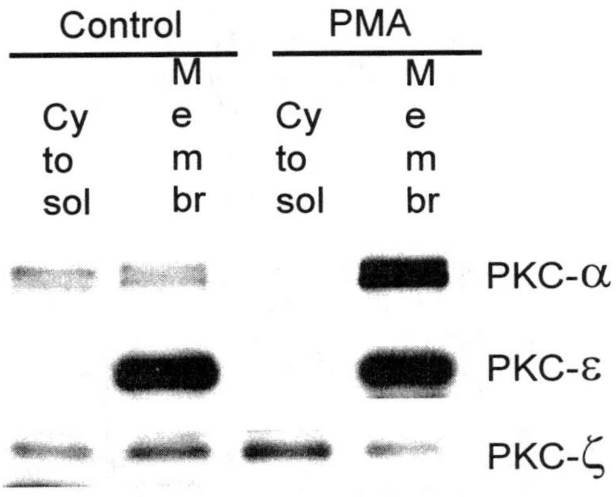

Figure 6. Subcellular localization of PKC isoforms endothelial cells assayed by Western blotting. cells were pretreated with either vehicle (control: DMSO, 10 min) or PMA (200 nM for 10 min) and washed free of culture media with HBSS. Lysates prepared, and cytosolic and membrane fractions were as described in "Materials and Methods." Western analysis was performed using isoform-specific antibodies.

analysis was performed using isoform-specific PKC antibodies. would not be useful in determining whether PKC–ε and PKC–ζ are activated by fluid shear stress.

4.5. Measurement of PKC Activity by Histone Phosphorylation

Another method to measure PKC activity is by phosphorylation of a PKC substrate. Since specific substrates for each isoform are not available, we measured the activity of the PKC isoforms by immunoprecipitating each isoform and then performing an immune complex kinase assay with a universal PKC substrate, histone-H1. In this assay, PKC–α activity was inhibited by the addition of staurosporine, exclusion of Ca^{2+} (below basal levels or to basal levels with PMA stimulation; data not shown), or exclusion of both Ca^{2+} and cofactors (diolein and phosphatidylserine, Figure 7 A). Addition of PMA to the reaction mixture potentiated PKC–α activity. Activity of the PKC–ε isoform was also inhibited by staurosporine and removal of Ca^{2+} and cofactors, but was not affected by removal of Ca^{2+} alone (Figure 7B). Addition of PMA stimulated PKC–ε activity. The activity of PKC–ζ was not inhibited by staurosporine, removal of Ca^{2+}, or removal of both Ca^{2+} and cofactors (Figure 7C). Further, PMA added directly to the assay was unable to stimulate activity. These results confirm that endothelial cell PKC–ζ is a calcium-independent and phorbol ester-unresponsive PKC isoform.

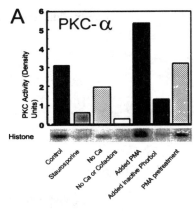

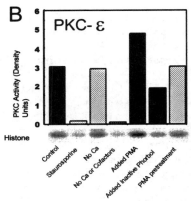

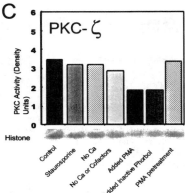

Figure 7. Measurement of PKC isoform activity under varying conditions by histone-H1 phosphorylation assay. Endothelial cells were washed in HBSS, lysates were prepared using assay-lysis buffer, PKC-isoforms were immunoprecipitated, and equal amounts of protein were assayed in an immune complex kinase reaction (as described in "Materials and Methods") containing histone-H1 and γ-32P-ATP at 30°C for 10 min. For some experiments 2 nM staurosporine, 200 nM PMA, or 200 nM inactive phorbol ester were added directly to the reaction mixture. Proteins were separated by SDS-PAGE and histone phosphorylation determined by autoradiogram and subsequent quantification by densitometry. Cells lysates used in the far right lane (PMA pretreatment) were treated with 200 nM PMA for 10 min prior to cell harvesting and immunoprecipitation.

Adding PMA to the reaction mixture stimulated activity of PKC-α and PKC-ε, but pretreating cells with PMA prior to immunoprecipitation failed to stimulate PKC activity as measured by histone phosphorylation (Figure 7 far right). These results suggest that immunoprecipitation separates PKC from cellular inhibitors and activators that regulate agonist-stimulated activity. In fact, no change in immunoprecipitated PKC activity was noted for any PKC isoform when cells were pretreated with PMA, fluid shear stress or thrombin (data not shown). Therefore, this assay is useful to characterize the effects of calcium, phorbol, and staurosporine *in vitro* on the separate isoforms but is not useful to measure the effects of physiological stimuli on intact cells.

4.6. PKC Antisense Oligonucleotides Are Specific and Effective

It appears that among the PKC isoforms present in endothelial cells, PKC-ε is the most likely isoform to mediate fluid shear stress ERK1/2 signaling. This conclusion is based on the findings that the PKC isoform is (1) phorbol ester responsive, (2) calcium-independent and (3) inhibited by staurosporine. Further, these data suggest that neither PKC-α nor PKC- is involved in this signaling process as PKC- is calcium-dependent and PKC-ζ is phorbol ester-unresponsive and resistant to inhibition by staurosporine. To establish the role of PKC- in fluid shear stress-mediated activation of ERK1/2, we decided to inhibit each expressed PKC isoform individually and measure changes in ERK1/2 activation. Since specific pharmacologic inhibitors of the separate PKC isoforms are currently unavailable, antisense phosphorothioate oligonucleotides and their corresponding scrambled controls for the different PKC isoforms were employed. Antisense oligonucleotides have previously been employed to inhibit expression of PKC- in mouse and human cell lines in an isoform-specific manner [37, 38]. HUVEC were transfected with antisense PKC- oligonucleotides for 6 hr, and the cells were harvested 3 days later for analysis. Protein levels for PKC- were reduced in a concentration dependent manner with reductions of 22±10%, 25±6% and 80±13% at 100, 300 and 1000 nM antisense PKC-ε oligonucleotide, respectively. Expression of PKC-α and PKC-ζ isoforms was not significantly affected at any concentration of antisense PKC-ε oligonucleotide, indicating that the antisense oligonucleotides were specific for PKC-ε. PKC-ε levels were not affected by treatment with 1000 nM scrambled PKC-ε oligonucleotides demonstrating minimal non-specific effects of the transfection protocol. Similar specificity and efficacy of 1000 nM antisense PKC-α and PKC-ζ oligonucleotides for their corresponding PKC isoforms was observed (data not shown).

4.7. Antisense PKC-ε Oligonucleotides Block Shear Stress-Mediated ERK1/2 Activation

Several studies have demonstrated that many PKC isoforms are able to activate ERK1/2 in a stimulus-specific manner, including PKC-α, PKC-ε, and PKC-ζ [39, 40] To determine the effect of inhibiting different PKC isoforms on ERK1/2 activation by fluid shear stress, cells treated with antisense PKC oligonucleotides were maintained in static culture or exposed to fluid shear stress. Antisense or scrambled PKC-α, -ε, -ζ oligonucleotide treatment did not affect baseline phosphorylation of ERK1/2 (Figure 8a, left three lanes). Antisense or scrambled PKC-α or –ζ oligonucleotides did not alter the ERK1/2 activation by fluid shear stress. However, in cells treated with antisense PKC-ε oligonucleotides fluid shear stress-mediated activation of ERK1/2 was completely inhibited (Figure 8a - far right). Scrambled PKC-ε oligonucleotide treatment had no effect on ERK1/2. Further, antisense PKC-ε oligonucleotides had no effect on bradykinin or EGF-induced ERK1/2 activation demonstrating that ERK1/2 was still capable of being activated through mechanisms independent of PKC-ε (Figure 8b). Treatment with antisense PKC-ε oligonucleotides inhibited PMA-induced ERK1/2 activation by only 35%. The inability of antisense PKC-ε oligonucleotides to completely inhibit PMA-induced ERK1/2 activation is likely due to PKC isoforms other than PKC-ζ that can also activate ERK1/2 in response to PMA.

These results show that PKC-ε is a component of a mechano-sensitive signal transduction pathway that leads to the activation of ERK1/2 in endothelial cells. Further, this pathway is specific for PKC-ε, as PKC-α and PKC-ζ are not required for the activation of ERK1/2. These results, combined with observations from other investigators that fluid shear stress stimulates changes in cellular physiology and gene expression [27], provide evidence that mechanical stimuli can activate signal transduction pathways in a manner similar to conventional agonist-receptor initiated signaling events. These results define a pathway for fluid shear stress-mediated ERK1/2 activation and establish a new function for PKC-ε in endothelial cells. Two upstream mechanisms for the activation of PKC-ε in response to fluid shear stress may be proposed based on previous studies. First, phospholipase C (PLC) is activated by fluid shear stress [28], resulting in the cleavage of

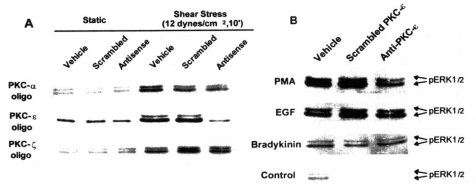

Figure 8. (A) Antisense PKC-ε oligonucleotides specifically inhibit ERK1/2 activation by fluid shear stress. HUVEC were treated with either 1000 nM antisense oligonucleotides or 1000 nM scrambled oligonucleotides against PKC-a,e, and -z isoforms for 6 hr before returning the cells to media with serum. Three days after transfection, endothelia cells were washed free of culture medium and maintained in static condition or exposed to 12 dynes/cm2 fluid shear stress for 10 min. Lysates were analyzed by Western blot using phosphospecific-ERK antibody. Western blots are representative from three separate HUVEC preparations. Antisense PKC-e oligonucleotide treatment completely blocked fluid shear stress mediated ERK1/2 activation while all other treatments did not affect ERK1/2 activation. (B) Effect of antisense PKC-e oligonucleotides treatment on ERK1/2 activation by various agonists. HUVEC were transfected with antisense PKC-e oligonucleotides as above. Three days after transfection, endothelial cells were either washed free of culture medium and exposed to either PMA (200 nM for 10 min), EGF (100 ng/mL for 5 min), or bradykinin (10 nM for 10 min) or received no treatment (control). Lysates were analyzed by Western blot using a phosphospecific-ERK antibody.

PIP$_2$ and generation of inositol 1,4,5-trisphosphate and diacylglycerol (DAG). PKC-ε is similar to the classical PKC isoforms in that it is activated by DAG [36] ; thus, one mechanism for activation of PKC-ε is through fluid shear stress-mediated generation of DAG. Second, other activators of PKC-ε such as phosphatidylinositol (3,4)-bisphosphate and phosphatidylinositol (3,4,5) trisphosphate, may be increased in endothelial cells in response to fluid shear stress. Reports show that both of these phosphoinositides, generated by PI 3-kinase activity, are potent and selective activators of the novel class of PKC isoforms and have little effect on the classical or atypical PKC isoforms [41]. To date, no studies have been published regarding changes in PI 3-kinase activity in response to fluid shear stress. Moriya et al. [42] reported that both the PI 3-kinase and the PLC pathway can activate PKC-ε in a cell-specific and stimulus-specific manner. The specificity of the PI 3-kinase pathway for the novel PKC isoforms suggests that analysis of PI 3-kinase activity in response to fluid shear stress will be a fruitful area for future studies.

5. Potential Fluid Shear Stress Sensors

A question of great importance in the field of mechanotransduction pertains to the identity of the primary mechanoreceptor(s) responsible for initiating signal transduction. Transduction of mechanical forces in anchorage-dependent cells is due to a combination of force transmission via the cytoskeletal elements and transduction of the physical forces to biochemical signals at mechanotransducer sites [15]. Based on the data presented above, the candidate mechanotransducer molecules should be responsive to fluid shear stress over the physiological range and result in the activation of a tyrosine kinases (e.g., c-Src), PKC, and ERK1/2. Due to their interaction with specific signaling molecules already implicated in signal transduction, we propose four candidates as likely mechanotransducers: integrin-matrix interactions, specialized membrane microdomains, ion channels, and G proteins (Figure 2).

In order to sense and transduce signals in response to fluid shear stress, endothelial cells must be anchored to their matrix [43]. Integrins are ubiquitous / heterodimeric transmembrane glycoproteins which act as adhesion receptors involved in the interaction between cells and extracellular matrix. Integrins play an important role in biological processes, including cell adhesion, cell migration, cell growth, tissue organization, blood clotting, inflammation, target recognition by leukocytes, and cell differentiation [44]. Studies performed by Dr. Ingber's group [45, 46] using magnetic torsion have demonstrated that integrins are capable of transducing mechanical stimuli to biochemical signals. A recent study by Muller *et al.* [47] showed that flow-induced vasodilation in coronary arteries, which is mediated by NO release, could be blocked with RGD peptides which compete with the matrix for integrin interactions. Similar attenuation of flow-induced vasodilation was obtained if a blocking antibody against the 3 integrin was employed, supporting the hypothesis that integrins are involved in the mechanotransduction of fluid shear stress. Integrins are also a particularly attractive candidate in that they have been reported to associate with PKC [33, 48] and c-Src-family tyrosine kinases [49]. Other studies by our laboratory have demonstrated that activation of 1 integrins (the predominant isoform on endothelial cells) with an activating antibody also stimulated ERK1/2, although at levels less than observed with fluid shear stress [26]. Further, human umbilical vein endothelial cells showed adhesion-mediated ERK1/2 activation when plated on a matrix of fibronectin, which engages β1 integrins, but showed no ERK1/2 activation when they adhered to matrix consisting of poly-L-lysine [43]. The relatively small magnitude of ERK1/2 stimulation by integrin activation does not preclude a key role for integrins in shear-mediated ERK1/2 activation; based on the importance of fluid shear stress to endothelial cell function and integrity, it is likely that redundant pathways with different mechanotransducer molecules mediate the full ERK/12 response to fluid shear stress.

Another possible candidate for the transduction of fluid shear stress into biochemical signals are caveolae, specialized domains of the plasma membrane that are rich in cholesterol. Because of their high cholesterol content, caveolae are more rigid than other portions of the plasma membrane. Caveolae are abundant in endothelial cells and have been implicated in transcytosis, ion movement across the membrane, and signal transduction [50] . The principal component of caveolae is a 21-24 kD integral membrane protein called caveolin. Caveolin seems to function as a scaffold for the recruitment and sequestration of signaling molecules. Among signaling molecules known to associate with caveolae are G proteins, c-Src-family tyrosine kinases, ras, PKC, eNOS [51] , shc, Grb2, mSOS, Raf-1, and ERK1/2 (see [52]). Caveolae represent an attractive site for mechanotransduction on the basis of their biophysical characteristics and interactions with signaling molecules. Experiments to determine the significance of caveolae and what effect changes in caveolae number may effect in fluid shear stress-mediated signaling should prove an exciting area for future research.

Recent data reported by Dr. Frangos' group [53] indicate that G proteins may act as primary mechanosensors in endothelial cells. This laboratory showed that treatment of endothelial cells with antisense G q oligonucleotides inhibited fluid shear stress-induced ras-GTPase activity, while scrambled oligonucleotide treatment had no effect. Another study reported that treatment of endothelial cells with pertussis toxin prevented fluid shear stress-mediated activation of ERK1/2 [22], also suggesting that G proteins are activated in response to fluid shear stress. Further, Frangos' group demonstrated that G proteins reconstituted in liposomes, in the absence of protein receptors, showed an increase in activity in response to fluid shear stress [54]. This fluid shear stress-mediated increase in G protein activity could be attenuated if the lipid bilayer was made more rigid by the addition of cholesterol, a significant finding in the context of caveolae as fluid shear stress signaling domains.

A common mechanism that has evolved to sense changes in mechanical stimuli are the mechanosensitive ion channels. These channels are widely distributed in tissues and participate in processes such as hearing, balance, and reflex contraction of smooth muscle and skeletal muscle. Endothelial cells exhibit ion channel responses to mechanical forces that are likely to participate in the signaling response to fluid shear stress. Several different mechanosensitive ion channels are present in endothelial cells, including a fluid shear stress-responsive potassium channel, and a stretch-activated calcium channel [27]. Studies have shown that blockade of mechanosensitive K^+ channels with barium chloride or tetraethylammonium blocked shear-mediated increases in NO production [55] and TGF-β release [56] , suggesting that transmembrane ion flux and intracellular ion homeostasis are important mediators of the endothelial cell response to fluid shear stress. However, efforts to clone the mechanosensitive K^+ channel from the endothelial cell have not yet been successful.

Based on the demonstrated importance of fluid shear stress to endothelial cell function and integrity, it is likely that each of these putative mechanoreceptors activates intracellular signaling pathways to effect the complete endothelial response to fluid shear stress. Differential coupling of signaling mechanisms and subsequent endothelial cell response to the individual fluid shear stress receptor "subtypes" may provide a flexibility to the endothelial cells in terms of responding to varying types and degrees of fluid shear stress.

References

[1]   R. Ross, The pathogenesis of atherosclerosis: A perspective for the 1990s., *Nature* **362** (1993) 801-809.

[2]   G. Helmlinger, Berk B.C., Nerem R.M., The calcium responses of endothelial cell monolayers subjected to pulsatile and steady laminar flow differ, *Amer J Physiol (Cell Physiol)* 269 (1995) C367-C375.

[3]   H.J. Hsieh, Li N.Q., Frangos J.A., Pulsatile and steady flow induces c-fos expression in human endothelial cells, *J Cell Physiol* . **154** (1993) 143-151.

[4]   J.A. Frangos, Eskin S.G., McIntire L.V., Ives C.L., Flow effects on prostacyclin production by cultured human endothelial cells., *Science* **227** (1985) 1477-1479.

[5]   D.N. Ku, Giddens D.P., Zarins C.K., Glagov S., Pulsatile flow and atherosclerosis in the human carotid bifurcation. Positive correlation between plaque location and low oscillating shear stress, *Arteriosclerosis* **5** (1985) 293-302.

[6]   T. Asakura, Karino T., Flow patterns and spatial distribution of atherosclerotic lesions in human coronary arteries, *Circ Res* **66** (1990) 1045-1066.

[7]   J.E. Moore, Jr., Xu C., Glagov S., Zarins C.K., Ku D.N., Fluid wall shear stress measurements in a model of the human abdominal aorta: oscillatory behavior and relationship to atherosclerosis, *Atherosclerosis* 110 (1994) 225-240.

[8]   P.M. Vanhoutte, Shimokawa H., Endothelium-derived relaxing factor and coronary vasospasm, *Circulation* **80** (1989) 1-9.

[9]   B.L. Langille, Graham J.J., Kim D., Gotlieb A.I., Dynamics of shear-induced redistribution of F-actin in endothelial cells in vivo, *Arterioscler Thromb* **11** (1991) 1814-1820.

[10]   K. Nishida, Harrison D.G., Navas J.P., Fisher A.A., Dockery S.P., Uematsu M., Nerem R.M., Alexander R.W., Murphy T.J., Molecular cloning and characterization of the constitutive bovine aortic endothelial cell nitric oxide synthase, *Journal of Clinical Investigation* **90** (1992) 2092-2096.

[11] S.P. Janssens, Shimouchi A., Quertermous T., Bloch D.B., Bloch K.D., Cloning and expression of a cDNA encoding human endothelium-derived relaxing factor/nitric oxide synthase [published erratum appears in J Biol Chem 1992 Nov 5;267(31):22694], *J Biol Chem* **267** (1992) 14519-14522.

[12] W.C. Sessa, Harrison J.K., Barber C.M., Zeng D., Durieux M.E., D'Angelo D.D., Lynch K.R., Peach M.J., Molecular cloning and expression of a cDNA encoding endothelial cell nitric oxide synthase, *J Biol Chem* **267** (1992) 15274-15276.

[13] M.J. Kuchan, Frangos J.A., Role of calcium and calmodulin in flow-induced nitric oxide production in endothelial cells, *Am J Physiol* **266** (1994) C628-C636.

[14] I. Fleming, Bauersachs J., Busse R., Calcium-dependent and calcium-independent activation of the endothelial NO synthase, *J Vasc Res* **34** (1997) 165-174.

[15] B.C. Berk, Corson M.A., Peterson T.E., Tseng H., Protein kinases as mediators of fluid shear stress stimulated signal transduction in endothelial cells: a hypothesis for calcium-dependent and calcium-independent events activated by flow, *J Biomech* **28** (1995) 1439-1450.

[16] M.A. Corson, James N.L., Latta S.E., Nerem R.M., Berk B.C., Harrison D.G., Phosphorylation of endothelial nitric oxide synthase in response to fluid shear stress, *Circ Res* **79** (1996) 984-991.

[17] S.L. Pelech, Sanghera J.S., MAP kinases: charting the regulatory pathways, *Science* **257** (1992) 1355-1356.

[18] H. Tseng, Peterson T.E., Berk B.C., Fluid shear stress stimulates mitogen-activated protein kinase in endothelial cells, *Circ Res* **77** (1995) 869-878.

[19] J.Y. Shyy, Lin M.C., Han J., Lu Y., Petrime M., Chien S., The cis-acting phorbol ester "12-O-tetradecanoylphorbol 13-acetate"-responsive element is involved in shear stress-induced monocyte chemotactic protein 1 gene expression, *Proc Natl Acad Sci U S A* **92** (1995) 8069-8073.

[20] M. Uematsu, Navas J.P., Nishida K., Ohara Y., Murphy T.J., Alexander R.W., Nerem R.M., Harrison D.G., Mechanisms of endothelial cell NO synthase induction by shear stress, *Circulation* **88** (1993) I-184.

[21] L. Yi-Shuan, John Y.-J., Shyy S., The cytoplasmic kinase pathways are involved in the shear stress-induced gene expression., *Circulation* **92** (1995) I-1.

[22] H. Jo, Sipos K., Go Y.-M., Law R., Rong J., McDonald J.M., Differential effect of shear stress on extracellular signal-regulated kinase and N-terminal Jun kinase in endothelial cells, *J Biol Chem* **272** (1997) 1395-1401.

[23] D. Kaiser, Freyberg M.A., Friedl P., Lack of hemodynamic forces triggers apoptosis in vascular endothelial cells, *Biochem Biophys Res Commun* **231** (1997) 586-590.

[24] S. Dimmeler, Haendeler J., Rippmann V., Nehls M., Zeiher A.M., Shear stress inhibits apoptosis of human endothelial cells, *FEBS Lett* **399** (1996) 71-74.

[25] O. Traub, Yan C., Berk B.C., In vitro simulation of shear stress and mitogen-activated protein kinase responses to shear stress in endothelial cells, in *Mechanical Forces and the Endothelium ed. P.I. Lelkes, London.* (1998)

[26] T. Ishida, Peterson T.E., Kovach N.L., Berk B.C., MAP kinase activation by flow in endothelial cells. Role of beta 1 integrins and tyrosine kinases, *Circ Res* **79** (1996) 310-316.

[27] P.F. Davies, Flow-mediated endothelial mechanotransduction, *Physiol Rev* **75** (1995) 519-560.

[28] M.U. Nollert, Eskin S.G., McIntire L.V., Shear stress increases inositol trisphosphate levels in human endothelial cells, *Biochem Biophys Res Commun* **170** (1990) 281-287.

[29] M.J. Kuchan, Frangos J.A., Shear stress regulates endothelin-1 release via protein kinase C and cGMP in cultured endothelial cells, *Am. J. Physiol.* **264** (1993) H150-156.

[30] P. Biswas, Abboud H.E., Kiyomoto H., Wenzel U.O., Grandaliano G., Choudhury G.G., PKC alpha regulates thrombin-induced PDGF-B chain gene expression in mesangial cells, *FEBS Lett* **373** (1995) 146-150.

[31] P.R. Girard, Nerem R.M., Endothelial cell signaling and cytoskeletal changes in response to shear stress, *Front Med Biol Eng* **5** (1993) 31-36.

[32] P.A. Watson, Function follows form: generation of intracellular signals by cell deformation, *FASEB J* **5** (1991) 2013-2019.

[33] O. Traub, Monia B.P., Dean N.M., Berk B.C., PKC-epsilon is required for mechano-sensitive activation of ERK1/2 in endothelial cells, *Journal Of Biological Chemistry* **272** (1997) 31251-31257.

[34] J. Shen, Luscinskas F.W., Connolly A., Dewey C.F.J., Gimbrone M.A.J., Fluid shear stress modulates cytosolic free calcium in vascular endothelial cells, *Am J Physiol* **262** (1992) C384-C390.

[35] R.V. Geiger, Berk B.C., Alexander R.W., Nerem R.M., Flow-induced calcium transients in single endothelial cells: spatial and temporal analysis, *Am. J. Physiol.* **262** (1992) C1411-1417.

[36] A.C. Newton, Protein kinase C: structure, function, and regulation, *J Biol Chem* **270** (1995) 28495-28498.

[37] N.M. Dean, McKay R., Condon T.P., Bennett C.F., Inhibition of protein kinase C-alpha expression in human A549 cells by antisense oligonucleotides inhibits induction of intercellular adhesion molecule 1 (ICAM-1) mRNA by phorbol esters, *J Biol Chem* **269** (1994) 16416-16424.

[38] N.M. Dean, McKay R., Inhibition of protein kinase C-alpha expression in mice after systemic administration of phosphorothioate antisense oligodeoxynucleotides, *Proc Natl Acad Sci U S A* **91** (1994) 11762-11766.

[39] K.J. Clark, Murray A.W., Evidence that the bradykinin-induced activation of phospholipase D and of the mitogen-activated protein kinase cascade involve different protein kinase C isoforms, *J Biol Chem* **270** (1995) 7097-7103.

[40] S.W. Young, Dickens M., Tavar'e J.M., Activation of mitogen-activated protein kinase by protein kinase C isotypes alpha, beta I and gamma, but not epsilon, *FEBS Lett* **384** (1996) 181-184.

[41] M. Liscovitch, Cantley L.C., Lipid second messengers, *Cell* **77** (1994) 329-334.

[42] S. Moriya, Kazlauskas A., Akimoto K., Hirai S., Mizuno K., Takenawa T., Fukui Y., Watanabe Y., Ozaki S., Ohno S., Platelet-derived growth factor activates protein kinase C epsilon through redundant and independent signaling pathways involving phospholipase C gamma or phosphatidylinositol 3-kinase, *Proc Natl Acad Sci U S A* **93** (1996) 151-155.

[43] M. Takahashi, Berk B.C., Mitogen-activated protein kinase (ERK1/2) activation by shear stress and adhesion in endothelial cells. Essential role for a herbimycin-sensitive kinase, *J Clin Invest* **98** (1996) 2623-2631.

[44] M.A. Schwartz, Schaller M.D., Ginsberg M.H., Integrins: Emerging paradigms of signal transduction, *Annu Rev Cell Dev Biol* **11** (1995) 549-599.

[45] N. Wang, Butler J.P., Ingber D.E., Mechanotransduction across the cell surface and through the cytoskeleton, *Science* **260** (1993) 1124-1127.

[46] D. Ingber, Integrins as mechanochemical transducers, *Curr Opin Cell Biol* **3** (1991) 841-848.

[47] J.M. Muller, Chilian W.M., Davis M.J., Integrin signaling transduces shear stress-dependent vasodilation of coronary arterioles, *Circ Res* **80** (1997) 320-326.

[48] R.W. Wrenn, Herman L.E., Integrin-linked tyrosine phosphorylation increases membrane association of protein kinase C alpha in pancreatic acinar cells, *Biochem Biophys Res Commun* **208** (1995) 978-984.

[49] K. Hamasaki, Mimura T., Morino N., Furuya H., Nakamoto T., Aizawa S., Morimoto C., Yazaki Y., Hirai H., Nojima Y., Src kinase plays an essential role in integrin-mediated tyrosine phosphorylation of Crk-associated substrate p130Cas, *Biochem Biophys Res Commun* **222** (1996) 338-343.

[50] J.E. Schnitzer, Liu J., Oh P., Endothelial caveolae have the molecular transport machinery for vesicle budding, docking, and fusion including VAMP, NSF, SNAP, annexins, and GTPases, *J Biol Chem* **270** (1995) 14399-14404.

[51] G. Garcia-Cardena, Oh P., Liu J., Schnitzer J.E., Sessa W.C., Targeting of nitric oxide synthase to endothelial cell caveolae via palmitoylation: implications for nitric oxide signaling, *Proc Natl Acad Sci U S A* **93** (1996) 6448-6453.

[52] J. Couet, Li S., Okamoto T., Ikezu T., Lisanti M.P., Identification of peptide and protein ligands for the caveolin-scaffolding domain. Implications for the interaction of caveolin with caveolae-associated proteins, *J Biol Chem* **272** (1997) 6525-6533.

[53] S.R.P. Gudi, Huver I.V., Taliana A.P., Boss G.R., Frangos J.A., Fluid flow-induced ras activation is mediated by Gaq in human vascular endothelial, *Faseb J* **11** (1997) A223.

[54] J.A. Frangos, Gudi S.R.P., Shear stress activates reconstituted G proteins in the absence of protein receptors by, *Faseb J* **11** (1997) A521.

[55] M. Uematsu, Ohara Y., Navas J.P., Nishida K., Murphy T.J., Alexander R.W., Nerem R.M., Harrison D.G., Regulation of endothelial cell nitric oxide synthase mRNA expression by shear stress, *Am J Physiol* **269** (1995) C1371-1378.

[56] M. Ohno, Cooke J.P., Dzau V.J., Gibbons G.H., Fluid shear stress induces endothelial transforming growth factor beta-1 transcription and production. Modulation by potassium channel blockade, *J Clin Invest* **95** (1995) 1363-1369.

Part III

Atherosclerosis

Vascular Endothelium: Mechanisms of Cell Signaling
J.D. Catravas et al. (Eds.)
IOS Press, 1999

ENDOTHELIAL DYSFUNCTION IN ATHEROSCLEROSIS

Allan D. Callow, MD, PhD
Whitaker Institute for Cardiovascular Research
Boston University School of Medicine
801 Albany Street, Room 117,
Boston, MA 02118, USA

1. Introduction

Atherosclerosis, through its multiple clinical manifestations is responsible for nearly 75% of all adult deaths in western societies and is the major cause of morbidity and mortality in males above 50 years of age and in women above 65. In the United States in 1992 all cardiovascular diseases combined claimed the lives of more than 440,000 males and 479,000 females compared to all forms of cancer which claimed 275,000 males and 246,000 females. The preponderance of cardiovascular disease as a cause of death holds true for males and females of Hispanic, Asian/Pacific Islander and Alaskan origin. From the ages of 35 - 74 the death rate from heart attack for black women is about two times that of white women and three times that of women of other races. At older ages women who have heart attacks are twice as likely as men to die from them within a few weeks. Twenty seven percent of men and 44 percent of women will die within one year after having a heart attack. [1]

Cardiovascular disease remains America I s number one cause of death and a leading cause of disability. More than 1 in 5 Americans suffer from cardiovascular diseases at an estimated cost of 259 billion dollars in 1997. About 13.7 million Americans, including 7 million under age 60, live with the effects of heart attack. Another 3.9 million Americans, more than 900,000 of whom are under age 60, suffer from the consequences of stroke, the main cause of permanent disability and the number 3 cause of death in the United States. Heart disease and stroke, both the consequence of atherosclerosis in the overwhelming majority of cases, represent 4 of the top hospital costs for all payers, excluding the complications of childbirth, and 4 of the top Medicare hospital costs. [2]

2. The Healthy Artery

Large arteries are classified as *elastic*, as for example the aorta and its iliac branches, and *muscular* which, while also serving a conduit function, are the direct supply lines to discrete regions and organs. The carotid arteries to the brain, and the vessels to the lungs, kidneys, viscera and extremities are examples of muscular arteries. The essential distinction is the amount of elastic versus muscular tissue within the artery. Elastic arteries store kinetic energy between heartbeats thus maintaining flow during diastole, the relaxation phase of the cardiac cycle. Muscular arteries contribute to flow maintenance, but by virtue of their larger smooth muscle component, they regulate pressure as well.

Vasoconstriction and dilation are the result of vascular smooth muscle response to mediators from several sources, most notably the endothelium of the vasculature.

From the interior or lumenal surf ace to the exterior, the layers of the arterial wall are the intima, the media and the adventitia. An internal elastic lamina separates the endothelium f rom the media, the muscular layer. The intima consists of a monolayer of endothelial cells and is the only cell type found in the normal intima. No better description of the special features and functions of the endothelium has been provided than Una Ryan's:

"----It has risen from being a ghostly substance, scarcely showing in early pathology or histology texts, of no known properties save that of lining blood vessels, to being a collection of cells endowed with pores that could be mathematically modeled but never seen, to possessing a rich array of enzymatic and processing properties. Its stature has grown to that of a metabolically active and responive tissue endowed with a diversity of enzymes, receptors, and transport molecules. It can be grown in culture and manipulated into postures it may never have to succumb to in vivo, its gene products have been cloned, and it has been made to reveal its relationships with other cells and molecules both near neighbors and distant targets. It is claimed as a regulator of blood pressure, a team player in hemostasis, a sparring partner with various blood cell types, and the dancing partner of the vas cular smooth muscle cell. At one time seen as the innocent victim of inflammatory attack we now know that it frequently calls the tune. It is both a target and a source of hormones, growth factors, vasoactive substances, hemostatic factors, and oxygen radicals. It binds complement components, can express receptors for immune reactions, present antigens, and can engulf and kill mnicroorganisms. It can be activated, excited and primed. Activated endothelium represents a remarkable amplification surface for local immune and inflammatory reactions and is able to initiate events that lead to closing off a vessel. Activation of endothelium plays a key role in the host response yet when inappropriately expressed can underlie much of vascular pathology. In fact it is likely that all diseases have a vascular etiology." [3]

The intermediate layer, the media is composed solely of smooth muscle cells and extracellular matrix which, together, comprise the major structural elements of the artery wall. The outermost layer, the adventitia consists of loosely woven connective tissue and contains multiple small vessels, nutrient to the outer two thirds of the vessel wall. These are known as vasa vasorum. The intima receives its nutrients from the blood within the vessel lumen.

The ability to isolate and culture endothelial cells f rom a variety of organs and species provided the opportunity to study their complex interactions with a myriad of stimuli. Hemostasis, thrombogenesis, inf lammatory and immune reactions are among their many participations. The quiescent endothelial cell has a slow turnover time, is antithrombogenic, and growth inhibiting. The perturbed endothelial cell becomes prothrombogenic, promotes smooth muscle cell growth and enhances leucocyte attachment. The activities of the endothelial cell can be thought of as those rendered by the individual cell and those rendered by the group of cells assembled to form an endothelial layer. In the latter setting the endothelial layer serves as a selective barrier organized to protect the intravascular contents and the extravascular milieu. The first line of defense in protecting of the integrity of the arterial wall is the endothelial layer.

Table 1. A Partial Listing of Adhesion Molecules and Cytokines Produced by or Reacting with the Endothelial Cell:

ENDOTHELIAL CELL PRODUCT	ENDOTHELIAL CELL ACTIVITY/FUNCTION
THROMBOSIS AND MATRIX REMODELING	
Platelet activating inhibitor uPA, tPA	Inhibits uPA and tPA
	Activate plasminogen to plasmin: fibrinolysis
Collagenase	Matrix degradation
Tissue factor	Extrinsic factor coagulation cofactor
Vitronectin	An integrin
LEUCOCYTE-ENDOTHELIAL INTERACTIONS	
ELAM-1, endothelial leucocyte adhesion molecule	Adhesion molecule of selectin family
ICAM-1	Adhesion molecule of immunoglobulin super gene family; binds ligands on PMNS, mono cytes, lymphocytes
GMP 140	Adhesion molecule
MHC-1 & 2	Major histocompatibility complex. Interacts with cytotoxic T cells
Il-6	B cell growth factor
Il-8	Neutrophil chemotactic factor
MCP	Monocyte chemotactic factor
Il-lB	Inflammatory cytokine
VASCULAR TONE AND PLATELET INTERACTIONS	
COX 1 & 2	Synthesis of PGI-2 & PGE-2
NO synthase	Synthesis of nitric oxide [EDRF] [relaxing factor]
Endothelin	Vasoconstrictor & growth factor
GROWTH FACTORS	
M-CSF, GM-CSF	Induce monocyte and macrophage colony formation
Platelet-derived growth factor [PDGF]	Smooth muscle cell mitogen. Induces cyclooxygenase expression in smooth muscle cells
Transforming growth factor [TGF-B]	Growth promoter and inhibitor
Basic fibroblast growth FACTOR [FGF-B]	Mitogen for many cell types

uPA: urokinase-type plasminogen; tPA: tissue-type plasminogen; M-CSF: Monocyte colony stimulating factor; GM: Granulocyte monocyte colony stimulating factor.

The metabolic organization of the arterial wall is such that the endothelial cell acts in concert with the smooth muscle cell. A balance exists between the two in the normal or quiescent arterial wall. The injured endothelial layer, as a consequence of high blood cholesterol levels, or hypoxia, or a host of other changes generates mitogens and other molecules which directly influence smooth muscle cell behaviour. Vasorelaxant and vasoconstrictor substances act in concert to mediate vascular tone and platelet activity. The expression and function of these factors are impaired in the hypercholesterolemic animal and in human atherosclerosis. Endothelial vasomotor dysfunction is especially prominent in coronary and peripheral arteries, and when severe, may be associated with local production of thrombin, platelet aggregation, and severe vasoconstriction. Oxidative stress may be increased due to an increase in production of reactive oxygen species. Impaired EDRF activity may be potentiated by oxidized low density liprotein [LDL cholesterol]. Also altered in the hypercholesterolemic state are fibrinolysis, recruitment of monocytes to the arterial wall by adhesion molecules, and control of intimal growth, all endothelial responsibilities.

Table 2. A Partial Listing of Endothelial Activation Programs

STIMULUS	RESPONSE
Interleukin-1, tumor necrosis	Increase leucocyte adhesion molecules, induce nitric oxide synthesis, decrease growth, Increase cytokine growth factor expression Increase prostanoid production
Thrombin	Increases PDGF, E-selectin production
Platelet activating factor	Increases P-selectin expression [minutes]
Interferon gamma	Increases ICAM-1 expression Induces nitric oxidesynthesis Increases histocompatibility gene expression
Heparin-binding growth	Stimulate smooth muscle cell proliferation
Shear	Activates an inward-rectifying K channel
Stretch	Activates a non-selective ion channel
Hypoxia	Increases PDGF gene expression Induces specific hypoxia-related genes of unknown function
unknown f unction	

PDGF: platelet-derived growth factor; FGF: fibroblast growth factors; ICAM-1: intercellular adhesion molecules

Table 3. A Partial Listing of Smooth Muscle Activation Programs

STIMULUS	RESPONSE
Platelet-derived growth factor	Increases growth of smooth muscle cells; Stimulates migration; Increases matrix synthesis
Interleukin-1, tumor necrosis factor	Increases growth; Increases cytokine, growth factor expression: PDGF, BFGF, Il-8, MCAF, CSFS; Induces nitric oxide synthesis
Interferon gamma	Decreases growth; Induces nitric oxide; synthesis; Increases histocompatibility gene expression
Heparin-binding growth factors [acidic & basic FGF]	Increase growth
Transforming growth factor -B	Increases interstitial; collagen synthesis; Variable effects on growth
Stretch	Increases matrix synthesis
Crush injury	Releases BFGF

MCAF: monocyte chemoattractant and stimulating factor; [6]

3. Atherosclerosis and Diet

Atherosclerosis is a systemic disease with segmental manifestations. The widespread, generalized distribution of atherosclerosis throughout the body is masked by the focal distribution of the symptomatic lesions. Thus, the gradual restriction of blood f low to a lower extremity results in limited skeletal muscle function and pain on exercise followed by disappearance of the pain of walking upon rest, i.e., intermittent claudication. Angina pectoris, episodic pain in the chest, is the consequence of insufficient blood flow to the myocardium attempting to respond to increased demand as occasioned by exercise. The coronary arteries are the locale of the atherosclerotic process. The stroke syndrome may be more complicated, but the typical atherosclerotic stroke is the result of narrowing of a critical artery to the brain, usually the cervical carotid or its branches, with reduced flow to an intracranial vessel, the consequence of thrombosis or embolism. The dramatic, often crippling effects of reduced blood flow in these organs direct attention to their vessels of supply. The remainder of the body's conduit arteries are usually ignored despite the likely presence of atherosclerotic lesions in various stage of development within them. These latter vessels and their lesions remain incognito until symptoms appear.

That a link between elevated blood lipids and atherosclerosis probably existed was suspected from obervations that the incidence of ischemic heart disease, its morbidity and mortaliy, were markedly reduced during World Wars I and II. In post-World War I Germany, in World War II Norway, and as an aftermath of the prolonged siege of Leningrad during World War II, populations which suffered severe dietary restrictions, cardiac disease was not the most frequent cause of death. [4,5]. Based on several decades of clinical observations, conventional opinion identifies several factors that are associated with an increased incidence and level of severity of atherosclerotic occlusive disease. These are:

> hyperlipidemia
> hypertension
> cigarette smoking, and
> family history-cultural as well as genetic items

Of lesser power, but nonetheless of substantial influence are:

> obesity
> diabetes mellitus, and
> a sedentary life style

Chlamydia sp.,Cytomegalovirus, Helicobacter pylorii and Pneumoniae gingivalis have been discovered in atherosclerotic plaques or sera of patients with coronary artery disease or have otherwise come under suspicion. Much additional study is needed to rank their precise role and importance.

4. Pathogenesis of Atherosclerosis

Atherosclerosis is the result of an injury or injuries to endothelial and smooth muscle cells, the exposure to which continues for many years. The cellular response to the injury builds over decades. It is widely accepted that hypercholesterolemia is the major risk factor for most individuals with tobacco use, diabetes, obesity and a sedentary life style serving as accelerating and intensifying, but not primary risks. The low density lipoprotein particle enters the vessel wall from the circulating blood, undergoes oxidation, and exerts a profound but still incompletely understood influence on the cells of the arterial wall, particularly the endothelial cell.

Various adhesion molecules, presumably responding to blood lipids, serve to attract, fasten, and aid penetration of the endothelial layer by circulating monocytes. Oxycholesterol presumably alters the integrity of the monocyte/macrophage which has penetrated the endothelium and subendothelial layer. Macrophages, by engulfing lipid particles, become converted to the fat-laden foam cell, which ultimately engorges fat to its death.

Smooth muscle cells, to a lesser extent, may follow this same foam cell formation and also die. Thus the central portion of the plaque consists of a lipid pool, smooth muscle cells and macrophage foam cells, the remnants of dead and dying cells and free cholesterol often in the form of crystals. At the shoulders of the plaque inflammatory cells, chiefly T lymphocytes, are found denoting an inflammatory component to atherogenesis. Overlying the mound of cholesterol and cellular debris is a fibrous cap all of which together form the atheroma. Calcium, usually as carbonate, may be found in advanced plaques. various adhesion molecules and cytokines have been identified in the process of foam cell development and death, together with proteases which lead to degradation of the extracellular matrix. In time the endothelium and fibrous cap may undergo erosion, with extrusion of plaque contents into the bloodstream. The plaque itself may develop a fracture or fissure setting the stage for intraplaque and intravascular thrombosis. Central to this scenario is the important concept of the interactions of the various cells with each other, the genes they carry and the gene products they express. If the reaction of one cell is on another this is a paracrine stimulus and response. Autocrine denotes stimulus and response restricted to the same cell. These oversimplifications serve to illustrate the extremely complex interrelatedness of the cellular and molecular events occurring in the microcosm of the arterial wall. [7,8,9,10,11,12].

Not all fatty streaks develop into fibrous plaques and not all intermediate plaques proceed to erosion and thrombosis. Reasons for this spectrum of plaque "hibernation 11 or progression are not clear. Yet, it is apparent that certain arteries such as the coronary, the carotids and the ilio-femoral system are far more vulnerable to advanced plaque formation and progression to symptoms than are others such those of the upper extremity, the pulmonary vessels and those of the abdominal and pelvic viscera. Two fundamental clinical observations are worth noting:

> 1) atherosclerosis is a widespread systemic disease with the majority of affected vessels and their plaques remaining asymptomatic throughout life, and 2) segmental, that is symptomatic, lesions usually develop preferentially at flow dividers such as bifurcations of vulnerable arteries.

5. Recent Research Reports

Lp(a), "Lp little a", is associated with premature atherosclerosis, early by-pass vein occlusion and the accelerated atherosclerosis of cardiac transplants. Its atherogenicity mechanism is not well understood but may be due to its interference with plasminogen activation as well as its atherogenic potential as a lipoprotein particle after receptor-mediated uptake. Yacoub and his associates demonstrated that Lp(a) stimulates production of vascular cell adhesion molecules 1 (VCAM-1) and E-selectin in cultured human coronary artery endothelial cells (HCAEC). This effect resulted from a rise in intracellular free calcium induced by Lp(a) and could be inhibited by the intracellular calcium chelator BAPTA/AM. Involvement of the LDL and VLDL receptors in Lp(a) activation of HCAEC were ruled out since Lp(a) induction of adhesion molecules was not prevented by an antibody (IgGC7) to the LDL receptor or receptor-activating protein, an antagonist of ligand binding to the VLDL receptor. "Because leucocyte recruitment to the vessel wall appears to represent one of the important early events in atherogenesis, this newly described endothelial cell-activating effect of Lp(a) places it at a crucial juncture in the initiation of atherogenicdiseasell.[13]

It is generally believed that the importance of high density lipoproteins [HDL], the so-called "good" cholesterols as contrasted "bad" cholesterol, LDL, relates to the ability of HDL to protect against the development of coronary heart disease. In addition to the recognized ability of HDL to promote the efflux of cholesterol from foam cells, and reducing the atherogenicity of LDLs by inhibiting their oxidation, Barter et al provide evidence that HDLs may be additionally antiatherogenic by virtue of their ability to inhibit the expression of adhesion molecules on endothelial cells. They have previously reported that HDLs inhibit the cytokine-induced expression adhesion molecules in endothelial cells. [14] In this report HDLs collected from a number of different human subjects were analyzed to detect whether different preparations of HDLs vary in their ability to inhibit expression of vascular cell adhesion molecule-1 (VCAM-1) in human umbilical vein endohelial cells activated by tumor necrosis factor-a . Different populations of HDLs differed markedly in their abilities to inhibit VCAM-L expression without regard to changes in apolipoprotein (apo) A-1 or cholesterolconcentrations.   The mechanisms remain to be elucidated [15]

Amorino and Hoover report a four to eightfold increase in levels of the metalloproteinaseMMP-9 protein and its MRNA after 18 hours incubation of human umbilical vein endothelial cells with the human monocytic cell line THP-1. Levels of another metalloproteinase MMP-2 were unaffected. Endothelial cells, through the release of soluble factors and through direct contact with monocytic cells regulate monocytic metalloproteinase production by endothelial cells and provide implications for atherogenesis. [16]

Using rabbits and high-low cholesterol diets, in conjunction with ballon injury of the intima, Libby and Shoen and their groups demonstrated that lipid lowering resulted in the appearance of mature intimal smooth muscle cells (SMCS) and reduced levels of platelet-rerived growth factor-B in the arterial intima, a factor known to suppress smooth muscle myosin expression. Lipid lowering favors accumulation of mature Smcs in the atherosclerotic intima in association with reduced levels of matrix metalloproteinase- 3 and -9 compared with Baseline and High groups.[17]

Gimbrone et al studied the history of cell migration, cell division and cell loss from the surface of a continuously monitored high shear environment in an in vitro system with high shear gradients caused by a surface protuberance.Individual endothelial cells were tracked with time-lapse video microscopy.In contrast to a uniform laminar flow field in which cells were observed to continually rearrange their relative position with no net migration, in a disturbed flow field there was a net migration directed away from the region of high shear gradient. In addition, cell division increased in the vicinity of the flow separation whereas cell loss was increased upstream and downstream in regions where shear gradient diminishes. These data suggest a steady cell proliferation-migration-losscycle and indicate that local shear stress gradient may play a key role in the morphological remodeling of the vascular endothelium in vivo. [18]

References

[1] American Heart Association, Heart and Stroke Facts: 1996 Statistical Supplement, American Heart Association, Age-Adjusted Death Rates for Major Cardiovascular Diseases. United States: 1940-1992.
[2] American Heart Association, 1998, Dallas TX.
[3] Ryan, US. Endothelial Cells. Preface. Vol 1. Ed. US Ryan CRC Press , Boca Raton, FL. 1988
[4] Brozek, J. 1946, Medical aspects of semistarvation in Leningrad (Siege of 1941-1942). Am Eve Soviet Med, 4: 790
[5] Strom, A. 1951, Mortality from circulatory disease in Norway, Lancet, 1: 126
[6] Libby, P, Schoen, F., 1993, Cardiovasc Path
[7] Amer Heart ASSOC Special Report. A Definition of Advanced Types of Atherosclerotic Lesions and a Histological Classification of Atherosclerosis, 1995. Amer Heart Assoc., Dallas TX.
[8] Stary, HC. The histologic classification of atherosclerotic lesions in human coronary arteries. In: Fuster V, Ross, R, Topel E. Eds. Atherosclerosis and Coronary Artery Disease. LippincottRaven, Phila. 1996

[9]   Furchgott RF, Zawadzki JV. 1980; The obligatory role of endothelial cells in the relaxation of arterial smooth muscle by acetylcholine. Nature; 288: 373-376

[10] Ignarro Li et al, 19 8 9; Endothelium-derived relaxing factor produced and released f rom artery and vein is nitric oxide. Nat; Proc Natl Acad Sci (USA) 84: 9265-9269

[11] Ross R, 1993; The pathogenesis of atherosclerosis: a perspective for the 1990s. Nature; 362: 801-809

[12] Shepherd JT et al. 1994; Report of the task force on vascular medicine. Circulation; 89: 532-535

[13] Allen S, Khan S, Tam S, Koschinsky M, Taylor P and Yacoub M 1998. Expression of adhesion molecules by Lp(a) : a potential novel mechanism for its atherogenicity. FASEB; 12: 1765-1776

[14] Cockerill, GW, Rye K-A, Gamble JR, Vadas MA, Barter PJ. 1995; High density lipoproteins inhibit cytokine-induced expression of endothelial cell adhesion molecules. Arterioscler Thromb Vasc Biol. 15: 1987-1994

[15] Ashby DT, Rye K-A, Clay MA, Vadas MA, Gamble JR, Barter PJ. 1998; Arterioscler vasc Biol Thromb; 18: 1450-1455

[16] Amorino GP, Hoover RL. 1998; Interactions of monocytic cells with human endothelial cells stimulate monocytic metalloproteinase production; Am J Path; 152 (1) 1909-207

[17] Aikawa M, Rabkin E, Voglic SA, Shing H, Nagai R, Schoen F, Libby P; 1998; Lipid lowering promotes accumulation of mature smooth muscle cells expressing smooth muscle myosin heavy chain isoforms in rabbit atheroma, Circ Res. 83: 1015-1026

[18] Tardy Y, Resnick N, Nagel T, Gimbrone MA Jr., 1997; Shear street gradients remodel endothelial monolayers in vitro via a cell prolif eration-migration-loss cycle. Arterioscler Thromb Vasc Biol. 11: 3102-3106.

Vascular Endothelium: Mechanisms of Cell Signaling
J.D. Catravas et al. (Eds.)
IOS Press, 1999

GENETIC FACTORS IN CORONARY HEART DISEASE

Kåre Berg
Institute of Medical Genetics, University of Oslo and Department of Medical Genetics,
Ullevål University Hospital
Oslo, Norway

Abstract

The importance of genetic factors in the etiology of coronary heart disease (CHD) is evident from familial aggregation of coronary heart disease cases and high heritability of its risk factors or protective factors. Also, associations have been reported between CHD and DNA polymorphisms in several functional candidate genes, including the apolipoprotein B gene, the low density lipoprotein receptor gene and the cholesteryl ester transfer protein gene. Recently, interest has focused on the variability gene concept as well as gene-gene interaction, in studies on CHD risk factors.

Lp(a) lipoprotein, a separate class of serum lipoprotein particles, under strict genetic control is now a well established independent CHD risk factor. In addition to its atherogenic/thrombogenic properties, Lp(a) lipoprotein may have important effects on the endothelium.

Hyperhomocysteinemia is a "new" risk factor and genes involved in folate metabolism are therefore functional candidate genes with respect to CHD. Hyperhomocysteinemia is an interesting example of a risk factor, which is under the influence of genes as well as environmental factors, and where change of diet can have a very favourable effect.

The rapidly increasing knowledge on the genetics of CHD is expected to lead to preventive and therapeutic measures tailored to the individual.

1. Familial Aggregation of Coronary Heart Disease Cases

It has been known since the late 1930s that premature coronary heart disease (CHD) together with high cholesterol level and tendon xanthomas exhibit aggregation of cases in families typical of autosomal dominant traits. It was, however, widely held that genetic factors would only rarely cause CHD. The changes in frequency of CHD in this century were by many workers believed to exclude a genetic contribution to the etiology of myocardial infarction or angina pectoris. The favored view was that CHD was a disease resulting exclusively from an unhealthy diet or unhealthy lifestyle.

Attention became focused on the importance of genetic factors in CHD only after the discovery in the 1970s that familial hypercholesterolemia is caused by mutant genes for the low density lipoprotein (LDL) receptor (LDLR).

An important study was published by Nora [1]. These workers showed beyond any reasonable doubt that having a first degree relative with premature CHD is a risk factor in its own right. They uncovered strong evidence of high heritability of CHD, even after cases of monogenic hyperlipidemias had been removed from the patient series. The conclusions of Nora et al. are in agreement with several other studies focusing on familial occurrence of CHD as a risk factor [reviewed in 2-5].

2. Heritability of Risk Factors or Protective Factors With Respect To Coronary Heart Disease

Classical twin studies as well as studies on offspring of monozygotic (MZ) twins (whereby problems inherent in the classical twin method are eliminated), as well as other family studies have uncovered significant heritability of several well established risk factors or protective factors with respect to CHD. Thus, total cholesterol, high density lipoprotein (HDL) cholesterol (HDLC) as well as triglycerides exhibit significant heritability which, however, may become less pronounced in high age [6]. Apolipoprotein levels, blood pressure, body mass index and homocystein all exhibit heritabilities between 0.51 and 0.76 whereas heritability of Lp(a) lipoprotein level is very close to unity and heritability of fibrinogen level is low (0.27), but significant (Table 1) [for review of heritability of CHD risk factors or protective factors, see 2,3,4,6,7].

Table 1.
Estimates of heritability (h^2) of selected risk factors or protective factors with respect to coronary heart disease [extracted from 7]

Variable	h^2	Variable	h^2
Total cholesterol	0.68	Systolic blood pressure	0.64
Fasting triglycerides	0.46	Diastolic blood pressure	0.51
Apolipoprotein B	0.64	Body mass index	0.76
Apolipoprotein A-I	0.55	Fibrinogen	0.27
Apolipoprotein A-II	0.68	Homocyst(e)ine	0.53
Lp(a) lipoprotein	1.0		

3. Nature, Nurture and Coronary Heart Disease

Once the importance of genetic factors in the etiology of CHD (in cases other than familial hypercholesterolemia) had been irrefutably documented, it was, at the intellectual level, not difficult to understand how environmental factors as well as genetic factors could be of importance in the etiology of one and the same disease. The obvious explanation is that dietary, life-style or other environmental factors, preferentially cause CHD in people with a genetic predisposition. This insight immediately suggested that it could become important to identify the susceptible state for many disorders, in order to be able to efficiently modify disease risks.

The early discoveries of strong genetic effects on CHD risk factors and on the disease itself were based on techniques for twin and family analyses and methods from the field of quantitative genetics. These studies provided very little in the way of hope that individual genes responsible for genetic effects on risk factors or disease would soon be identified. The only genes available for testing were random genetic markers such as blood groups but extensive studies were conducted with these tools and positive and highly reproducible disease associations were uncovered. More targeted approaches were, however, started in the 1970s and have flourished in the last 12-15 years.

4. Candidate Gene Approaches

The term "*candidate gene*" is frequently used about today's highly specific and targeted approaches to identify individual genes. A candidate gene approach is either a "*positional candidate gene approach*" or a "*functional candidate gene approach*". In the former, one knows from other studies (for example from lod score studies in families) that a given gene is in one specific area of the genome. Its position is known and the challenge is to find the gene in question in the area where it has to be. If the area is very large, identifying the right gene among many genes and stretches of non-coding DNA sequences can be a formidable task (thus, it took about 10 years from the approximate position of the gene causing Huntington's chorea became known, until it was successfully cloned and characterized).

A functional candidate gene is a gene whose protein product is in one way or the other involved in, or believed to be involved in structures or functions related to a normal trait or disorder under study. Thus, with respect to CHD, a functional candidate gene is any gene expressed in atherosclerotic lesions, or whose protein product is involved in:
- Lipoprotein structure or metabolism
- Thrombogenesis, thrombolysis or fibrinolysis
- Regulation of blood flow in coronary arteries
- Regulation of blood pressure
- Reverse cholesterol transport
- Regulation of growth of atherosclerotic lesions
- Early development of coronary arteries

The term "candidate gene" was coined after the event of DNA polymorphisms in the beginning of the 1980s. However, the possible role of "candidate genes" with respect to CHD had already been examined in the 1970s with some success. Thus, the association between CHD and a high level of Lp(a) lipoprotein [81 was discovered already in 1974 [91 and the relationship between cholesterol levels and homospecific allotypes in apolipoprotein B (apoB), expressed as the Ag allotypes of LDL was discovered in 1976 [10]. Accordingly, the validity of the functional candidate gene approach was evident already by the mid-1970s. In the late 1970s, the genetic polymorphism of apolipoprotein E (apoE) was detected and soon shown to be associated with serum cholesterol level [For review of the road from association studies with random genetic markers to functional candidate gene studies, see 11].

5. Associations between Coronary Heart Disease Risk and Dva Polymorphisms in Functional Candidate Genes

Studies on CHD risk factors, applying the functional candidate gene approach have been conducted on numerous genes whose protein product was believed to be related to atherogenesis/thrombogenesis, as relevant genes were cloned and genetic variants became available for testing. Thus, numerous studies have been conducted on polymorphisms in the apob gene and an association between variants in an XbaI polymorphism and lipid levels has been found in sufficiently many studies to be considered a true biological phenomenon. The same polymorphism also exhibits direct association with myocardial infarction [12].

Early studies on the LDLR function in families conducted in our laboratory, suggested the existence of frequent, normal alleles at the LDLR locus that affect lipid level (in addition to the major mutations causing the rare disease familial hypercholesterolemia) [13]. This finding was confirmed at the DNA level several years later by Pedersen in our group [14].

A TaqI polymorphism (the "B polymorphism") in the cholesteryl ester transfer protein (CETP) gene exhibits significant association with HDLC and apolipoprotein A-I (apoA-I) levels [15]. There is renewed interest in this polymorphism since it was recently reported that "IB2B2" homozygotes with CHD did not benefit from Pravastatin treatment whereas the other two genotypes had a beneficial effect with respect to progression of atherosclerosis [16].

Many other associations between candidate genes and risk factors or overt disease have been reported but far from all have been unambiguously confirmed. The effect of genes belonging to normal polymorphisms is usually of a moderate size but combinations of several genes acting in an unfavorable direction will still be clinically important.

6. The Variability Gene Concept

Data in the literature suggest that in addition to high absolute levels of risk factors, the amount of variability in some risk factors could also be of importance with respect to CHD risk. In laboratory animals, including rabbits, differences between strains with respect to lipid responses to dietary changes have been known for many years. The "high responder" or "low responder" property is a permanent characteristic of a given strain and almost certainly a genetic trait. Evidence for the existence of "high responder" and "low responder" traits in man has also been reported, together with evidence that the responder characteristic is a trait that persists in a given individual, at least over many years [17].

MZ twins offer a possibility to identify genes that have an effect on risk factor variability. The within-pair difference in a continuous variable in MZ twins of one genotype in a genetic polymorphism could be compared with the within-pair difference in MZ twins of a different genotype. Genes with a restrictive effect on risk factor variability would result in a lower within-MZ-pair difference in pairs possessing the restrictive genotypes than in those lacking them.

Our early studies with random genetic markers [18] strongly suggested that this concept is valid. One of the observed "variability gene" effects was readily confirmed in a second study [19], and in 1986 we launched the "variability gene concept" [20].

Variability genes with respect to different lipoprotein parameters have since been observed in apolipoprotein genes. There are, for example, variability genes with respect to cholesterol in an EcoRI polymorphism in the APOB gene and also in a polymorphism at the CETP locus. Several workers have now published variability gene effects on lipoprotein parameters, in response to changes in lipid intake. Such effects have also been found in response to variation in fiber intake.

Although the vast majority of papers on genetic markers and CHD risk factors focuses on relationships between markers and absolute risk factor levels ("level genes"), interest in the variability gene concept is growing and data that are already in the literature substantiate the essential correctness of the variability gene concept [For review of the variability gene concept, see 21].

7. Lp (A) Lipoprotein – A Unique, Inherited Risk Factor

Serum levels of Lp(a) lipoprotein [8] are determined by the LPA locus near the end of the long arm of chromosome 6. Its level is stable in healthy people, yet there is an almost 1000-fold difference between individuals with respect to Lp(a) lipoprotein concentration. The concentration is under strict genetic control in healthy people. Berg and co-workers [91 detected a definite association between Lp(a) lipoprotein and premature CHD, and this has since been confirmed in numerous studies [for review of studies of Lp(a) lipoprotein as a CHD risk factor, see 22]. In the review by Djurovic and Berg [22], ten out of thirteen prospective studies and numerous case-control studies were found to clearly confirm high Lp(a) lipoprotein level as a CHD risk factor, Technical problems and/or inadequate awareness of the lability of the Lp(a) lipoprotein may explain why some workers have failed to detect the relationship between a high Lp(a) lipoprotein level and CHD, the inadequacy of some of the commercially available test kits probably being of significance [23].

Evidence supporting an important role of Lp(a) lipoprotein in cardiovascular disease originates from several different fields of research. For example, transgenic mice possessing CDNA representing the LPA gene develop lipid lesions in their aortae, on a normal or a lipid enriched diet. This suggests that the affinity of Lp(a) lipoprotein to vascular walls resides in the apo(a) part of the molecule, since mice have extremely little LDL that apo(a) could become attached to (in humans, the Lp(a) polypeptide chain is attached to apob in LDL particles). The experience with these transgenic mice also suggest that free apo(a) must have some affinity to lipid, since the lesions clearly accepted lipid stain and therefore contained lipids (Berg et al. in preparation).

The extensive evidence confirming the importance of Lp(a) lipoprotein in the etiology of CHD and other atherosclerotic/ thrombotic disorders includes:
- Numerous case/control studies of CHD
- Several prospective studies of CHD
- Case/control studies of other atherosclerotic diseases
- Studies relating Lp(a) lipoprotein level to degree of atherosclerosis
- Studies on re-stenosis of cardiac vessels after angioplasty
- Studies demonstrating presence of Lp(a) lipoprotein in atherosclerotic lesions
- Studies indicating that Lp(a) lipoprotein may interfere with thrombolytic/fibrinolytic processes
- Studies suggesting that Lp(a) lipoprotein may stimulate growth of vascular smooth muscle cells
- Other studies on effects of Lp(a) lipoprotein on phenomena or functions (such as endothelial functions) that could be related to atherogenesis/thrombogenesis
- Studies on arterial lesions in LPA transgenic mice

The reasons for the association between CHD and Lp(a) lipoprotein are not fully known. However, the Lp(a) lipoprotein is atherogenic in the sense that it is present in atherosclerotic lesions, and several laboratory studies have indicated that Lp(a) lipoprotein may interfere with thrombolytic/fibrinolytic processes, probably because of the similarity of apo(a) to plasminogen, a much smaller protein (the LPA gene developed from the plasminogen gene and has numerous repeats of a structure corresponding to "kringle IV", in plasminogen). Furthermore, Lp(a) lipoprotein has been shown to stimulate proliferation of vascular smooth muscle cells *in vitro*. There is support in the literature for a relationship between Lp(a) lipoprotein and endothelial function, endothelial-dependent vasodilation being altered in people with a high Lp(a) lipoprotein level. Finally, Lp(a) lipoprotein has been shown to affect expression of the endothelin gene in cultures of human umbilical vein endothelial cells [24].

8. Hyperhomocysteinemia, A "New" Risk Factor

Several studies have shown that a high level of serum/plasma homocystein is associated with CHD. Although it has not been confirmed in all studies, the total amount of data clearly favor a role of hyperhomocysteinemia in the etiology of CHD. Homocystein level is partly determined by genes [25] and genes whose products are involved in folate metabolism are therefore candidate genes with respect to CHD risk. This includes the genes for cystathionine beta-synthase (CBS), methylene-tetra-hydrofolate reductase (MTHFR), and methionine synthase (MS).

Polymorphisms have been uncovered in genes of importance in folate metabolism, and at least one polymorphism is associated with level of homocystein. There is one paper where the same polymorphism is reported to exhibit direct correlation with clinical CHD but this has not been unequivocally confirmed. Doubtless, the area of hyperhomocysteinemia and genes contributing to it will remain a focus of research to fully uncover the role of hyperhomocysteinemia and relevant genes in the etiology of CHD. Most importantly, hyperhomocysteinemia may be reduced by folate intake. This makes hyperhomocysteinemia a CHD risk factor where genetics and diet could be of equal importance (homocysteine level in healthy people exhibits a heritability of 0.53, see Table 1). Dietary changes should make it possible to remove the portion of CHD risk that is not determined by genes in an unchangeable manner.

9. Gene - Gene Interactions

It is well documented that presence of the apoE4 allele of the apoE polymorphism, significantly increases cholesterol level. The series of Pedersen and Berg [14] that uncovered effect on total and LDL cholesterol of normal alleles at the LDLR locus were also examined with respect to apoE genotypes. It was found that the total series exhibited the well established effect on cholesterol level of the apoE4 allele. However, this effect was totally obliterated in the presence of a normal allele at the LDLR locus detected as a variant in a PvuII polymorphism [26]. This is the first example of a significant effect on CHD risk factors of gene-gene interaction between normal polymorphisms in functional candidate genes.

10. Concluding Remarks

A rich tapestry of genetic factors of importance for development of CHD is unfolding. This will doubtless increase our understanding of disease processes and eventually lead to therapeutic progress, possibly with individually tailored therapeutic approaches. However, the new knowledge should be utilized already at the present time to identify those at particularly high CHD risk in order to make it possible for them to take advantage of all disease-preventing options available. The new genetic knowledge underlines the importance of developing preventive measures tailored to the individual, in addition to preventive efforts directed towards the total population.

Acknowledgements

Work in the author's laboratory was supported by the Norwegian Council on Cardiovascular Disease, Anders Jahres Foundation for the Promotion of Science and the Research Council of Norway.

References

[1]   J.J. Nora, R.H. Lortscher, R.D. Spangler, A.H. Nora and W.J. Kimberling. Genetic-epidemiologic study of early-onset ischemic heart disease. Circulation 61 (1980) 503-508.

[2]   K. Berg, Genetics of coronary heart disease. In: A.G. Steinberg, A.G. Bearn, A.G. Motulsky & B. Childs (eds.). Progress in Medical Genetics. New Series, Vol. V. ISBN: 0-7216-1074-9. W.B. Saunders Co., Philadelphia, 1983, pp. 35-90.

[3]   K. Berg, Genetics of coronary heart disease and its risk factors. In: K. Berg (ed.). Medical Genetics: Past, Present, Future. ISBN: 0-8451-5027-8. Alan R. Liss, Inc., New York, 1985, pp. 351-374.

[4]   K. Berg, Genetics of atherosclerosis. In: A.G. Olsson (ed.). Atherosclerosis. Biology and Clinical Science. ISBN: 0 443 03169 X. Churchill-Livingstone, Edinburgh, 1987, pp. 323-337.

[5]   Y. Friedlander, Familial clustering of coronary heart disease: a review of its significance and role as a risk factor for the disease. In: U. Goldbourt, U. de Faire, K. Berg (eds.). Genetic Factors in Coronary Heart Disease. ISBN 0-7923-2752-7. Kluwer Academic Press, Dordrecht/Boston/London, 1994, pp. 37-53.

[6]   U. de Faire and N. Pedersen, Studies of twins and adoptees in coronary heart disease. In: U. Goldbourt, U. de Faire, K. Berg (eds.). Genetic Factors in Coronary Heart Disease. ISBN 0-7923-2752-7. Kluwer Academic Press, Dordrecht/Boston/London, 1994, pp. 55-68.

[7]   K. Berg, Genetic and environmental factors in the development of cardiovascular disease. In: M.-M. Galteau, G. Siest, J. Henry (eds.). Biologie prospective. ISBN: 2-7420-0013-5. Comptes Rendus du 8e Colloque de Pont-a-Mousson, John Libbey Eurotext, Paris, 1993, pp. 471-480.

[8]   K. Berg, A new serum type system in man - the Lp system. Acta path microbial scand 59 (1963) 369-382.

[9]   K. Berg, G. Dahlén and M.H. Frick, Lp(a) lipoprotein and pre-β_1 lipoprotein in patients with coronary heart disease. Clin Genet 6 (1974) 230-235.

[10]   K. Berg, C. Hames, G. Dahlén, M.H. Frick and I. Krishan, Genetic variation in serum low density lipoproteins and lipid levels in man. Proc Natl Acad Sci (USA) 73 (1976) 937-940.

[11]   K. Berg, From random genetic markers to candidate genes in association and linkage studies of coronary heart disease and its risk factors. In: U. Goldbourt, U. de Faire, K. Berg (eds.). Genetic Factors in Coronary Heart Disease. ISBN 0-7923-2752-7. Kluwer Academic Publishers, Dordrecht/Boston/London, 1994, pp. 301-308.

[12]   M. Bøhn and K. Berg, The XbaI polymorphism at the apolipoprotein B locus and risk of atherosclerotic disease. Clin Genet 46 (1994) 77-79.

[13]   K. Maartmann-Moe, P. Magnus, W. Golden and K. Berg, Genetics of the low density lipoprotein receptor: III. Evidence for multiple normal alleles at the low density lipoprotein receptor locus. Clin Genet 20 (1981) 113-129.

[14]   J.C. Pedersen and K. Berg, Normal DNA polymorphism at the low density lipoprotein receptor (LDLR) locus associated with serum cholesterol level. Clin Genet 34 (1988) 306-312.

[15]   I. Kondo, K. Berg, D. Drayna and R. Lawn, DNA polymorphism at the locus for human cholesteryl ester transfer protein (CETP) is associated with high density lipoprotein cholesterol and apolipoprotein levels. Clin Genet 35 (1989) 49-56.

[16]   J.A. Kuivenhoven, J.W. Jukema, A.H. Zwinderman, P. de Knijff, R. McPherson, A.V.G. Bruschke, K.I. Lie and J.J.P. Kastelein, The role of a common variant of the cholesteryl ester transfer protein gene in the progression of coronary atherosclerosis. New Engl J Med 33 (1998) 86-93.

[17]   M.B. Katan, A.C. Beynen, J.H.M. De Vries and A. Nobels, Existence of consistent hypo- and hyperresponders to dietary cholesterol in man. Amer J Epidemiol 123 (1986) 221-234.

[18]   K. Berg, Twin studies of coronary heart disease and its risk factors. Acta Genet Med Gemellol 33 (1984) 349-361.

[19]   K. Berg, Variability gene effect on cholesterol at the Kidd blood group locus. Clin Genet 33 (1988) 102-107.

[20] K. Berg, Normal genetic lipoprotein variations and atherosclerosis. In: C.R. Sirtori, A.V. Nichols
      (eds.).   Human Apolipoprotein Mutants. ISBN: 0-306-42370-7. Plenum Publishing Corporation,
      New York, 1986, pp. 31-49.
[21] K. Berg, Gene - environment interaction: variability gene concept. In: U. Goldbourt, U. de Faire, K.
      Berg (eds.). Genetic Factors in Coronary Heart Disease. ISBN: 0-7923-2752-7. Kluwer Academic
      Publishers, Dordrecht/Boston/London, 1994, pp. 373-383.
[22] S. Djurovic and K. Berg, Epidemiology of Lp(a) lipoprotein: its role in atherosclerotic/thrombotic
      disease. Clin Genet 52 (1997) 281-292.
[23] K. Berg, Confounding results of Lp(a) lipoprotein measurements with some test kits. Clin Genet 46
      (1994) 57-62.
[24] K.E. Berge, S. Djurovic, H.J. Muller, P. Aleström and K. Berg, Studies on effects of Lp(a) lipoprotein
      in gene expression in endothelial cells in vitro. Clin Genet 52 (1997) 314-325.
[25] K. Berg, M.R. Malinow, P. Kierulf and D. Upson, Population variation and genetics of plasma
      homocyst(e)ine level. Clin Genet 41 (1992) 315-321.
[26] J. Pedersen and K. Berg, Interaction between low density lipoprotein receptor (LDLR) and
      apolipoprotein E (apoe) alleles contributes to normal variation in lipid level. Clin Genet 35 (1989)
      331-337.

Vascular Endothelium: Mechanisms of Cell Signaling
J.D. Catravas et al. (Eds.)
IOS Press, 1999

ROLE OF CAVEOLAE IN MECHANOTRANSDUCTION

Victor Rizzo and Jan E. Schnitzer

Dept. Pathology
Harvard Medical School
Beth Israel Deaconess Medical Center
Boston, MA 02215, USA

Abstract

The mechanisms by which fluid forces generated by circulating blood are detected and converted by endothelia into a sequence of biological responses are presently unknown. Our recent work has focused primarily on what effects hemodynamic factors such as fluid shear stress and vascular pressure may have on the endothelium as it exists in its native setting in vivo. We report that significant mechano-signaling can occur at the luminal endothelial cell surface. The mechanotransduction activated by increased flow and pressure in situ occurs not diffusely over the cell plasmalemma, but instead quite selectively in specialized invaginated microdomains called caveolae. Increased vascular flow and pressure induces a rapid regionalized protein phosphorylation cascade at the luminal cell surface that requires intact caveolae and involves local translocation of key signaling molecules, ultimately leading to activation of the Ras-Raf-MAP kinase pathway. Moreover, endothelial cell nitric oxide synthase (eNOS), as well as other molecules responsive to flow, reside on the cell surface in caveolae. Consistent with the hypothesis that caveolae have an important role in mechanotransduction, eNOS activity in caveolae is quite sensitive to changes in vascular flow and pressure and appears to be regulated by the caveolar coat protein, caveolin. Thus, caveolae appear to have the molecular machinery required for mediating rapid flow-induced responses as seen in endothelium and seems to be flow-sensing organelles converting mechanical stimuli into chemical signals transmitted into the cell. Models of how caveolae may function in mechanotransduction are discussed as well as the mechanisms of mechanotransduction via single molecules or multiple effectors located in microdomains.

1. Background

The vascular endothelium is continually challenged by hemodynamic forces such as pressure and shear stress which play important roles in the acute and chronic regulation of vascular tone [6] and vessel remodeling [35, 78] as well as in the development of various vascular diseases [6, 46, 60]. The endothelium is uniquely positioned between the blood and tissue compartments to receive directly the fluid forces generated by the blood flowing through the vasculature. These forces invoke unique responses within endothelial cells and serve to modulate their intrinsic structure and function [6]. In vitro experiments designed to mimic the forces imposed on the endothelium in vivo, by using human and animal cultured endothelial cell monolayers have demonstrated the importance of flow in determining cell morphology [14], activating second messenger signaling pathways [4, 30,

40, 63], releasing vaosactivators such as nitric oxide [13, 16], and inducing the expression of specific genes [44, 60]. Although many of these observations were made in endothelial cell subjected to only changes in laminar shear stress, it is becoming apparent that both increased pressure and stretch can elicit many of the same endothelial cell responses to shear stress using what seems to be similar mechanisms [6, 7, 81].

Endothelial responses to flow can be distinctly grouped based on a temporal order of events. Initial changes in flow or shear stress conditions rapidly induce the release of vasorelaxants, such as nitric oxide (NO) [33] and prostacylins (i.e. PGI$_2$) [13] and downregulation of endothelin-1 [10, 43], a potent vasoconstrictor, which together serve to acutely regulate vascular tone. On the other hand, sustained changes in hemodynamic conditions cause morphological [14] and metabolic [6] adaptations within the endothelium. Both the acute and chronic endothelial cell responses to flow have been shown to involve the activation of second messenger signaling cascades, the initiation of which remains a central question.

The earliest known changes to occur within the endothelium following fluid-mechanical stimulation is the activation of stretch or mechanosensitive ion channels [36, 56]. Flow imposed on bovine aortic endothelial cells grown in microcapillary tubes rapidly caused the opening of inward rectifying potassium (K$^+$) channels resulting in a hyperpolarization of the cell membrane [56]. Channel blockade prior to induction of flow prevents the usual increase in transforming growth factor-β1 [54]and downregulation of endothelin-1 mRNA expression [45]. Although these data provide evidence for K$^+$ channel activation in the mechanotransduction pathways leading to an endothelial cell response to flow, G-protein activation and elevation of guanosine 3',5'–cyclic monphosphate (cGMP) appear to mediate potassium channel activation [55] suggesting that these channels lie downstream from a primary mechanoreceptor.

Many of the early flow-induced and shear-related responses described in the literature share a similarity to those that often follow ligand-receptor binding, such as activation of typical receptors coupled to G-proteins. Human umbilical vein endothelial cells (HUVEC) subjected to fluid flow showed rapid activation of their membrane associated heterotrimeric G-proteins [25]. In addition, purified G-proteins reconstituted into phospholipid vesicles appear to be activated by shear forces, suggesting inherent mechanosensing capabilites of the G-protein when embedded alone in the phospholipid bilayer as well as mediation of mechanotransduction by the lipid bilayer itself [24]. Furthermore, prostacyclin release [3] and platelet-derived growth factor gene expression [27] appear to require G-protein activation as does flow-induced NO production [33]. These data cumulatively suggest a prominent role for G-proteins in mechanotransduction of fluid-mechanical forces.

Currently, much more is known about the more distal aspects of the mechanotransduced signaling cascade, namely the effect of flow on molecular events at or near the nucleus [45, 60]. Transcription factors such as nuclear factor kappa B (NF-kB) and activator protein 1 (AP-1), upon activation, are translocated to the nucleus where they bind to DNA recognition sites and thereby regulate transcription. Shear stress has been shown to stimulate the formation of both NF-kB and AP-1 complexes with DNA of cultured bovine aortic endothelial cells [27]. In addition, exposure to flow induced expression of the immediate early response genes (IERGs) c-myc, c-fos and c-jun, [26, 34] which, in turn, can further regulate gene expression. Flow-induced gene expression results from the interaction of transcription factors with a shear stress response element corresponding to a 6-bp component originally described in the promoter region of PDGF-B gene [59]. This sequence has been identified in a number of other genes including eNOS, TGF-β1 and endothelin-1 and appears to be part of a more general mechanism involved in the regulation of endothelial gene expression by fluid-mechanical stimuli.

These nuclear event are regulated, in part, by the MAP kinase pathway, a convergence point for many of the second messenger signaling pathways. Phosphorylation of both 42- and 44- kDa MAP kinases (ERK 1/2) occurrs in both cultured bovine aortic [29] and umbilical vein endothelial cells [82] within 5-15 min of exposure to increased fluid shear stress.   Recently, expression of either mutant Gα$_{i2}$ or a dominant negative Ras prevented shear dependent activation of ERK 1/2 cultured in bovine aortic endothelial cells [30]. Other members of the MAP kinase family such as N-terminal Jun Kinase (JNK) however, seem to be regulated by an alternative mechanism requiring at least 30 min exposure to flow and phosphatidlylinositide 3-kinase   rather than G-proteins as an upstream effector [23]. Although MAP kinases has been shown to be stimulated in cultured endothelial cells subjected to shear stress, the initial sensor of fluid mechanical forces and precise cell surface relay leading to MAP kinase activation in endothelium remains unknown.

2. Past Models

Research over the past 15 years has deciphered many of the mechanisms by which the endothelium respond to hemodynamic pressure and shear stress. However, a key missing element is the flow-sensing mechanism or mechanoreceptor purported to exist in the endothelial cell. One interesting site for mechanotransduction may be the focal adhesion sites which are quite evident in endothelial cells, at least in culture, and serve to tether the cell to the underlying substratum. Focal adhesion complexes have been shown to play a role in the adaptations of endothelial cell monolayers in culture to flow and may serve as a potential mechanosenory site.   These sites undergo remodeling when shear stress is applied to the luminal surface of cultured endothelial cells and realign in the direction of flow [22]. Cytoskeletal elements similarly rearrange and form stress fibers parallel to flow suggesting an association with focal adhesions [22]. In addition, several cytosolic proteins localized to focal adhesions, particularly focal adhesion kinase [67] and paxillin [83], undergo phosphorylation and initiate signal-transduction events in response to flow. Although focal adhesion complexes, especially in cultured endothelial cells, can clearly play a role in the cellular responses to flow, the signaling events at these sites typically manifest rather slowly, after 10-60 min of exposure to increased flow [2]. These observation are consistent with the concept that signals mediating quite rapid endothelial cell responses to flow are generated at a sites other than focal adhesion complexes.

A model which serves to reconcile forces recieved at the cell surface with signaling events originating primarily inside the cell such as the nucleus or even those occurring at focal adhesion sites has been described by Ingber and co-workers [28]. Based on the observation that cells are under tension, the tensegrity model suggests that a structural system exists within cells for direct communication of regulatory information from the cell surface to other areas within the cell. When tension is changed, the interconnected structural system rapidly rearranges to a new position. Therefore, direct shear-induced mechanotransduction in endothelial cells is explained by activation of a cell surface coupler which transmits the forces it experiences via cytoskeletal elements to be distributed either focally or throughout the cell including sites remote from the externally applied stress, such as focal adhesion complexes. Although this model provides an integrated view of mechanotransmission, individual components, particularly those with mechanosensing capabilities, remain to be identified.

3. New Approach to Studying Mechanotransduction in Situ

The importance of flow in determining cellular morphology, gene expression and activation of second messenger pathways has clearly been demonstrated [6] in culture systems designed to mimic the forces imposed on the endothelium. Although these experiments have greatly enhance our understanding of endothelial cell response to flow, removal of endothelial cells from their native environment and grown in culture can and does induce very significant phenotypic changes (i.e., appearance of stress fibers, loss of caveolae) which may introduce potential artifacts into the experimental system. Thus, there is a need for experimental data performed in vivo and in situ, where the endothelium exists under more native physiological conditions, to study flow-mediated regulation of vascular endothelium.

A modern concept of force transduction through the endothelium may include activation of a putative cell surface receptor, be it a single molecule or a complex of elements, resulting in force transmission throughout the cell via signal transduction mechanisms. A functioning cell surface mechanoreceptor may therefore, be located at a site where stress acts directly or can be efficiently transmitted. It is the luminal surface of the endothelium that is directly exposed to the circulation and is logically expected to be a critical interface directly involved in the transmission of fluid forces to the cell. Therefore, the existence of a flow sensing, mechanotransducing element on the luminal endothelial cell surface seems logical.

A distinct structure present on the cell surface of many endothelia in vivo and even in culture are the smooth, flask-shaped invaginations called caveolae. Recent studies have garnered great interest in caveolae because of their apparent role in transport [73] and signaling [1, 41, 42]. We, and others, have shown that many key signaling molecules reside concentrated within caveolae and become activated upon binding receptors in caveolae [39, 42, 68, 79]. Some of these signaling molecules have been implicated in rapid endothelial cell responses to flow which lead us to propose in 1995 that caveolae may serve as mechanotransductin site at the cell surface [69]. For instance, both Ca^{2+}-ATPase and IP3-activated channels, which may mediate flow-induced calcium influxes, are enriched in endothelial caveolae [15, 72]. Moreover, G-proteins which may modulate shear-sensitive K^+ channels and PLC generation of IP3 and DAG in mechanically stimulated endothelial cells are also present in caveolae [70]. The localization of signaling molecules within a small invaginated microdomain is likely to provide the proximity necessary for rapid, efficient and specific propagation of signals to downstream targets.

We have developed a technology to rapidly isolate and analyze the luminal endothelial cell surface membrane and its caveolae directly from whole tissue [71, 72]. This procedure provides a unique opportunity to assess mechantransduction at the endothelial cell surface in situ and also to establish the presence of, and possibly even identify, a discrete flow-sensor associated with the luminal cell surface. In our in situ model, vascular fluid flow is achieved by perfusion of a mammalian Ringer's solution at 37 C through the rat lung in situ at a predetermined rates, pressures and times of delivery using a variable speed pump. Pressure and flow rates are measured during lung perfusions with flow rates producing pressures in the normal physiological range. Rates of 4-5 ml/min produce pressures of 8-10 mmHg and 10 ml/min and 12 ml/min resulting in pressures of 18-20 mmHg and 22-24 mmHg, respectively. At the conclusion of the perfusion experiments, the vasculature is immediately cooled to 10 C by perfusion with 20mM MES-buffered saline (2-[N-morpholino]ethanesulfonic acid) [71]. The luminal endothelial cell plasma membranes and then their caveolae are then rapidly purified using an *in situ* silica coating procedure described previously [71]. Briefly, a positively charged colloidal silica solution is perfused through the rat lung vasculature to selectively coat the luminal endothelial cell plasma membranes. Cross-linking of the silica particles by subsequent perfusion with polyacrylic acid creates a stable adherent silica pellicle that marked this specific membrane of interest. This coating firmly attaches to the plasma membrane greatly increases its density and thus permits purification by centrifugation of the silica-coated endothelial cell plasma membranes (P) from the whole lung homogenates (H). The silica-coated membrane pellets have many associated caveolae and display ample enrichment for various endothelial cell surface markers while being markedly depleted in molecules associated with other tissue structures [68, 71]. The attached caveolae can be sheared away from P and purified by sucrose gradient flotation [71, 72]. A membrane band (V) which is easily detected at a density of 15-20% sucrose contains a homogeneous population of caveolae amply enriched in caveolar markers and greatly depleted in noncaveolar markers [68, 71, 72]. The remaining silica-coated membrane pellet stripped of caveolae is labeled P-V.

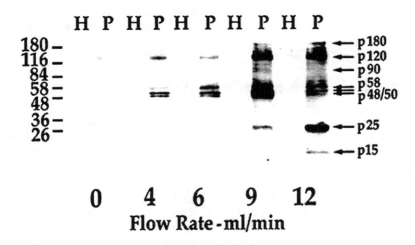

Figure 1 - Flow-induced tyrosine phosphorylation of proteins on the luminal endothelial cell surface in site. Rat lungs were perfused for 10 min at the indicated flow rate prior to purification of the luminal endothelial cell plasma membrane (P) from whole tissue homogenates (H). Western analysis indicates a flow-dependent protein-tyrosine phosphorylation easily detected in the purified plasma membranes but not the whole tissue homogenates. Arrows denote proteins phosphorylated by flow [62].

Using this approach, we found that increased fluid flow through the rat lung vasculature in situ induces tyrosine phosphorylation of several proteins on the luminal endothelial cell surface. Figure 1 shows that the flow-induced phosphorylation was difficult to detect in the starting whole lung homogenates (H) but became quite evident when the luminal endothelial cell plasma membranes (P) were purified, consistent with the known enrichment of endothelial cell surface proteins [71]. As seen in figure 1, increasing flow and pressure stimulates protein-tyrosine phosphorylation detected at the luminal endothelial plasma membrane (P). Both the number of proteins phosphorylated and the degree to which they become phosphorylated increases significantly on the luminal endothelial cell surface [62]. It seems that normal flow maintains a basal level of endothelial cell surface stimulation in situ because under no flow conditions the detected phosphorylation was minimal. This induced protein-tyrosine phosphorylation occurs very rapidly. It required only 1 min to achieve a maximum response.

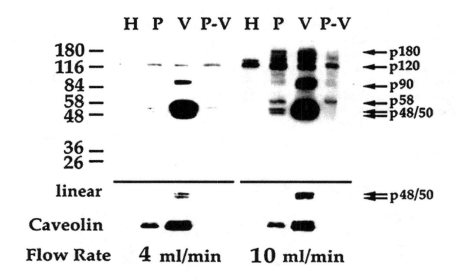

Figure 2 - Analysis of protein-tyrosine phosphorylation in caveolae. Subfractionation of purified plasma membrane (P) into caveolae (V) and membranes stripped of caveolae (P-V) was performed following rat lung perfusions at 4 or 10 ml/min. Western blot analysis of proteins from each fraction demonstrated a significant level of phosphorylated proteins (arrows) within the caveolae. Antibodies to caveolin demonstrate a 20-fold enrichment in caveolae. (H: rat lung homogenates) [62].

These rapid phosphorylation events do not occur generally over the whole endothelial cell surface but rather in very distinct plasmalemmal microdomains, the caveolae. Subfractionation to purify caveolae showed that the majority of the proteins rapidly phosphorylated in response to enhanced flow are found in the caveolae as illustrated in Figure 2. The total protein-tyrosine phosphorylation in the caveolae was 8-20 fold greater than elsewhere in the cell thereby suggesting that caveolae are major sites for flow-induced mechanosensory phosphorylation. Although our tests so far indicate that our isolation procedure yields a homogeneous population of caveolae [68, 71, 72], immuno-affinity isolations were also performed with antibodies to phosphotyrosine residues as well as caveolin. On the isolated caveolar fraction to be certain that even a low level of contaminant was not responsible for the observed signal. Indeed, both caveolin and flow-induced phosphorylated proteins were found in the same vesicle, namely caveolae. Interestingly, under low flow and pressure conditions (8-10 mmHg), only 20% of the purified caveolae were found to have sufficient tyrosine phosphorylation to be in the bound fraction of the immunoisolates. However, after doubling flow and pressure in situ, nearly 95% of the caveolin-coated caveolae contain proteins that have been tyrosine-phosphorylated [62]. This finding is in stark contrast to the more restrictive stimulation of caveolae by growth factors [42] where only half of the caveolae in the purified caveolar fraction exhibited protein-tyrosine phosphorylation after PDGF treatment of the endothelium. Mechanical stimulation from increased vascular flow and pressure causes quite rapid and rather selective tyrosine phosphorylation of proteins in caveolae.

For the first time, it appears quite clear that significant mechanotransduction does indeed occur in tissue at the luminal endothelial cell surface [62]. More specifically, this "acute flow-sensing" appears to occur in the caveolae. Yet, as discussed earlier, a significant gap still exists between the distal aspects of the mechanotransduced signaling cascade leading to alteration in gene expression and the more proximal signaling events occuring at or near the plasma membrane. To begin to address this gap, we have examined flow activation of an effector of the MAP kinase pathway and the upstream effectors of this pathway. Increasing flow through the rat lung vasculature does indeed activate ERK 1/2 in a time-dependent manner. Activation occurs as early as 30 seconds reaching a maximal increase of 15-fold at 3 min. Furthermore, Raf appears to be activated with rapid translocation to the plasma membrane, particularly to its caveolae [62]. Similar flow-induced increases are readily seen for other molecules including Ras, Src-like nonreceptor tyrosine kinases (Lyn, Src and Yes but not Lck) and 14-3-3 but not ACE, β-actin, PLC-γ or caveolin. It appears that mechanical forces can stimulate key signaling molecules in caveolae, resulting in localized signal transduction with activation of the Ras/Raf/MAP kinase pathway and perhaps other signaling pathways. Caveolae may provide a bridge between the cell surface and nucleus using the Ras/Raf/MAP kinase pathway as the linker.

4. Elimination of Organized Caveolae Disrupts Efficient Mechanotransduction

The organization or compartmentalization of molecules within caveolae appear to be necessary for efficient mechanotransduction. Cholesterol is a very important component of caveolae that is to be required to maintain the structural integrity of this vesicular complex. Caveolin binds cholesterol [50] and forms an oligomeric cage around caveolae [49, 64]. Induced expression of caveolin in cells without caveolae causes caveolae formation [12]. Cholesterol binding agents, such as filipin, sequester cholesterol, remove it from plasma membranes, and cause reversible disassembly of caveolae to effectively disperse proteins normally found in caveolae over the cell surface [65, 74]. Interestingly, PDGF signaling occurs in caveolae and filipin-induced disassembly of caveolae can greatly inhibit PDGF-induced signaling in caveolae [42]. In our in situ rat lung model, filipin significantly reduces the flow-dependent tyrosine phosphorylation detected on the endothelial cell surface as well as the activation of MAP kinase [62]. Filipin does not have intrinsic kinase inhibitory activity nor can it reduce vanadate-stimulated protein tyrosine phosphorylation [42]. Furthermore, we can not purify caveolae after perfusing filipin which is consistent with past work showing nearly complete loss of caveolar invaginations on the cell surface [65, 74]. A very recent report confirms our in situ findings that filipin inhibits mechanical stimulation of the MAP kinase pathway induced by fluid shearing of cultured endothelial cells [58]. Interestingly, filipin inhibition was selective for the more rapid MAP kinase response than for the slower responding Jun kinase pathway.

It appears that the disruption by filipin of caveolae as an organized subcompartment of the plasmalemma prevents the efficient and rapid conversion of the mechanical stimulus into a transduced signaling cascade leading to MAP kinase activation. One must consider that the interaction of filipin with cholesterol and/or the ability of filipin to remove cholesterol from membranes such as caveolae may directly or indirectly disrupt caveolae function that is dependent on caveolins affinity for cholesterol. The depolymerization of caveolin may cause caveolae to disassemble and release compartmentalized signaling molecules to a more random plasmalemmal distribution [65, 74]. Or, perhaps, filipin may directly affect caveolins ability to regulate key signaling molecules. Either way, the result is a lack of effecient mechanotransduction apparently from a de-sensitization of signaling stimulated by hemodynamic stresses. This response is rapid (sec to min), occurs in caveolae and ultimately activates the Ras/Raf/MAP kinase pathway in a way that is distinct from other slower cellular signaling responses. Lastly, one must bear in mind that other cholesterol dependent microdomains, such as those rich in GPI-anchored proteins and glycolipids while distinct from caveolae [71], are also sensitive to filipin and possibly responsive to mechanical stimulation.

5. eNOS and Other Mechanosensing Molecules in Caveolae

Nitric oxide (NO) has been identified as an endothelial relaxing factor [16, 48, 57] which is released by changes in flow   [5, 32, 51, 66]. The mechanisms of this basic cardiovascular response leading to activation of eNOS to generate NO has remained elusive, especially in vivo.   Based on the short half-life of NO and the physiological effects that activate NO production such as shear stress, it is somewhat perplexing that in culture, eNOS appears to reside primarily in the Golgi and cytoplasmic compartments [51, 75]. When appropriately lipid acylated, eNOS can be targeted to membrane subfractions rich in caveolin and therefore assumed to be specialized plasmalemmal vesicles called caveolae [20, 76]. Although caveolin at the cell surface is quite specific for caveolae, it can also be quite abundant in the trans-Golgi network, at least in cultured cells [8]. One may expect that, at least for the flow responsive pool of eNOS, the enzyme would reside at the endothelial cell surface, especially the surface which is directly exposed to the forces of the circulation in vivo and not within an intracellular compartment far removed from these forces.

Recently, eNOS has been shown to be present in various caveolar isolates [20, 76] but not in another [80]. It can associate with the caveolar coat protein, caveolin, both in cultured endothelial cell lysates [9, 20] and in recombinant protein-protein assays [19, 31, 47]. In vitro recombinant protein-protein interaction studies suggest that caveolin may inhibit the functional activity of eNOS [19, 31, 47]. The physiological relevance of this ability to associate as recombinant proteins in the test tube however, remains undefined, especially under physiological conditions experienced in vivo.

We have looked very carefully at eNOS localization as it exists in endothelium in vivo as well as examined the regulation and mechanism of eNOS activation under changing hemodynamic conditions in vivo [61]. In our system, eNOS is amply present on the luminal endothelial cell surface, primarily in caveolae, as detected by its enrichment in caveolae purified by subcellular fractionation [20, 61] and by immuno-gold electron microscopy [61]. The presence of eNOS within luminal plasma membrane caveolae has also been confirmed by rapid immuno-affinity isolation of the caveolae fraction with a high affinity monoclonal antibody to caveolin that, unlike other antibodies, recognizes oligomeric caveolin on intact caveolae [53]. Nearly all of the eNOS and caveolin detected were contained in the same immunoisolated vesicles [61]. It is important to note that, with time, eNOS as well as other signaling molecules dissociate from the caveolae into solution. Therefore, rapid immunoisolation is a necessity. This dissociation may partially explain the absence of eNOS in the caveolar isolates described in the one past report [80].

The presence of eNOS in caveolin-coated caveolae does not necessarily confer functionality. We looked at eNOS activity in the caveolae and found it to be significantly greater than that detected in the other membrane subfractions including the plasma membrane as a whole [61]. More importantly, incremental increases in vascular flow and pressure activates the eNOS activity found in caveolae very rapidly in just 1 min [61]. Within this time period period, the caveolar content of eNOS did not change with increasing flow, demonstrating that the observed enhancement of eNOS activity was not caused by flow-induced recruitment of eNOS to the caveolar compartment but rather an increase in eNOS enzymatic activity found in the caveolae.

The importance of caveolin association with eNOS became more clear in our in situ experiments that show that rapid activation of caveolar eNOS is associated with eNOS dissociation from caveolin and its rapid association with calmodulin [61]. However, the actual mechanism by which pressure or shear stress causes this caveolae dissociative-associative process resulting ultimately in activation of eNOS remains undefined. Changes in hemodynamic forces may directly cause a conformational change to the overall oligomeric structure of caveolin (see discussion below). The physical perturbation of the caveolar substructure (caveolin, other oligomer or protein, or lipid milieu) may therefore influence the physical arrangement of signaling molecule present within caveolae and known to associate with caveolin. One possible senario therefore, would be a force-induced change in the conformation of caveolin which translates into the physical release of eNOS, as well as possibly other signaling molecules. Once removed from caveolin's inhibitory clamp and available for interaction with positive effectors such as calmodulin, eNOS becomes active. Alternatively or perhaps in addition, because hemodynamic forces have been shown to regulate calcium fluxes within endothelium [21] and may be required for the acute activation of eNOS [11], changes in pressure or shear stress may regulate calcium signaling molecules known to be concentrated within caveolae [15, 72]. Focal increase in calcium concentration may have profound influence on the activation of calcium-dependent molecules, such as eNOS. From the current data, it appears that hemodynamic forces transmit through caveolae to release eNOS from its inhibitory association with caveolin, apparently to allow more complete activation by calmodulin and other possible effectors such as Hsp90 [17]. At a minimum, the current data demonstrate a physiologically relevant mechanotransduction event occuring directly in caveolae at the luminal endothelial cell surface in situ. Hence, caveolae appear to function as flow-sensing organelles rapidly transducing mechanical stimuli that regulate eNOS activity.

Caveolae contain many other molecules implicated in rapid endothelial cell responses to flow. For instance, the production of prostacyclin and nitric oxide in endothelial cells is mediated by flow activation of G-proteins, ion channels, intracellular calcium, inositol trisphosphate, and protein kinases (see reviews [6, 16]). Many of these "response effectors" may be found in caveolae[42]. Flow-induced calcium fluxes [21, 77] also exist at the cell surface as well as stretch-activated Ca^{2+} or K^+ channels [36, 56]. G proteins may modulate shear-sensitive K^+ channels [56] or PLC to generate IP_3 and diacylglycerol in mechanically stimulated endothelial cells [63] which may lead to elevated intracellular calcium and activation of PKC. Consistent with these functional findings, Ca^{2+}-ATPase and IP_3-activated channels on the endothelial cell surface reside concentrated in caveolae [72].Although we have found that many G-proteins are present in caveolae [70], it is interesting that so far only Gq resides quite concentrated in caveolae [53]. PKC and PLC are in caveolae and PLC- is translocated to caveolae from the cytosol with increased flow (our unpublished observations). Thus, it appears that the caveolae have the necessary molecular machinery required for converting mechanical stimuli at the cell surface into the rapid chemical responses seen in the endothelium.

6. Current Model Incorporating Caveolae in Mechanotransduction

These recent results support a model of mechanotransduction occurring through the caveolae via localized tyrosine phosphorylation events activating at least the downstream Ras-Raf-MAP kinase pathway ultimately to turn on gene transcription. The question remains, however, as to how the caveolae are able to detect and transmit changes in hemodynamic forces directed at the endothelial cell surface. Perhaps it is the overall molecular structure of these unique plasma membrane microdomains.   Caveolae formation appears to depend upon the ability of caveolin to self-associate into oligomers, thus forming a substructural protein coat of caveolae [49, 64]. Caveolin also has been shown to interact directly with lipid-anchored signaling molecules, many of which have been implicated in mechanotransduction including Ras, G proteins, Src -like kinases [38]

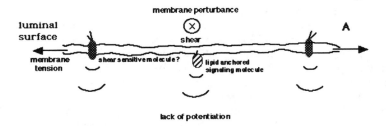

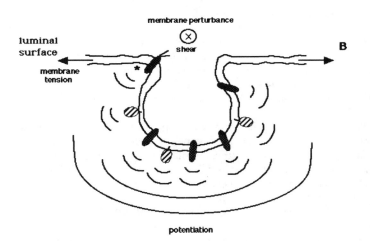

Figure 3 - Model incorporating caveolae in mechanotransduction. A) Mechanosensing signaling molecules organized diffusely over the cell surface, whether transmembrane or lipid anchored, may be activated by appropriate stresses to create signaling "noise" but not enough to reach a critical threshold of activity needed to propagate an effective signal into the cell. **B)** Mechanical forces may active transmembrane proteins with "antenae sensors" (*) or perturb the overall lipid environment to activate, directly or indirectly, multiple signaling molecules known to reside in or near caveolae. Necessary substrates as well as the overall proximity of individually activated mechanosensing molecules, all concentrated in a small region of the plasma membrane, may in the end, contribute to more efficient signal activation. Thus, activation in a localized fashion may attain the necessary threshold for conversion of mechanical stimuli into a chemical signal which amplifies and propagates into the cell.

and eNOS [18, 19, 31, 47]. Caveolin also has lipid-binding properties, particularly with cholesterol, which appears essential for maintaining caveolar form and function [65, 74]. In addition, we recently reported that dynamin forms an oligomeric structural collar around the neck of caveolae that clearly functions in the fission and internalization of

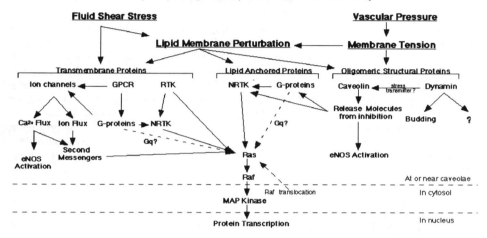

Figure 4 - Rapid mechanotransduction cascade initiated at multiple mechanosensory sites. Diagram shows the influence of two major hemodynamic stressors at the cell surface at or near caveolae. Fluid shear stress can directly affect a shear sensing surface moelecule exposed at the cell surface, probably but not necessarily a transmembrane protein (with its mechanosensing "antenae") such as ion channels, G-protein coupled receptors (GPCR) or receptor tyrosine kinases (RTK). Alternatively or perhaps in addition, shearing may directly perturb the lipids in the membrane. Similarly, perturbation of the lipid membrane may be caused indirectly by changes in membrane tension as a result of intravascular pressure fluctuations. Changes at the lipid membrane may change the microenvironmental milieu surrounding any membrane protein which may be important for those proteins functionally dependent on lipid interaction such as caveolin, RTK, ion channels, heterotrimeric G-proteins, non-receptor tyrosine kinases (NRTK) and eNOS. For example, changes in hemodynamic forces may exert an effect on these membrane proteins by altering the surrounding concentration of lipids and serve either to directly activate these lipids and/or lipid anchored proteins (G-proteins and NRTK) or to cluster substrates near shear sensitive effectors. Additionally, tension causing changes in membrane structure may induce conformational changes to oligomeric proteins such as dynamin and caveolin. The activation of dynamin may initiate caveolar budding events which may serve to regulate endothelial sensitivity to hemodynamic forces (see text) or transmit stressors from regions which lie adjacent to these forces (caveolar neck) to caveolin. Conformational changes to caveolin may release and thereby activate caveolin associated signaling molecules such as eNOS, G-proteins and NRTK. G-proteins in turn, may directly activated Ras and NRTK which itself can also activate Ras. Ultimately, Raf translocation to the caveolae from the cytosol binds to activated Ras in caveolae which can then activate MAP kinase leading to altered gene expression. Ion channel, which are activated directly as mechanosensing transmembrane molecules or indirectly by GPCR, may permit localized inward calcium or other ion fluxes leading to calcium-dependent eNOS activation and/or activation of second messengers that affect the Ras/Raf/MAP kinase pathway for induced protein transcription. In the end, it is a series of parallel chemical signaling events within the cell (as indicated by the arrows) mediated through caveolae that result in an organized and efficient propagation of a mechanical stimuli.

caveolae [52] but also may participate in hemodynamic stressors in caveolae for other functions including transmitting mechanotransduction.

The polymerization of caveolin and its association with cholesterol to create the invaginated form of caveolae [65] as well as the presence of dynamin at the caveolar neck [52] may set up a molecular structure capable a detecting physical stresses as well as induced alterations at the plasma membrane [62]. Because hemodynamic forces are known to impose a strain on caveolae which can distort them [37], one can envision a role for each or even all of these structural caveolar molecules in mechanotransduction. We have hypothesized that the oligomeric form of caveolin may act as a loaded tension-bearing coiled spring [62]. Stresses acting at the membrane (i.e., membrane tension) increase the strain on the oligomeric caveolin cage which may effectively alter the conformation of caveolin sufficiently to release associated signaling molecules. This release from the inhibitory caveolin clamp would contribute to localized activation of these signaling molecules resulting in the propagation of the Ras/Raf/MAP kinase signaling cascade. Alternatively or in addition, perhaps, molecules which reside closer to the luminal plasma membrane proper (i.e. the neck region of the caveolae) are positioned more suitably for sensing changes in fluid shear forces. Thus, molecules such as dynamin or molecules associated with dynamin at the neck (other proteins and/or lipids) could then propagate pressure or shear forces into the caveolae resulting in direct or indirect activation of key caveolar signaling molecules such as Ras, eNOS or even ion channels. It remains unclear whether stressed-induced signaling is derived from a single entity endowed with the potential to initiate the observed signaling events or a composite of several signaling and structural proteins located in or near the caveolae that have the ability to mechanotransduce collectively.

It appears that the vascular endothelium has developed an efficient means of regulating cell surface signaling events by concentrating a variety of signaling molecules and their immediate substrates within a small invaginated microdomain which seems to provide the necessary proximity for rapid and specific propagation of signals to downstream targets. Hemodynamic forces acting on the endothelium resolve into blood pressure stressors perpendicular to the fluid flow creating endothelial cell plasma membrane tension and transmural forces into the cell. In addition, a tangential force creates a frictional component or shear stress at the endothelial cell surface. Changes in both vascular pressure or fluid shear stress can exert tension on the entire lipid membrane leading to membrane alterations including perturbation of caveolar structure. Many cell surface molecules with "flow-sensing" capabilities may exist that by themselves may be mechanosensitive or have sensors which extend out into the circulating fluid environment capable of detecting changes in shear. In addition, mechanosensing may come from perturbation of lipids leading to an effect on signaling molecules. Caveolae have a specialized lipid milieu which may impart particular properties to the caveolae, thereby creating a structure sensitive to mechanical forces. Without compartmentalization however, the activation of signaling molecules organized diffusely over the cell surface may not result in the attainment of a key localized threshold of activity which may emanate random, yet induced, "noise" rather than propagate an effective, amplified and meaningful signal into the cell. These concepts are depicted schematically in Figure 3 and 4.

Our preference at this time, as depicted in Figure 4, is that many molecules may sense mechanical forces received at the plasma membrane. Caveolar components with the potential to directly detect changes in flow or even physical alterations in membrane structure as a result of changing hemodynamic forces are transmembrane proteins (ion channels, G-protein coupled receptors or receptors with tyrosine kinase activity), lipid anchored proteins (G-proteins, non-receptor tyrosine kinases and eNOS) and the caveolin oligomer itself. Mechano-activation of membrane proteins may lead to specific ion fluxes,

G-protein activation as well as activation of both receptor and non-receptor tyrosine kinases. Additionally, lipid anchored molecules such as G-proteins, eNOS and non-receptor tyrosine kinases can be directly activated by changes in membrane tension. In addition, it seems likely, based on their association with caveolin, that these signaling molecules become functional upon release from caveolin's inhibitory clamp, a process that may depend upon the structural integrity of oligomeric caveolin. Hence, one must also consider that caveolin interactions may be a way to prevent over sensitivity of these signaling molecules which may be especially problamatic when concentrated in microdomains. Once activated, these molecules propagate a signaling cascade through protein tyrosine phosphorlation to the Ras/Raf/MAP kinase pathways which ultimately influence protein transcription. In the end, these components, although potentially able to detect hemodynamic forces individually, may require appropriate organization and positioning on the cell surface in order to effectively and orderly transmit mechanical forces into the cell.

Vesicular trafficking may also be important in signaling and mechanotransduction. The ability of caveolae to bud from the cell surface into the cell may move the signal originating in or near caveolae to new intracellular sites which may serve to either enhance, reduce or otherwise change the overall signaling event. Although our observations do not indicate a loss of caveolin at the cell surface after flow stimulation up to 10 min [62], it is possible that internalization of caveolae does indeed occur with efficient recycling, thereby maintaining levels constant for caveolin/caveolae at the cell surface. It is interesting to speculate then that an enhancement or reduction of the number of cell surface caveolae is a means by which endothelial cells can modulate their "sensitivity" to mechanical force.

The data implicating caveolae in mechanosensing provide a new focus for defining the molecular events mediating mechanotransduction in endothelium. It remains to be seen whether the caveolae act as flow-sensing organelles on the endothelial cell surface through their structure and overall organization or just contain a single flow-sensing transmembrane protein that on its own is sufficient to initiate signaling events organized in the caveolae. With the molecular machinery capable of converting mechanical stimuli at the cell surface into the rapid chemical responses seen in the endothelium, the perturbation of caveolae by mechanical shear can result in organized and amplified signals transduced into the cell. Although defining exact molecular mechanisms awaits further experimentation, caveolae, as specialized plasmalemmal subcompartments acting as acute mechanotransduction centers, appear to be necessary to convert mechanical signals rapidly and efficiently into a localized cascade of phosphorylation and translocation events perpetuating the signal into the cell.

References

[1]   Anderson, R. G. W. Caveolae:where incoming and outgoing messengers meet. (1993)*Proc. Natl. Acad. Sci.* **90** 10909-10913.

[2]   Berk, B. C., M. A. Corson, T. E. Peterson, and H. Tseng. Protein kinases as mediators of fluid shear stress stimulated signal transduction in endothelial cells: A hypothesis for calcium-dependent and calcium- independent events activated by flow. (1995) *J Biomechanics* **28** 1439-1450.

[3]   Berthiaume, F., and J. A. Frangos. Flow-induced prostacyclin production is mediated by a pertussis toxin-sensitive G protein. (1992) *FEBS* **308** 277-279.

[4]   Bhagyalakshmi, A., F. Berthiaume, K. M. Reich, and J. A. Frangos. Fluid shear stress stimulates membrane phospholipid metabolism in cultured human endothelial cells. (1992) *J Vasc Res* **29** 443-449.

[5]   Cooke, J. P., E. Rossitch, N. A. Andon, L. Loscalzo, and V. J. Dzau. Flow activates an endothelial potassium to release an endogenous nitrovasodilator. (1991) *J. Clin. Invest.* **88** 1663-1671.

[6]   Davies, P. F. Flow-mediated endothelial mechanotransduction. (1995) *Physiol Rev* **75** 519-560.

[7]   Du, W., I. Mills, and B. E. Sumpio. Cyclic strain causes heterogeneous induction of transscription factors, AP-1, CRE binding protein and NF-kB, in endothelial cells: species and vascular bed diversity. (1995) *J. Biomechanics* **28**: 1485-1491.

[8]   Dupree, P., R. G. Parton, G. Raposo, T. V. Kurzchalia, and K. Simons. Caveolae and sorting in the trans-Golgi network of epithelia cells. (1993) *EMBO J.* **12** 1597-1605.

[9]   Feron, O., L. Belhassen, L. Kobzik, T. W. Smith, R. A. Kelly, and T. Michel. Endothelial nitric oxide synthase targeting to caveolae. (1996) *J. Biol. Chem.* **37** 22810-22814.

[10]   Flaherty, J. T., J. E. Pierce, D. J. Ferrans, W. K. Patel, W. K. Tucker, and d. L. Fry. Endothelial nuclear pattern in the canine arterial tree with particular reference to hemodynaimc events. (1972) *Circ. Res.* **30** 23-33.

[11]   Forstermann, U., J. S. Pollock, H. H. Schmidt, M. Heller, and F. Murad. Calmodulin-dependent endothelium- derived relaxing factor synthase activity is present in the particulate and cytosolic fractions of bovine aortic endothelial cells. (1991) *Proc. Natl. Acad. Sci.* **88** 1788-1792.

[12]   Fra, A. M., E. Williamson, K. Simons, and R. G. Parton. Detergent-insoluble glycolipid microdomains in lymphocytes in the absence of caveolae. (1994) *J. Biol. Chem.* **269** 30745-30748.

[13]   Frangos, J. A., S. G. Eskin, L. V. McIntire, and C. L. Ives. Flow effects on prastacyclin production by cultured human endothelial cells. (1985) *Science* **227** 1477-1479.

[14]   Franke, R.-P., M. Grafe, H. Schnittler, D. Seiffge, C. Mittermayer, and D. Drenckhahn. Induction of human vascular endothelial stress fibers by fluid shear stress. (1984) *Nature* **307** 648-649.

[15]   Fujimoto, T. Calcium pump of the plasma membrane is localized in caveolae. (1993) *J. Cell Sci.* **120** 1147.

[16]   Furchgott, R. F., and P. M. Vanhoutte. Endothelium-derived relaxing and constricting factors. (1988) *FASEB J.* **3** 2007-2018.

[17]   Garcia-Cardena, G., R. Fan, V. Shah, R. Sorrentino, G. Cirino, A. Papapetropoulos, and W. C. Sessa. Dynamic activation of endoethelial nitric oxide synthase by Hsp90. (1998) *Nature* **392** 821-824.

[18]   Garcia-Cardena, G., R. Fan, D. F. Stern, J. Liu, and W. C. Sessa. Endothelial nitric oxide synthase is regulated by tyrosine phsophorylation and interacts with caveolin-1. (1996) *J. Biol. Chem.* **271** 27237-27240.

[19]   Garcia-Cardena, G., P. Martasek, B. S. Siler-Masters, P. M. Skidd, J. Couet, S. Li, M. P. Lisanti, and W. C. Sessa. Dissecting the interaction between nitric oxide synthase (NOS) and caveolin. (1997) *J. Biol. Chem.* **272** 25437-25440.

[20]   Garcia-Cardena, G., P. Oh, J. Liu, J. E. Schnitzer, and W. C. Sessa. Targeting of nitric oxide synthase to endothelial cell caveolae via palmitoylation: Implications for nitric oxide signaling. (1996) *Proc Natl Acad Sci USA* **93** 6448-6453.

[21]   Geiger, R. V., B. C. Berk, R. W. Alexander, and R. M. Nerem. Flow-induced calcium transients in single endothelial cells: spatial and temporal analysis. (1992) *Am J Physiol* **262** C1411-C1417.

[22]   Girard, P. R., and R. M. Nerem. Shear stress modulates endothelial cell morphology and F-actin organization through the regulation of focal adhesion-associated proteins. (1995) *J Cell Physiol* **163** 179-193.

[23]   Go, Y.-M., H. Park, M. C. Maland, V. M. Darley-Usmar, B. Stoyanov, R. Wetzker, and H. Jo. Phosphatidylinositide 3-kinasey mediates shear stress-dependent activation of JNK in endothelial cells. (1998) *Am. J. Physiol.* **274** (in press).

[24]   Gudi, S., J. P. Nolan, and J. A. Frangos. Modulation of GTPase activity of G proteins by fluid shear stress and phosplipid composition. (1998) *Proc. Natl. Acad. Sci.* **95** 2515-2519.

[25]   Gudi, S. R. P., C. B. Clark, and J. A. Frangos. Fluid flow rapidly activates G proteins in human endothelial cells. (1996) *Circ. Res.* **79** 834-839.

[26]   Hsieh, H.-J., N.-Q. Li, and J. A. Frangos. Pulsatile and steady flow induces c-*fos* expression in human endothelial cells. (1993) *J Cell Physiol* **154** 143-151.

[27]   Hsieh, H.-J., N.-Q. Li, and J. A. Frangos. Shear-induced platelet-derived growth factor gene expression in human endothelial cells is mediated by protein kinase C. (1992) *J Cell Physiol* **150** 552-558.

[28]   Ingber, D. E. Tensegrity: the architectural basis of cellular mechanotransduction. (1997) *Annu. Rev. Physiol.* **59** 575-99.

[29]   Ishida, T., T. E. Peterson, N. L. Kovach, and B. C. Berk. MAP kinase activation by flow in endothelial cells. (1996) *Circ. Res.* **79** 310-316.

[30] Jo, H., K. Sipos, Y.-M. Go, R. Law, J. Rong, and J. M. McDonald. Differential effect of shear stress on extracellular signal- regulated kinase and N-terminal jun kinase in endothelial cells. (1997) *J. Biol. Chem.* **272** 1395-1401.

[31] Ju, H., R. Zou, V. J. Venema, and R. C. Venema. Direct interaction of endothelial nitric oxide synthase and caveolin-1 inhibits synthase activity. (1997) *J. Biol. Chem.* **272** 18522-18525.

[32] Kuchan, M. J., and J. A. Frangos. Role of calcium and calmodulin in flow-induced nitric oxide production in endothelial cell. (1994)*Am. J. Physiol.* **266** C628-C636.

[33] Kuchan, M. J., H. Jo, and J. A. Frangos. Role of G proteins in shear stress-mediated nitric oxide production by endothelial cells. (1994) *Am J Physiol* **267** C753-C758.

[34] Lan, Q., K. O. Mercurius, and P. F. Davies. Stimulation of transciption factors NF kB and AP-1 in endothelial cells subjected to shear stress. (1994) *Biochem. Biophys. Res. Commun.* **201** 950-956.

[35] Langille, B. L., and F. O'Donnel. Reduction in arterial diameter produced by chronic decrease in blood flow are endotheium-dependent. (1986) *Science* **231** 405-407.

[36] Lansman, J. B., T. J. Hallam, and T. J. Rink. Single stretch-activated ion channels in vascular endothelial cells as mechanotransducers? (1987) *Nature* **325** 811-813.

[37] Lee, J., and G. W. Schmid-Schonbein. Biomechanics of skeletal muscle capillaries: hemodynamic resistance, endothelial distensibility and pseudopod formation. (1995) *Ann. Biomed. Eng.* **23** 226-246.

[38] Li, S., J. Coute, and M. P. Lisanti. Src tyrosine kinases, Ga subunits, and H-Ras share a common membrane-anchored scaffolding protein, caveolin. (1996) *J. Biol. Chem.* **271** 29182-29190.

[39] Li, S., T. Okamoto, M. Chun, M. Sargiacomo, J. E. Casanova, S. H. Hansen, I. Nishimoto, and M. P. Lisanti. Evidence for a regulated interaction between heterotrimeric G proteins and caveolin. (1995) *J. Biol. Chem.* **270** 15693-15701.

[40] Li, Y.-S., J. Y.-J. Shyy, S. Li, J. Lee, B. Su, M. Karin, and S. Chein. The ras-jnk pathwat is involved in shear-induced gene expression. (1996) *Mol. Cell. Biol.* **16** 5947-5954.

[41] Lisanti, M. P., P. E. Scherer, Z. Tang, and M. Sargiacomo. Caveolae, caveolin and caveolin-rich membrane domains: a signalling hypothesis. (1994) *Trends Cell Biol.* **4** 231-235.

[42] Liu, J., P. Oh, T. Horner, R. A. Rogers, and J. E. Schnitzer. Organized endothelial cell surface signal transduction in caveolae distinct from glycosylphophatidylinositol-anchored protein microdomains. (1997) *J. Biol. Chem.* **272** 7211-7222.

[43] Malek, a. M., a. L. Greene, and S. Izumo. Regulation of enothelin-1 gene by fluid shear stress is transcriptionally mediated and independent of protein kinase C and cAMP. (1993) *Proc. Natl. Ac. Sci.* **90** 5999-6003.

[44] Malek, A. M., and S. Izumo. Control of endothelial cell gene expression by flow. (1995) *J Biomechanics* **28** 1515-1528.

[45] Malek, A. M., and S. Izumo. Role of tyrosine kinase, intracellular calcium release and mechanosensitive channels in endothelial shear stress transduction. (1993) *Circulation* **88** 0976.

[46] Melkumyants, A. M., S. A. Balashov, and V. M. Khayutin. Control of arterial lumen by shear stress on endothelium. (1995)*NIPS* **10** 204-210.

[47] Michel, J. B., O. Feron, K. Sase, P. Prabhakar, and T. Michel. Caveolin vs. calmodulin. (1997) *J. Biol. Chem.* **272** 25907- 25912.

[48] Moncada, S., M. W. Radomski, and R. M. J. Palmer. (1988) *Biochem. Pharmacol.* **37** 2495-2501.

[49] Monier, S., R. G. Parton, F. Vogel, J. Behlke, A. Henske, and T. V. Kurzchalia. VIP21-caveolin, a membrane protein constituent of the caveolar coat, oligomerizes *in vivo* and *in vitro*. (1995) *Mol. Biol. Cell* **6** 911-927.

[50] Murata, M., J. Peranen, R. Schreiner, F. Wieland, T. V. Kurzchalia, and K. Simons. VIP21/caveolin is a cholesterol-binding protein. (1995) *Proc. Natl. Acad. Sci. USA* **92** 10339-10343.

[51] O'Brien, H. A., H. N. Young, J. M. Pobey, and J. V. Furness. (1995) *Histochem.* **103** 221-225.

[52] Oh, P., P. D. McIntosh, and J. E. Schnitzer. Dynamin at the neck of caveolae mediates their budding to form transport vesicles by GTP-driven fission from the plasma membrane of endothelium. (1998) *J Cell Biol.* **141** 101-114.

[53] Oh, P., and J. E. Schnitzer. Towards understanding the basics of purifying caveolae. (1997) *Mol. Biol. Cell* **8** 207A.

[54] Ohno, M., J. P. Cooke, and G. H. Gibbons. Shear-stress induced TGF-b1 gene transcription via a flow-activated potassuim channel. (1993) *Circulation* **88** 0975.

[55] Ohno, M., G. H. Gibbons, V. J. Dzau, and J. P. Cooke. Shear stress elevates endothelial cGMP. Role of a potassium channel and G-protein coupling. (1993) *Circulation* **88** 193-197.

[56] Olesen, S.-P., D. E. Clapham, and P. F. Davies. Haemodynamic shear stress activates a K^+ current in vascular endothelial cells. (1988)*Nature* **331** 168-170.

[57] Palmer, R. M., A. G. Ferrige, and S. Moncada. Nitric oxide release accounts for the biological activity of endothelium-derived relaxing factor. (1987) *Nature* **327** 524-526.

[58] Park, H., M.-Y. Go, P. L. St-John, M. C. Maland, M. P. Lisanti, D. R. Abrahamson, and H. Jo. Plasma membrane cholesterol is a key molecule in shear stress-dependent activation of extracellular signal-regulated kinase. (1998) *J. Biol. Chem.* **273** (in press).

[59] Resnick, N., T. Collins, W. Atkinson, D. T. Bonthron, C. F. Dewey, and M. A. Gimbrone. Platelet-derived growth factor B chain promoter contains a cis-acting fluid shear-stress responsive element. (1993) *Proc. Natl. Acad. Sci.* **90** 4591-4595.

[60] Resnick, N., and M. A. Gimbrone. Hemodynamic forces are complex regulators of endothelial gene expression. (1995) *FASEB J* **9** 874-882.

[61] Rizzo, V., D. P. McIntosh, P. Oh, and J. E. Schnitzer. Flow activates eNOS in caveolae at the luminal cell surface of endothelium in situ with rapid caveolin dissociation and calmodulin association. (1998) *J. Biol. Chem.* (in press).

[62] Rizzo, V., A. Sung, P. Oh, and J. E. Schnitzer. Rapid mechanotransduction in situ at the luminal cell surface of the microvascular endothelium and its caveolae. (1998) *J. Biol. Chem.* **273** 26323-26329.

[63] Rosales, O. R., and B. E. Sumpio. Changes in cyclic strain increase inositol triphosphate and diacylglycerol in endothelial cells. (1992) *Am J Physiol* **262** C956-C962.

[64] Rothberg, K. G., J. E. Heuser, W. C. Donzell, Y. S. Ying, J. R. Glenney, and R. G. Anderson. Caveolin, a protein component of caveolae membrane coats. (1992) *Cell* **68** 673-682.

[65] Rothberg, K. G., Y.-S. Ying, B. A. Kamen, and R. G. W. Anderson. Cholesterol controls the clustering of the glycophospholipid-anchored membrane receptor for 5-methltetrahydrofolate. (1990) *J. Cell Biol.* **111** 2931-2938.

[66] Rubanyi, G. M., J. C. Romero, and P. M. Vanhoutte. Flow-induced release of endothelium-derived relaxing factor. (1986)*Am. J. Physiol.* **250** H1145-H1149.

[67] Schaller, M. D., B. C.A., B. S. Cobb, R. R. Vines, A. B. Reynolds, and J. T. Parsons. pp125FAK, a structurally distinctive protein-tyrosine kinase associated with focal adhesions. (1992) *Proc. Natl. Acad. Sci.* **89** 5192-5196.

[68] Schnitzer, J. E. The endothelial cell surface and caveolae in health and disease. In: *Vascular Endothelium: Physiology, Pathology and Therapeutic Opportunities*, edited by G. V. R. Born and C. J. Schwartz. Stuttgart: Schattauer, 1997, p. 77-95.

[69] Schnitzer, J. E. Molecular architecture of endothelial caveolae: Possible stress-sensing organelles. (1995) *Ann. Biomed. Eng.* **23** S34.

[70] Schnitzer, J. E., J. Liu, and P. Oh. Endothelial caveolae have the molecular transport machinery for vesicle budding, docking, and fusion including VAMP, NSF, SNAP, annexins, and GTPases. (1995) *J Biol Chem* **270** 14399-14404.

[71] Schnitzer, J. E., D. P. McIntosh, A. M. Dvorak, J. Liu, and P. Oh. Separation of caveolae from associated microdomains of GPI-anchored proteins. (1995) *Science* **269** 1435-1439.

[72] Schnitzer, J. E., P. Oh, B. S. Jacobson, and A. M. Dvorak. Caveolae from luminal plasmalemma of rat lung endothelium: microdomains enriched in caveolin, Ca^{2+}-ATPase, and inositol trisphosphate receptor. (1995) *Proc. Natl. Acad. Sci. USA* **92** 1759-1763.

[73] Schnitzer, J. E., P. Oh, and D. P. McIntosh. Role of GTP hydrolysis in fission of caveolae directly from plasma membranes. (1996) *Science* **274** 239-242.

[74] Schnitzer, J. E., P. Oh, E. Pinney, and J. Allard. Filipin-sensitive caveolae-mediated transport in endothelium: Reduced transcytosis, scavenger endocytosis, and capillary permeability of select macromolecules. (1994) *J Cell Biol* **127** 1217-1232.

[75] Sessa, W. C., G. Garcia-Cardena, J. Liu, A. Keh, J. S. B. Pollock, J., S. Thiru, I. M. Braverman, and K. M. Desai. (1995) *J. Biol. Chem.* **270** 17641-17644.

[76] Shaul, P. W., E. J. Smart, L. J. Robinson, Z. German, I. S. Yuhanna, Y. Ying, R. G. W. Anderson, and T. Michel. Acylation targets endothelial nitric-oxide synthase to plasmalemmal caveolae. (1996) *J Biol Chem* **271** 6518-6522.

[77] Shen, J., F. W. Luscinskas, A. Connolly, C. F. J. Dewey, and M. A. J. Gimbrone. Fluid shear stress modulates cytosolic free calcium in vascular endothelial cells. (1992)*Am J Physiol* **262** C384-C390.

[78] Skalak, T. C., and R. J. Price. The role of mechanical stresses in microvascular remodeling. (1996) *Microcirculation* **3** 143-165.

[79] Song, K. S., S. Li, T. Okamoto, L. A. Quilliam, M. Sargiacomo, and M. P. Lisanti. Co-purification and direct interaction of Ras with caveolin, an integral membrane protein of caveolae microdomains. (1996) *J. Biol. Chem.* **271** 9690-9697.

[80] Stan, R.-V., W. G. Roberts, D. Predescu, K. Ihida, L. Saucan, Ghitescu, L., , and G. E. Palade. Immunoisolation and partial characterization of endothelial plasmalemmal vesicles (caveolae). (1997) *Mol. Biol. Cell* **8** 595-605.

[81] Sumpio, B. E., M. D. Widmann, J. Ricotta, M. A. Awolesi, and M. Watase. Increased ambient pressure stimulates proliferation and morphologic changes in cultured endothelial cells. (1994) *J. Cell. Physiol.* **158:** 133-139.

[82] Tseng, H., T. E. Peterson, and B. C. Berk. Fluid shear-stress stimulated mitogen-activted protein kinase in endothelial cells. (1995) *Circ. Res.* **77** 869-878.

[83] Turner, C. E., J. R. Glenny, and K. Burridge. Paxillin: a new vinculin-binding protein present in focal adhesions. (1990) *J. Cell Biol.* **111** 1059-1068.

Part IV

Hypertension / NOS

Vascular Endothelium: Mechanisms of Cell Signaling
J.D. Catravas et al. (Eds.)
IOS Press, 1999

ENDOTHELIN AND PULMONARY HYPERTENSION

Suzanne Oparil, M.D. and Yiu-Fai Chen, Ph.D.
The University of Alabama at Birmingham
Division of Cardiovascular Disease, Vascular Biology and Hypertension Program
Birmingham, Alabama 35294-0007, U.S.A.

Abstract

Biochemical and molecular biological evidence indicates that endothelin-1 (ET-1) and its receptors are selectively upregulated in the lung during exposure to hypoxia, while functional evidence indicates that ET-1 is a major mediator of hypoxia-induced pulmonary vasoconstriction and vascular remodeling. Hypoxia stimulates ET-1 gene transcription and peptide synthesis in cultured endothelial cells, and plasma ET-1 levels are increased in patients with primary pulmonary hypertension and in humans exposed to high altitude, while immunoreactive ET-1 and ET-1 mRNA levels are increased in pulmonary artery endothelial cells of patients with primary pulmonary hypertension. Rats exposed to normobaric hypoxia exhibit increased pulmonary artery pressure, increased ET-1 peptide levels in plasma and lung, and selective increases in steady-state ET-1 and ET-A and ET-B receptor mRNA levels in lung but not in organs perfused by the systemic vasculature. The observations that both ET-1 and its major vascular smooth-muscle cell receptor are upregulated in response to hypoxia suggest that ET-1 may be a mediator of hypoxia-induced pulmonary hypertension. Moreover, hypoxic pulmonary vasoconstriction and vascular remodeling can be prevented and reversed by administration of either an ET-A-selective or a combined ET-A and ET-B receptor antagonist. These findings support the hypothesis that endogenous ET-1 plays a major role in hypoxic pulmonary vasoconstriction/hypertension, right heart hypertrophy, and pulmonary vascular remodeling and further suggest that ET-receptor blockers may be useful in the prevention and treatment of hypoxic pulmonary hypertension in humans.

1. Introduction

Hypoxia has a major influence on vascular smooth muscle tone, generally causing vasoconstriction in pulmonary arteries and vasodilation in systemic arteries of intact animals [1-3] (Figure 1). This is reflected in a rapid (seconds to minutes) increase in pulmonary artery pressure and a decrease in systemic arterial pressure, with a corresponding increase in pulmonary and decrease in systemic vascular resistance during acute hypoxic exposures. Cardiac output and heart rate increase initially, then fall below baseline (normoxic) values. All of these alterations are rapidly reversible upon return to a normoxic environment. Hypoxia augments the contractile responses of isolated blood vessels to a variety of vasoconstrictor agents [4-8], indicating that hypoxia induced vasoconstriction can be mediated by autocrine/paracrine factors within the vessel wall, and is not dependent on circulating hormones or neural transmitters.   Removal of the endothelium greatly attenuates or abolishes hypoxia induced vasoconstriction in a variety of vascular preparations [7,8]. For example, the presence of an intact endothelium has been shown to be necessary for hypoxia induced contractions in porcine main pulmonary arteries studied_*in vitro* [3]. Although main pulmonary arteries are not primarily responsible for hypoxic vasoconstriction *in vivo*, this finding suggests that the endothelium

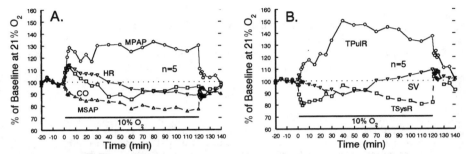

Figure 1. Hemodynamic responses to 120 min hypoxic exposure (10%O_2, 1 atm) in 11-12 wk old male Sprague-Dawley rats. Data are normalized by baseline values measured at 21% O_2. Each line represents an average value for 5 animals. A. Hemodynamic measurements. MPAP, mean pulmonary arterial pressure; HR, heart rate; CO, cardiac output; MSAP, mean systemic arterial pressure. B. Calculated values. TPulR, total pulmonary vascular resistance= MPAP/CO; TSysR, total systemic vascular resistance=MSAP/CO; SV, stroke volume=CO/HR.

and endothelium derived vasoconstrictor factor(s) play a role in the pulmonary vascular response to hypoxia. The observations that hypoxic vasoconstriction in the rat is abolished by experimental insults such as hyperoxia that damage endothelial cells [9] and that hypoxia induced pulmonary hypertension in the rat is associated with a reversible (on return to a normoxic environment) loss of endothelium derived relaxing factor (EDRF) activity in pulmonary vessels [10] confirm this interpretation.

The structure(s) of the endothelium derived, hypoxia induced vasoconstrictor substance(s) were not elucidated by these early studies, which employed bioassay techniques. It was shown, however, that inhibitors of cyclo-oxygenase, lipoxygenase and phospholipase A_2, of adrenergic, serotonergic and histaminergic receptors, and of endothelium-derived relaxing factor did not affect hypoxia induced vasoconstriction, excluding these classes of compounds from consideration [11]. A subsequent study showed that conditioned medium from cultured bovine aortic endothelial cells causes slowly developing and sustained constriction of isolated rings of canine, porcine or bovine coronary arteries [12]. The vasoconstrictor principle in this system has been characterized as a peptide and named endothelium-derived contracting factor (EDCF) [12]. More recently, Yanagisawa et al identified a novel potent vasoconstrictor peptide in the conditioned medium from cultured porcine aortic endothelial cells [13]. This peptide, endothelin (ET), is the most potent vasoconstrictor peptide known. Enhanced ET release from isolated rat mesenteric arteries perfused under hypoxic conditions has been reported [14], although bioassay data have disputed the candidacy of ET as a mediator of endothelium-dependent hypoxic vasoconstriction in isolated blood vessels [15].

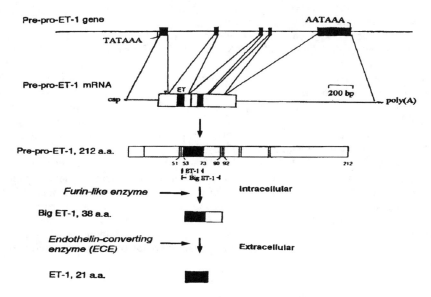

Figure 2. The pathway for generation of endothelin (ET)-1, including structural organization of the human pre-pro-endothelin-1 (PPET-1) gene and mRNA. Exons are indicated by filled boxes, introns and 5'- and 3'-flanking sequences are indicated by lines. The locations of the putative TATA box, TATAAA, and poly(A) addition signal AATAAA are indicated. The structural organization of the mRNA is presented above the schema of the gene structure.

2. Endothelin and Endothelin Receptors

ET is a 21-amino acid peptide that contains two intramolecular disulfide bonds and has a high level of structural homology with sarafotoxin S6b [13,16]. Four distinct genes which encode four isoforms of ET, ET-1, ET-2, ET-3 and VIC (Vasoactive Intestinal Contractor or endothelin-) [17] and the cDNAs for at least two distinct ET receptors have been cloned and characterized [18-20] (for review, see [21-23]). The ET-1 isoform is the most widely distributed, being found in many organs of a variety of species and in the culture media of endothelial and epithelial cells derived from these organs. The biologically active 21-amino acid ET-1 peptide is synthesized from a larger precursor by a process that involves four proteolytic cleavages [21] (Figure 2). Following removal of the signal peptide, cleavage of the Lys-Arg bond at the NH_2 terminal of the mature ET sequence and of an Arg-Arg or Lys-Arg bond at position 92-93 (pig) or 91-92 (man) is accomplished by a dibasic-amino acid-pair-specific endopeptidase, giving rise to a 39-amino acid (in pig; 38 amino acid in man) intermediate designated big ET. A membrane-bound neutral metalloendopeptidase, endothelin converting enzyme (ECE), then converts big ET to the biologically active 21 amino acid peptide ET. In endothelial cells, removal of the signal peptide and generation of big ET are accomplished within the cytoplasm, while conversion of big ET to ET occurs in the extracellular space. ECE is inhibited by the chelating agents EDTA, EGTA and o-phenanthroline, and by the neutral metalloendopeptidase inhibitor phosphoramidon [24,25]. Big ET lacks biological activity in vitro but has a pressor effect equivalent to that of ET in vivo because of conversion to ET by ECE; the pressor effect of big ET can be inhibited by phosphoramidon [26].

A full length cDNA encoding rat prepro ET-1 has been used as a probe to analyze the tissue distribution of prepro ET-1 mRNA in the rat by Northern analysis [27]. Prepro ET-1 mRNA is most abundant in lung. The brain, eye, uterus, stomach, submandibular gland and small intestine also contained relatively large amounts of prepro ET-1 mRNA. Smaller amounts of prepro ET-1 mRNA are detected in heart, kidney, adrenal gland, liver, spleen and testis. The gene transcript distribution is concordant with the previously described tissue distribution of immunoreactive ET-1 in the rat [28]. Since ET-1 receptors and pharmacologic actions of ET-1 have also been described in these tissues, it is likely that ET-1 acts locally to mediate its biological effects [27].

The human preproendothelin-1 gene contains five exons and four intervening sequences [29] (Figure 2). The first exon contains the 5 -untranslated region and sequences encoding the first 22 amino acids of preproendothelin including most, if not all, of the hydrophobic leader sequence. The second exon encodes sequences corresponding to the 21 amino acids of endothelin, and the third exon encodes the endothelin-like peptide. The fourth exon contains sequences for the preproendothelin residues 131-178. The fifth exon contains the 34 carboxyl-terminal amino acids of preproendothelin and the 3 -untranslated region.

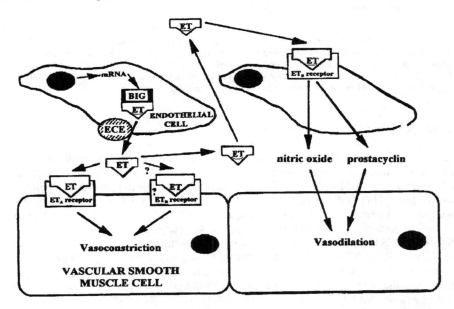

Figure 3. Vascular actions of endothelin-1 (ET). BIG ET, big endothelin-1; ECE, endothelin converting enzyme. (23)

The biological activity of ET is transduced by binding to and activation of receptors that are distributed widely in mammalian tissues [30] (Figure 3). Cross-linking experiments with ^{125}I-labeled ET's have identified multiple subtypes of the ET receptor [31,32]. The cDNA's coding for two subtypes of ET receptor, ET_A (selective for ET-1) and ET_B (nonselective, exhibiting similar affinities for ET-1, ET-2 and ET-3), were originally cloned from bovine [33] and rat [34] lung tissue, and, more recently, from a variety of other species and cell types. These receptors appear to share important structural features: they contain seven membrane-spanning domains and are rich in -helix, N-linked glycosylation sites at the N-terminal outer membrane domain and potential phosphorylation sites in the C-terminal cytoplasmic domains, consistent with a family of G protein-coupled receptors [33]. The physiological effects of the ET's are mediated through these cell surface receptors coupled to intracellular G-proteins and second messenger systems, including phospholipase C, the phosphoinositide cascade, intracellular calcium fluxes, phospholipase A_2 and the arachidonic acid cascade [35,36]. ET-1 has mitogenic effects on smooth muscle cells [37,38] and stimulates c-fos and c-myc expression in vitro [39], and thus may play a role in the initiation of cell proliferation in the vasculature.

ET-A mRNA is expressed in medial smooth muscle layers of blood vessels, atrial and ventricular myocardium, and cultured rat and human vascular smooth muscle cells (VSMCs) [40-43]. ET-A receptors mediate the vasoconstrictor and positive inotropic effects of ET in these tissues [44-47]. Expression of ET-A mRNA is highest in lung and the cardiac atrium and ventricle [48, 49]. In human pulmonary tissue, ET-A receptors are located on both resistance and conduit arteries [44,50]. Competitive binding studies in human main pulmonary artery show a predominance (~90%) of ET-A receptors [50]. However, the relative proportion of ET-A vs. ET-B receptors in human and rat pulmonary resistance vessels is uncertain. Activation of ET-A receptors by ET-1 has mitogenic effects on VSMCs and fibroblasts and stimulates c-fos and c-myc expression, and thus may play a role in the initiation of cell proliferation and remodeling in the vasculature [45,51-53]. ET-B receptors are found in multiple cell types, including endothelial and VSMC, glia, epithelial cells of the choroid plexus, ependymal cells, myocardium, glomerular endothelial cells, and epithelial cells of Henle's loops [44-47,54,55]. ET-B mRNA levels are highest in the cerebellum and also high in lung [48, 49]. ET-B receptors have been classified into $ET-B_1$ and $ET-B_2$ subtypes, which mediate endothelium-dependent vasorelaxation and VSMC dependent vasoconstriction, respectively [46,56]. In addition, the ET-B receptor is important for the clearance of ET-1 from the circulation, and administration of a selective ET-B receptor antagonist has been shown to increase circulating ET-1 levels via blockade of ET-1 clearance receptors [57,58]. A third ET receptor subtype (ET-C) has been identified in anterior pituitary and Xenopus laevis, but function of these receptors is unclear [59].

ET-1 elicits both pressor and depressor responses. The pressor response is chiefly mediated by ET-A receptors on VSMC and the depressor response by ET-B receptors on endothelial cells. Recently, however, It has been demonstrated that both ET-A and ET-B receptors are present on VSMC and mediate vascular contraction [47,61-64]. The contributions of ET-A and ET-B receptors to the contractile effects of ET-1 differ depending on the species and vascular bed studied [47,61-64]. In general, it appears that ET-B receptors have a high affinity but low capacity (density), whereas ET-A receptors have a lower affinity but are present in higher density in blood vessel walls [61]. Therefore, the contributions of both ET-A and ET-B receptors may be important for vasoconstriction and proliferation of VSMCs. The vasodilator effect of ET-1 is mediated mainly by activation of ET-B receptors on endothelial cells, which results in the formation of prostacyclin and nitric oxide, mediators of endothelium-dependent vasorelaxation [46,47,65]. ET-1-induced vasoconstrictor and vasodilator responses occur mainly in small vessels, not in large vessels such as human internal mammary artery and porcine coronary artery [66].

2.1. Role of ET-1 in the Pathogenesis of Pulmonary Hypertension

Elevated levels of ET-1 have been associated with a number of disease conditions characterized by pulmonary hypertension, including persistent pulmonary hypertension of the newborn [67,68], adult respiratory distress syndrome [69], chronic obstructive lung disease (COPD) [70], bronchial asthma [71], primary and secondary pulmonary hypertension [72-74], sepsis [75], lung tumors [76] and congestive heart failure, including pulmonary edema [77]. Studies performed in our laboratory demonstrated that rats exposed to hypoxia developed pulmonary hypertension with medial hypertrophy of the pulmonary arteries and right atrial and ventricular hypertrophy associated with selective increases in both ET-1 levels and ET-1 and ET-A and ET-B receptor mRNA expression in lung [48,49,78]. Short-term (48 hr) exposure of rats to normobaric hypoxia significantly increased pulmonary artery pressure, plasma ET-1 concentrations and ET-1 mRNA levels in the lung but not in organs supplied by the systemic vascular bed [78]. Short term hypoxic exposure was also associated with selective increases in ET-1 peptide and ET-A mRNA levels in lung; ET-B mRNA levels were unchanged [48]. Both ET-A and ET-B receptor steady state mRNA levels were increased in thoracic aorta, left atrium and right ventricle and tended to be increased in right atrium of hypoxia exposed rats compared to air controls. No change in expression of steady state mRNA levels for either ET receptor was seen in organs perfused by the systemic vascular bed. In no case were ET receptor mRNA levels in hypoxic rats reduced below air control levels, despite elevations in local and/or circulating ET-1. These results confirm our previous observation that hypoxia leads to selective stimulation of ET-1 gene expression and ET-1 synthesis in the pulmonary vasculature of the rat. This, in addition to our finding of upregulation of ET-A receptor steady state mRNA levels in the hypoxia adapted lung, is consistent with the hypothesis that a selective increase in synthesis and release of ET-1 from main pulmonary artery and more distal sites in lung could account for hypoxic pulmonary hypertension.

Subsequent experiments tested the hypothesis that exposure to chronic normobaric hypoxia (10% O_2 for 4 wks) is associated with increased circulating ET-1 levels and selective increases in ET-1 and ET-A and ET-B receptor gene transcript levels in lung and main pulmonary artery of rats with hypoxia-induced pulmonary hypertension [49]. Chronic hypoxic exposure was associated with increases in pulmonary artery pressure, right ventricular weight, plasma ET-1 levels, ET-1 mRNA in lung and pulmonary artery and ET-1 stores and ET-A and ET-B receptor mRNA levels in lung. ET-A and ET-B receptor mRNA levels were increased in thoracic aorta and all four heart chambers. No change in either ET-1 or ET receptor mRNA levels was seen in organs perfused by the systemic vascular bed except for liver, where ET-A receptor mRNA levels were decreased. These findings are consistent with the hypothesis that a selective increase in synthesis and release of ET-1 from the main pulmonary artery and more distal sites in lung could account for selective hypoxic pulmonary vasoconstriction, pulmonary vascular remodeling and the maintenance of chronic hypoxia-induced pulmonary hypertension via paracrine effects on pulmonary VSMCs.

To test this hypothesis, we examined the effects of a variety of selective ET-A receptor antagonists, including BQ-123 [cyclo(D-Trp-D-Asp-Pro-D-Val-Leu] (79-81); A-127722[trans-trans-2-(4-methoxyphenyl)-4-(1,3)-benzodioxol-5-yl0-1-((N,N-dibutylamino) carbonylmethyl)pyroolidine-3-carboxylic acid] (47,82) and TBC11251 (thiophene-3-sulfonamide, Texas Biotechnology Corp.) (83); and the combined ET-A/ET-B receptor antagonist bosentan {R0-470203, 4-tert-butyl-N-[6-(2-hydroxy-ethoxy)-5-(2-methoxy-phenoxy)-2,2'-bipyrimidin-4-yl]-benzenesulfonamide} (84,85) on the development and

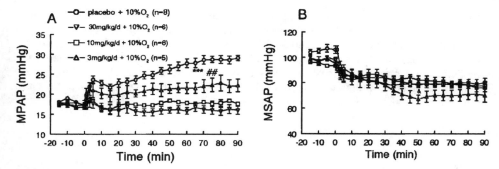

Figure 4. Effects of short-term pretreatment with A-127722 (3, 10, and 30 mg/kg/day), via drinking water for 2 days) on A) mean pulmonary arterial pressure (MPAP), and B) mean systemic arterial pressure in rats before and during short-term exposure to normobaric hypoxia (10% O_2 for 90 min). Results are means±SEM. ******* Significant difference between hypoxia+placebo and hypoxia+A-127722 (10- and 30-mg/kg/day) groups, $p < 0.001$. ## Significant difference between hypoxia+placebo and hypoxia+A-127722 (3-mg/kg/day) group, $p < 0.01$. (82)

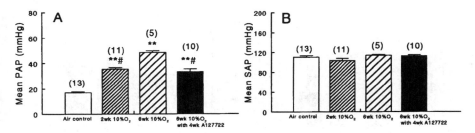

Figure 5. Effects of A-127722 (10 mg/kg/day via drinking water for 4 weeks after 2 weeks of prior hypoxic adaptation) on A) mean pulmonary arterial pressure (MPAP) and B) mean systemic arterial pressure. Two-wk 10% O_2 and 6-wk 10% O_2, placebo groups with 2 weeks and 6 weeks hypoxic exposure, respectively. Six-wk 10% O_2 + 4-wk A-127722, group in which A-127722 was administered for 4 weeks during continued exposure to hypoxia after 2-wk period of hypoxic adaptation. Results are means±SEM (n). Numbers in parentheses, number of rats. ** Significantly different from air control group, $p < 0.01$. # Significantly different from 6-wk 10% O_2 group, $p < 0.05$. (82)

maintenance of hypoxia-induced pulmonary hypertension and vascular remodeling in the rat. Pretreatment with all four ET receptor antagonists completely blocked the pulmonary vasoconstrictor response to acute hypoxia (Figure 4), while chronic treatment prevented the development of chronic hypoxia-induced pulmonary hypertension, attenuated the associated right heart hypertrophy, and prevented the remodeling of small (50-100 m) pulmonary arteries without altering systemic arterial pressure [79,81-84]. Further, institution of BQ-123, A-127722, or bosentan treatment after 2 wks of hypoxia reversed established hypoxia-induced pulmonary hypertension, right heart hypertrophy, and pulmonary vascular remodeling despite continuing hypoxic exposure (Figures 5 and 6) [79,82,84]. Similar observations have been made in other experimental models of pulmonary hypertension, such as the fawn-hooded rat, a strain which develops spontaneous pulmonary hypertension [86], the monocrotaline-treated rat, a model of pulmonary hypertension caused by vascular endothelial damage [87,88], and in lambs with a vascular shunt between the ascending aorta and main pulmonary artery, a model with increased pulmonary blood flow-induced pulmonary hypertension [89]. These findings support the hypothesis that endogenous ET-1 plays a major role in hypoxic pulmonary vasoconstriction, hypertension, right heart hypertrophy and pulmonary vascular remodeling and strongly suggest that ET-A receptor blockade may be useful in the treatment of hypoxic pulmonary hypertension in humans. Further study is needed to define the role of the ET-B receptor in these processes.

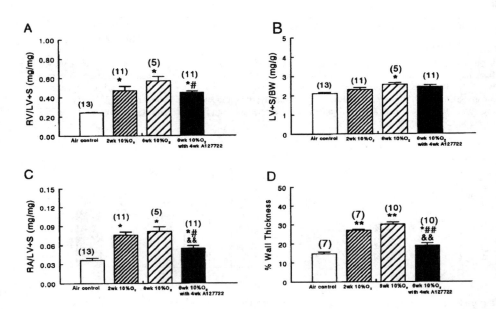

Figure 6. Effects of A-127722 (10 mg/kg/day via drinking water for 4 weeks) on A) right ventricular (RV) weights [normalized for left ventricle+septum (LV+S) weights], B) LVS/body weights (BW) ratios, C) right atrial (RA)/LV+S ratios and D) % wall thickness [(2 x medial wall thickness)/external diameter] x 100] after 2 weeks of hypoxic adaptation. Two-wk 10% O$_2$ and 6-wk 10% O$_2$, placebo groups with 2 weeks and 6 weeks hypoxic exposure, respectively. Six-wk 10% O$_2$ + 4-wk A-127722, group in which A-127722 was administered for 4 weeks during continued exposure to hypoxia after 2-week period of hypoxic adaptation. Results are means±SEM (n). Numbers in parentheses, number of rats. Significantly different from air control group: * p<0.05, ** p<0.01. Significantly different from 6-wk 10% O$_2$ group: # p < 0.05. Significantly different from 2-wk 10% O$_2$ group: && p<0.01. [82]

2.2. ET-1 and ET Receptors are Hypoxia Response Genes

Several lines of evidence have begun to elucidate the cellular and molecular mechanisms by which hypoxia induces ET-1 gene expression. Exposure to hypoxia has been shown to increase transcription of the ET-1 gene and secretion of ET-1 into the media from cultured human vascular endothelial cells, including pulmonary microvessel, coronary artery, umbilical arterial and venous endothelial cells (90-93). The induction of ET-1 by hypoxia in vitro occurred exclusively in early passage endothelial cells [90,93], and was prevented by treatment with the protein synthesis inhibitor cycloheximide, mimicked by treatment with transition metals (e.g. Co^{++} or Ni^{++}) and antagonized by NO or CO [91-94], indicating that ET-1 induction by hypoxia requires new protein synthesis, and may involve a heme-containing pathway in O$_2$ sensing [90-93]. ET-1 induction by hypoxia is not affected by inhibitors of protein kinase C, protein kinase A, calcium-calmodulin dependent protein kinase or cyclic GMP dependent protein kinase, but basal expression is decreased and hypoxic induction is eliminated by treating cells with tyrosine kinase-selective inhibitors, indicating that a protein kinase step is implicated in both basal and induced expression of the ET-1 gene [90]. The stimulatory effects of low O_2 tension on ET-1 mRNA levels are reversible on return to a normoxic environment. Nuclear runoff experiments showed that ET-1 mRNA levels was increased 8-12 fold in cultured human umbilical vein endothelial cells exposed to 1-0.5% O_2 for 6-24 hrs compared to cells cultured under normoxic conditions [90,91]. The half-life of the ET-1 transcript, assessed by actinomycin-D chase experiments, was <30 min under both conditions, indicating that the hypoxia-induced increase in steady state ET-1 mRNA levels was due to increased transcription rather than increased message stability.

Similar increases in mRNA levels and transcription rates for the B chain of platelet derived growth factor (PDGF-B) have been observed in human umbilical venous endothelial cells cultured under hypoxic conditions (0-3% O_2) for periods of 24 hrs or more [92]. Compared to the ET-1 response, the PDGF-B response was delayed (onset 24 hrs vs. 1 hr for ET-1) and occurred only with severe hypoxia (pO_2 20-45 vs. 60-80 mmHg for ET-1). In contrast, transcript levels of other endothelial cell-derived growth factors, including PDGF A-chain, transforming growth factor- (TGF), granulocyte-macrophage colony-stimulating factor, basic fibroblast growth factor (bFGF), von Willebrand factor (vWF), sodium-potassium ATPase and -actin, were not affected by hypoxia [92]. The selective responsiveness of the genes for the vasoconstrictor/growth factors ET-1 and PDGF-B to hypoxia suggests that overproduction of these peptides by pulmonary vascular endothelial cells may contribute to the smooth muscle hypertrophy and remodeling of the pulmonary vasculature characteristic of chronic hypoxic pulmonary hypertension. The earlier and more sensitive response of ET-1 to hypoxia makes it a likely candidate as an important regulator of regional blood flow in response to acute changes in O_2 tension, as well as an important mediator of VSMC hypertrophy and architectural remodeling in chronic hypoxia.

Studies currently in progress in our laboratory are designed to define the cis-regulatory element(s) involved in amplifying transcription of the ET-1 gene in endothelial cells in response to hypoxia and to identify and clone the hypoxic transcription activator protein(s). We have recently determined that the 5'-flanking region of the human ET-1 gene contains a hypoxia response element. Initial explorations of the effects of hypoxia on the promoter activity of the human ET-1 gene were carried out in transgenic mice harboring a LUC reporter gene driven by a 2.45 kb human ET-1 gene promoter -2459 to +165 bp from the transcriptional start site (Figure 7) [95].

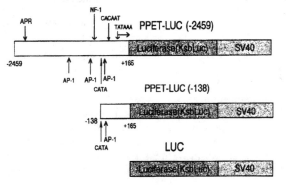

Figure 7. Schematic diagram of pre-pro-endothelin (PPET)-1/luciferase (LUC) constructs used for transfection experiments and the generation of transgenic mice. A 2624- or 303-bp fragment excised from the human PPET-1 gene was ligated to the LUC expression vector KsbLUC to create PPET-1/LUC (-2459) and PPET-1/LUC (-138), respectively. APR, acute phase response element; AP-1 activator protein 1, fos/jun binding site; NF-1, nuclear factor (NF)-B-1 binding site. GAGA, CACAAT, and TATAAA are conserved motifs typically found in or near promoters.

We have examined the effects of hypoxia on the promoter activity of the ET-1 gene in the prepro-ET-1/-2459/LUC transgenic mice. In the initial experiment, heterozygotes were exposed to hypoxia (10%O$_2$) or room air for 24 hrs and LUC activity in various organs was measured [95]. The 2.45 kb human prepro-ET-1 promoter was active in numerous tissues, and tissue LUC activity was increased by hypoxic exposure.

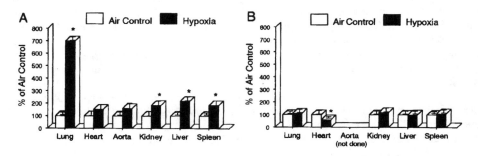

Figure 8. Effects of hypoxia on luciferase (LUC) activity in mice expression the A) human PPET-1/LUC (-2459) construc or B) a promoterless LUC construct. Mice expressing the PPET-1/LUC (-2459) transgene were exposed to room air or hypoxic (10% O2 for 24 hr) conditions. PPET-1 promoter activity was assessed by LUC reporter gene expression. LUC activity is reported as degree of increase±SEM from hypoxic tissues compared with normoxic tissue from n=6 mice. * p<0.05, compared with air control.

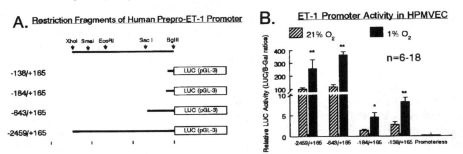

Figure 9. Transcriptional analysis following transfection of human pulmonary microvascular endothelial cells (HPMVEC) with recombinant human pre-pro-ET-1 promoter/LUC DNA constructs. A) Four different restriction fragments were subcloned 5' to the LUC reporter gene in a pGL3 vector. B) The constructed plasmids were transfected into HPMVEC by the lipofection method. A cytomegalovirus (CMV) promoter-driven-β-galactosidase (β-Gal) gene was cotransfected for assessment of transfection efficiency. Transfected cells were expressed as LUC/ -Gal activity ratios in cell extracts. Results are expressed as means±SEM; n=number of plates from three independent transfection experiments. * p<0.05; ** p<0.01, compared to their respected normoxic groups.

As predicted, the magnitude of the increase was greater (7 fold) in lung than in any other organ (Figure 8). These data indicate that the 2.45 kb promoter region of the human ET-1 gene in the 5'-flanking region adjacent to the transcriptional start site contains cis-regulatory sequence(s) that mediate a hypoxia-inducible response. The selectivity of hypoxic stimulation of LUC activity for lung is consistent with the pattern of selective increase of ET-1 mRNA levels in rat lung in our previous studies and suggests that tissue specific hypoxia inducible transcription factor(s) in lung mediate the hypoxic response. Thus, these animals provide an excellent tool to study the regulation of ET-1 gene expression in vivo, particularly the mechanism of its organ specificity (for lung). By quantitating LUC activity, we can study ET promoter activity in response to diverse physiological and pathological stimuli in addition to hypoxia. Moreover, because the LUC assay is so sensitive, we can localize LUC protein and/or mRNA in tissue with precision. Further, this DNA construct and defined regions within it can be transfected into hypoxia responsive cells in vitro in order to define the cis-regulatory element(s) involved in amplifying transcription of the ET-1 gene in response to hypoxia and to identify and clone the hypoxia responsive transcription activator protein(s).

We have subcloned fragments of the 5'-flanking promoter of the human ET-1 gene into a pGL3 vector with a LUC reporter gene and transfected the constructed plasmids into cultured human pulmonary microvascular endothelial cells (HPMVEC) and hepatocytes by lipofection [93,96] (Figure 9). Exposure of transfected HPMVEC to 1% O_2 for 24 hrs resulted in a 3-fold elevation in LUC activity for construct containing the -138/ +165 sequence, indicating that there may be positive hypoxia response element(s) located between -138 bp and the transcription start site of the 5'-flanking region of the ET-1 promoter. More precise localization of these hypoxia response elements and characterization of the hypoxia-induced transcription activator(s) with which they interact are major goals of current research in our laboratory.

References

[1]   Holm P. Endothelin in the pulmonary circulation with special reference to hypoxic pulmonary vasoconstriction. Scandinavian Cardiovascular J Supplement 46:1040, 1997.
[2]   Kiely DG, Cargill RI, Struthers AD and Lipworth BJ. Cardiopulmonary effects of endothelin-1 in man. Cardiovas Res 33:378-386, 1997.
[3]   Holden WE and McCall E. Hypoxia-induced contractions of porcine pulmonary artery strips depend on intact endothelium. Exp Lung Res 7:101-112, 1984.
[4]   Detar R and Bohr DF. Contractile responses of isolated vascular smooth muscle during prolonged exposure to anoxia. Am J Physiol 222:1269-1277, 1972.
[5]   Vanhoutte PM. Effects of anoxia and glucose depletion on isolated veins of the dog. Am J Physiol 230:1261-1268, 1976.
[6]   Van Nueten JM and Vanhoutte PM. Effect of Ca^{2+} antagonist lidoflazin on normoxic and anoxic conditions of canine coronary arterial smooth muscle. Eur J Pharmacol 64:173-176, 1980.
[7]   DeMey JG and Vanhoutte PM. Heterogenous behavior of the canine arterial and venous wall. Circ Res 51:439-477, 1982.
[8]   DeMey JG and Vanhoutte PM. Anoxia and endothelium-dependent reactivity of the canine femoral artery. J Physiol 335:65-74, 1983.
[9]   Newman JH, McMurtry IF and Reeves JT. Blunted pulmonary pressor responses to hypoxia in blood perfused, ventilated lungs isolated from oxygen toxic rats: Possible role of prostaglandins. Prostaglandins 22:11-20, 1981.
[10] Adnot S, Raffestin B, Eddahibi S, Braquet P and Chabrier PE. Loss of endothelium-dependent relaxant activity in the pulmonary circulation of rats exposed to chronic hypoxia. J Clin Invest 87:155-162, 1991.
[11] Rubanyi GM and Vanhoutte PM. Hypoxia releases a vasoconstrictor substance from the canine vascular endothelium. J Physiol 364:45-56, 1985.
[12] Hickey KA, Rubanyi GM, Paul RJ and Highsmith RF. Characterization of a coronary vasoconstrictor produced by endothelial cells in culture. Am J Physiol 248:C550-C556, 1985.
[13] Yanagisawa M, Kurihara H, Kumura S, Tomobe Y, Kobayashi M, Mitsui Y, Goto K and Masaki T. A novel potent vasoconstrictor peptide produced by vascular endothelial cells. Nature (London) 332:411-415, 1988.
[14] Rakugi H, Tabuchi Y, Nakamaru M, Nagano M, Higashimori K, Mikami H, Ogihara T and Suzuki N. Evidence for endothelin-1 release from resistance vessels of rats in response to hypoxia. Biochem Biophys Res Commun 169:973-977, 1990.
[15] Vanhoutte PM, Auch-Schwelk W, Boulanger C, Janssen PA, Katusic ZS, Komori K, Miller VM, Schini VB and Vidal M. Does endothelin-1 mediate endothelium-dependent contractions during anoxia? J Cardiovasc Pharmacol 13:S124-S128, 1989.

[16]   Takasaki C, Tamiya N, Bdolah A, Wolleberg Z, and Kochva E. Sarafotoxins S6: Several isotoxins from Atractaspis engaddensis (burrowing asp) venom that affect the heart. Toxicon 26:543-548, 1988.

[17]   Saida K, Mitsui Y and Ishida N. A novel peptide, vasoactive intestinal contractor, of a new (endothelin) peptide family. J Biol Chem 264:14613-14616, 1989.

[18]   Inoue A, Yanagisawa M, Takuwa Y, Kobayashi M and Masaki T. The human endothelin family: three structurally and pharmacologically distinct isopeptides predicted by three separate genes. Proc Natl Acad Sci USA 86:2863-2867, 1989.

[19]   Sakurai T, Yanagisawa M, Takuwa Y, Miyazaki H, Kimura S, Goto K and Masaki T. Cloning of cDNA encoding a nonisopeptide-selective subtype of the endothelin receptor. Nature (London) 348:732-735, 1990.

[20]   Arai H, Hori S, Aramori I, Ohkubo H and Nakanishi S. Cloning and expression of a cDNA encoding an endothelin receptor. Nature (London) 348:730-732, 1990.

[21]   Masaki T, Kimura S, Yanagisawa M and Goto K. Molecular and cellular mechanism of endothelin regulation. Implications for vascular function. Circulation 84:1457-1468, 1991.

[22]   Rubanyi GM, ed. Endothelin. Oxford University Press, New York, 1991.

[23]   Haynes WG and Webb DJ. Endothelin as a regulator of cardiovascular function in health and disease. J Hypertens 16:1081-1098, 1998.

[24]   Okada K, Miyazaki Y, Takada J, Matsuyama K, Yamaki T and Yano M. Conversion of big endothelin-1 by membrane-bound metalloendopeptidase in cultured bovine endothelial cells. Biochem Biophys Res Commun 171:1192-1198, 1990.

[25]   Ikegawa R, Matsumura Y, Tsukahara Y, Takaoka M and Morimoto S. Phosphoramidon, a metalloproteinase inhibitor, suppresses the secretion of endothelin-1 from cultured endothelial cells by inhibiting a big endothelin-1 converting enzyme. Biochem Biophys Res Commun 171:669-675, 1990.

[26]   Matsumura Y, Hisaki K, Takaoka and Morimoto. Phosphoramidon, a metalloproteinase inhibitor, suppresses the hypertensive effect of big endothelin-1. Eur J Pharmacol 185:103-106, 1990.

[27]   Sakurai T, Yanagisawa M, Inoue A, Ryan US, Kimura S, Mitsui Y, Goto K and Masaki T. cDNA cloning, sequence analysis and tissue distribution of rat preproendothelin-1 mRNA. Biochem Biophys Res Commun 175:44-47, 1991.

[28]   Matsumoto H, Suzuki N, Onda H and Fujino M. Abundance of endothelin-3 in rat intestine, pituitary gland and brain. Biochem Biophys Res Commun 164:74-80, 1989.

[29]   Inoue A, Yanagisawa M, Takuwa Y, Mitsui Y, Kobayashi M and Masaki T. The human preproendothelin-1 gene. Complete nucleotide sequence and regulation of expression. J Biol Chem 264:14954-14959, 1989.

[30]   Koseki C, Imai M, Hirata Y, Yanagisawa M and Masaki T. Autoradiographic distribution in rat tissues of binding sites for endothelin: a neuropeptide? Am J Physiol 256(Regulatory Integrative Comp Physiol 25):R858-R866, 1989.

[31]   Watanabe H, Miyazaki H, Kondoh M, Masuda Y, Kimura S, Yanagisawa M, Masaki T and Murakami K. Two distinct types of endothelin receptors are present on chick cardiac membranes. Biochem Biophys Res Commun 161:1252-1259, 1989.

[32]   Sugiura M, Snajdar RM, Schwartzberg M, Badr KF and Inagami T. Identification of two types of specific endothelin receptors in rat mesangial cell. Biochem Biophys Res Commun 162:1396-1401, 1989.

[33]   Arai H, Hori S, Aramori I, Ohkubo H and Nakanishi S. Cloning and expression of a cDNA encoding an endothelin receptor. Nature 348:730-732, 1990.

[34]   Sakurai T, Yanagisawa M, Takuwa Y, Miyazaki H, Kimura S, Goto K and Masaki T. Cloning of a cDNA encoding a non-isopeptide-selective subtype of the endothelin receptor. Nature 348:732-735, 1990.

[35]   Lin HY, Kaji EH, Winkel GK, Ives HE and Lodish HF. Cloning and functional expression of a vascular smooth muscle endothelin 1 receptor. 88:3185-3189, 1991.

[36]   Simonson MS, Wann S, Mene P, Dubyak GR, Sester M, Nakasato Y, Sedor JR and Dunn MJ. Endothelium stimulates phospholipase C, Na^+/H^+ exchange, c-fos expression and mitogenesis in rat mesangial cells. J Clin Invest 83:707-712, 1989.

[37]   Simonson MS and Dunn MJ. Cellular signaling by peptides of the endothelin gene family. FASEB J 4:2989-3000, 1990.

[38]   Nakaki T, Nakayama M, Yamamoto S and Kato R. Endothelin-mediated stimulation of DNA synthesis in vascular smooth muscle cells. Biochem Biophys Res Commun 158:880-883, 1989.

[39]   Hirata Y, Takagi Y, Fukuda Y and Marumo F. Endothelin is a potent mitogen for rat vascular smooth muscle cells. Arteriosclerosis 78:225-228, 1989.

[40] Brown LA, Nunez DJ, Brookes CI and Wilkins MR. Selective increase in endothelin-1 and endothelin A subtype in the hypertrophied myocardium of the aorto-venacaval fistula rat. Cardiovas Res 29:768-774, 1995.

[41] Hasegawa K, Fugiwara H, Doyama K, Inada T, Ohtani S, Fujiwara T and Hosoda K. Endothelin-1-selective receptor in the arterial intima of patients with hypertension. Hypertension 23:288-293, 1994.

[42] Molenaar P, O'Reilly G, Sharkey A, Kuc RE, Harding DP, Plumpton C, Gresham GA and Davenport AP. Characterization and localization of endothelin receptor subtypes in the human atrioventricular conducting system and myocardium. Cir Res 72:526-538, 1993.

[43] Newman P, Kakkar VV and Kanse SM. Modulation of endothelin receptor expression in human vascular smooth muscle cells by interleukin-1 beta. FEBS Letters 363:161-164, 1995.

[44] Goldie RG, Henry PJ, Knott PG, Self GJ, Luttmann MA and Hay DW. Endothelin-1 receptor density, distribution, and function in human isolated asthmatic airways. Amer J Respir & Critical Care Med 152:1653-1658, 1995.

[45] Hislop AA, Zhao YD, Springall DR, Polak JM and Haworth SG. Postnatal changes in endothelin-1 binding in porcine pulmonary vessels and airways. Am J Respir Cell & Molecular Biol 12:557-566, 1995.

[46] Masaki T. Possible role of endothelin in endothelial regulation of vascular tone. Annu Rev Pharmacol Toxicol 35:235-255, 1995.

[47] Opgenorth TJ. Endothelin receptor antagonism. Advances in Pharmacology 33:1-65, 1995.

[48] Li HB, Elton TS, Chen YF and Oparil S. Increased endothelin receptor gene expression in hypoxic rat lung. Am J Physiol 266:L553-L560, 1994a.

[49] Li HB, Chen SJ, Chen YF, Meng QC, Durand J, Oparil S and Elton TS. Enhanced endothelin-1 and endothelin receptor gene expression in chronic hypoxia. J Appl Physiol 73:1451-1459, 1994b.

[50] Russel FD and Davenport AP, Characterization of endothelin receptors in the human pulmonary vascularture using bosentan. J Cardiovasc Pharmacol 26 (S3):S346-S347, 1995.

[51] Bobik A, Grooms A, Millar JA, Mitchell A and Grinpukel S. Growth factor activity of endothelin on vascular smooth muscle. Am J Physiol 258:C408-C415, 1990.

[52] Brown KD and Littlewood CJ. Endothelin stimulates DNA synthesis in swiss 3T3 cells: synergy with polypeptide growth factors. Biochem J 263:977-980, 1989.

[53] Komuro I, Kurihara H, Sugiyama F, Takaku F and Yazaki Y. Endothelin stimulates c-fos and c-myc expression and proliferation of vascular smooth muscle cells. FEBS Lett 238:249-252, 1988.

[54] Deng LY, Li JS and Schiffrin EL. Endothelin receptor subtypes in resistance arteries from human and rats. Cardiovas Res 29:532-535, 1995.

[55] Noll G, Wenzel RR and Luscher TF. Endothelin and endothelin antagonists: potential role in cardiovascular and renal disease. Mol Cell Biochem 157:259-267, 1996.

[56] Sudjarwo SA, Hori M, Takai M, Urade Y, Okada T and Karaki H. A novel subtype of endothelin B receptor mediating contraction in swine pulmonary vein. Life Sci 53:431-437, 1993.

[57] Fukuroda T, Fujikawa T, Ozaki S, Ishikawa K, Yano M and Nishikibe M. Clearance of circulating endothelin-1 by ETB receptors in rats. Biochem Biophys Res Commun 199(3):1461-1465, 1994.

[58] Dupuis J, Goresky CA and Fournier A. Pulmonary clearance of circulating endothelin-1 in dogs in vivo: exclusive role of ETB receptors. J Appl Physiol 81(4):1510-1515, 1996.

[59] Karne S, Jayawickkreme CK and Lerners MR. Cloning and characterization of an endothelin-3 specific receptor (ET-C receptor) from Xenopus laevis dermal melanophores. J Bio Chem 268:19126-19133, 1993.

[60] Levin ER. Endothelins as cardiovascular peptides. Am J Nephrol 16:246-251, 1996.

[61] Luscher TF. Endothelin, endothelin receptors, and endothelin antagonists. Current Opinion in Nephrology and Hypertension 3:92-98, 1994.

[62] MacLean MR, McCulloch KM and Baird M. Endothelin ET-A and ET-B receptor mediatedvasoconstriction in rat pulmonary arteries and anterioles. J Cardiovasc Pharmacol 23:838-845, 1994.

[63] Schiffrin EL. Endothelin: Potential role in hypertension and vascular hypertrophy. Hypertension 25:1135-1143, 1995.

[64] Teerlink JR, Breu V, Sprecher U, Clozel M and Clozel JP. Potent vasoconstriction mediated by endothelin ET_B receptors in canine coronary arteries. Circ Res 74:105-114, 1994.

[65] Takayanagi R, Kitazumi K, Takasaki C, Ohnaka K, Aimoto S, Tasaka K, Ohashi M and Nawata H. Presence of non-selective type of endothelin receptor on vascular endothelium and its linage to vasodilation. FEBS letters 282:103-106, 1991.

[66] Seo B, Oemar BS, Siebenmann R, von Segesser L and Luscher TF. Both ETA and ETB receptors mediate contraction to ET-1 in human blood vessels. Circulation 89:1203-1208, 1994.

[67] Rosenberg AA, Kennaugh J, Koppenhafer SL, Loomis M, Chatfield BA and Abman SH. Elevated immunoreactive endothelin-1 levels in newborn infants with persistent pulmonary hypertension. J Pediatrics 123:109-114, 1993.

[68] Steinhorn RH, Millard SL and Morin FC 3rd. Persistent pulmonary hypertension of the newborn. Role of nitric oxide and endothelin in pathophysioogy and treatment. Clinics in Perinatology 22:405-428, 1995.

[69] Druml W, Steltzer H, Waldhausl W, Lenz K, Hammerle A, Vierhapper H, Gasic S and Wagner OF. Endothelin in adult respiratory distress syndrome. Am Rev Respir Dis 148:1169-1173, 1993.

[70] Ferri C, Bellini C, De Angelis C, De Siati L, Perrone A, Properzi G and Santucci A. Circulation endothelin-1 concentrations in patients with chronic hypoxia. J Clin Pathol 48:519-524, 1995.

[71] Ackerman V, Carpi S, Bellini A, Vassallin GM and Mattoli S. Constitutive expression of endothelin in bronchial epithelial cells of patients with symptomatic and asymptomatic asthma and modulation by histamine and interleukin-1. J Allergy & Clin Immunol 96:618-627, 1995.

[72] Giaid A, Yanagisawa M, Langleben D, Michel RP, Levy R, Shennib H, Kimura S, Masaki T, Duguid WP and Stewart DJ. Expression of endothelin-1 in the lungs of patients with pulmonary hypertension. New Eng J Med 328:1732-1739, 1993.

[73] Dupuis J, Cernacek P, Tardif J-C, Stewart DJ, Gosselin G, Dyrda I, Bonan R and Crepeau J. Reduced pulmonary clearance of endothelin-1 in pulmonary hypertension. Am Heart J 135:614-620, 1998.

[74] Cacoub P, Dorent R, Nataf P, Carayon A, Riquet M, Noe E, Piette JC, Godeau P and Gandjbakhch I. Endothelin-1 in the lungs of patients with pulmonary hypertension. Cardiovas Res 33:196-200, 1997.

[75] Cruzen NP, Kaddoura S, Griffiths MJ and Evans TW. Endothelin-1 in rat endotoxemia: mRNA expression and vasoreactivity in pulmonary and systemic circularions. Am J Physiol 272:H2353-2360, 1997.

[76] Giaid A, Hamid QA, Springall DR, Yanagisawa M, Shinmi O, Sawamura T, Masaki T, Kimura S, Corrin B and Polak JM. Detection of endothelin immunoreactivity and mRNA in pulmonary tumours. J Pathology 162:15-22, 1990.

[77] Rodman Stelzner TJ, Zamora MR, Bonvallet ST, Oka M, Sato K and O'Brien RF. Endothelin-1 increases the pulmonary microvascular pressure and causes pulmonary edema in salt solution but not blood-perfused rat lungs. J Cardio Pharmacol 20:658-663, 1992.

[78] Elton TS, Oparil S, Taylor GR, Hicks PH, Yang RH, Jin H and Chen YF. Normobaric hypoxia stimulates endothelin-1 gene expression in the rat. Am J Physiol 32:R1260-R1264, 1992.

[79] DiCarlo VS, Chen SJ, Meng QC, Durand J, Yano M, Chen YF and Oparil S. Endothelin-A receptor antagonist, BQ-123, prevents chronic hypoxia-induced pulmonary vascular remodelling in the rat. Am J Physiol 169:L690-L697, 1995.

[80] Ihara m, Noguchi K, Saeki T, Fukuroda T, Tauchida S, Kimura, S, Fukami T, Ishikawa K, Nishibike M and Yano M. Biological profile of highly potent novel endothelin antagonists selective for the ET-A receptor. Life Sci 50:247-255, 1991.

[81] Oparil S, Chen SJ, Meng QC, Elton TS, Yano M and Chen YF. Endothelin-A receptor antagonist prevents acute hypoxia induced pulmonary hypertension in the rat. Am J Phsyiol 268: L95-L100, 1995.

[82] Chen SJ, Chen YF, Opgenorth TJ, Wessale JL, Meng QC, Durand J, DiCarlo VS and Oparil S. The orally active nonpeptide endothelin A receptor antagonist A-127722 prevents and reverses hypoxia induced pulmonary hypertension and pulmonary vascular remodeling in Sprague-Dawley rats. J Cardiovasc Pharmacol 29:713-725, 1997.

[83] Chen SJ, Brock T, Stavros F, Okun I, Wu C, Chan F, Mong S, Dixon RAF, Oparil S and Chen YF. TBC11251, a highly selective endothelin-A receptor antagonist, prevents and reverses acute hypoxia-induced pulmonary hypertension in the rat. FASEB J 10(3):A104, #601, 1996.

[84] Chen SJ, Chen YF, Meng QC, Durand J, DiCarlo VS and Oparil S. The endothelin receptor antagonist bosentan prevents and reverses hypoxia induced pulmonary hypertension in the rat. J Appl Physiol 79:2122-2131, 1995.

[85] Clozel M, Breu V, Gray G, Kalina B, Loffler BM, Burri K, Cassal JM, Hirth G, Muller M, Neidhart W and Ramuz H.   Pharmacological characterization of bosentan, a new potent orally active nonpeptide endothelin receptor antagonist. J Pharmacol Exp Therap 270:228-235, 1994.

[86] Stelzner TJ, O'Brien RF, Yanagisawa M, Sakurai T, Sato K, Webb S, Zamora M, McMurtry I.F and Fisher JH. Increased lung endothelin-1 production in rats with idiopathic pulmonary hypertension. Am J Physiol 262:L614-L620, 1992.

[87] Mansoor AM, AM, Honda M, Saida K, Ishinaga Y, Kuramochi T, Maeda A, Takabatake T and Mitsui Y. Endothelin induced collagen remodelling in experimental pulmonary hypertension. Biochem Biophy Res Comm 215:981-986, 1995.

[88] Mathew R, Zeballos GA, Tun H and Gewitz MH. Role of nitric oxide and endothelin-1 in monocrotaline-induced pulmonary hypertension in rats. Cardiovas Res 30:739-746, 1995.

[89] Wong J, Reddy VM, Hendricks-Munoz K, Liddicoat JR, Gerrets R and Fineman JR. Endothelin-1 vasoactive responses in lambs with pulmonary hypertension and increased pulmonary blood flow. Am J Physiol 269:H1965-H1972.

[90] Bodi I, Bishopric NH, Discher DJ, Wu X and Webster KA. Cell-Specificity and signaling pathway of endothelin-1 gene regulation by hypoxia. Cardiovas Res 30:975-984, 1995.

[91] Kourembanas S, Marsden PA, McQuillan LP and Faller DV. Hypoxia induces endothelin gene expression and secretion in cultured human endothelium. J Clin Invest 88:1054-1057, 1991.

[92] Kourembanas S, McQuillan LP, Leung GK and Faller DV. Nitric oxide regulates the expression of vasoconstrictors and growth factors by vascular endothelium under both normoxia and hypoxia. J Clin Invest 92:99-104, 1993.

[93] Li HB, Chen YF, Elton TS and Oparil S. Hypoxia stimulates endothelin-1 gene expression in human pulmonary microvessel endothelial cells by a mechanism that involves a heme-containing protein. J Invest Med 43(S1):45A (abstract), 1995.

[94] Morita T and Kourembanas S. Endothelial cell expression of vasoconstrictors and growth factors is regulated by smooth muscle cell-derived carbon monoxide. J Clin Invest 96:2676-2682, 1995.

[95] Aversa CR, Oparil S, Chen YF, H Li, Sun SD, Caro J, Swerdel MRl, Monticello TM, DurhamSK, Minchenko A, Lira SA and Webb ML. Hypoxia stimulates human preproendothelin (PPET-1) promoter activity in transgenic mice. Am J Physiol 273:L848-L855, 1997.

[96] Li H, Chen YF and Oparil S. Identification of the hypoxia-response element in the 5'-flanking region of human endothelin-1 gene. FASEB J 10:A761, 1996.

Vascular Endothelium: Mechanisms of Cell Signaling
J.D. Catravas et al. (Eds.)
IOS Press, 1999

ENDOTHELIAL NITRIC OXIDE SYNTHASE REGULATION VIA PROTEIN-PROTEIN INTERACTIONS

Richard C. Venema
Vascular Biology Center, Medical College of Georgia
Augusta, Georgia 30912, U.S.A.

Abstract

Endothelial nitric oxide synthase (eNOS) participates in at least four different kinds of protein-protein interactions. The best-established example of an eNOS-interacting protein is that of Ca^{2+}/calmodulin (CaM). Using several different techniques, we have recently identified the bovine eNOS CaM-binding domain as residues 493-512. A peptide comprised of this sequence produces a Ca^{2+}-dependent electrophoretic mobility shift of CaM on 4 M urea gels. The peptide is also a potent inhibitor of the CaM-mediated activation of neuronal NOS and has a dissociation constant for CaM binding of 4.0 nM. Furthermore, substitution of the eNOS CaM-binding domain for that of inducible NOS (iNOS) in a chimeric iNOS protein produces a functional chimeric which (in contrast to wild-type iNOS) is both Ca^{2+} - and CaM-dependent. To investigate the subunit interactions of eNOS, we have expressed wild-type and mutant forms of the enzyme in the baculovirus system and examined the quaternary structure of the purified enzymes by low temperature SDS-PAGE. eNOS dimer formation requires incorporation of the heme prosthetic group but does not require myristoylation or CaM or tetrahydrobiopterin binding. In order to identify the domains in eNOS that are involved in subunit interactions, we have also expressed eNOS oxygenase and reductase domain fusion proteins in a yeast two-hybrid system. Analysis of subunit interactions in the two-hybrid system shows that eNOS dimer formation involves not only head to head interactions of oxygenase domeins but also tail to tail interactions of reductase domains and head to tail interactions between oxygenase and reductase domains. To examine the interaction of eNOS with the plasmalemmal caveolae structural protein, caveolin-1 we have investigated the eNOS-caveolin-1 interaction in an *in vitro* binding assay system using glutathione S-transferase (GST)-caveolin-1 fusion proteins and purified recombinant eNOS. We have also mapped the domains involved in the interaction using a yeast two-hybrid system. Results from both protein interaction assays show that both N- and C-terminal cytoplasmic domains of caveolin-1 interact directly with the eNOS oxygenase domain. Interaction significantly inhibits eNOS activity. Synthetic peptides corresponding to caveolin-1 membrane-proximal residues 82-101 and 135-156 also potently inhibit eNOS by interfering with the interaction of the enzyme with Ca^{2+}/CaM. A fourth protein-protein interaction in which eNOS participates is the interaction of the enzyme with a 90 kDa eNOS-associated protein which we have termed ENAP-1 (for endothelial nitric oxide synthase-associated protein 1). ENAP-1 coimmunoprecipitates with eNOS from endothelial cell lysates and undergoes cycles of tyrosine phosphorylation/dephosphorylation in cultured endothelial cells in response to the eNOS-activating agonist, bradykinin. The role of this phosphorylation event in eNOS regulation, however, has not yet been clearly defined.

1. Introduction

The obligatory role of the endothelium in mediating the vasorelaxant effects of acetylcholine on arterial smooth muscle was first described in 1980 [10]. The authors of this pioneering study proposed that vascular endothelial cells release a factor in response to acetylcholine stimulation that causes relaxation of the underlying vascular smooth muscle cells. Following this initial discovery, endothelium-dependent relaxation was demonstrated in many different vascular preparations, as well as in the intact organism, and was shown to occur in response to a variety of stimuli including acetylcholine, adenine nucleotides, thrombin, substance P, bradykinin, histamine, Ca^{2+} ionophores, and increased blood flow [24]. Although the identity of the substance released by the endothelium remained unknown for several years, it became referred to as endothelium-derived relaxing factor or EDRF [4]. Subsequent investigation revealed that EDRF was a very labile substance that was readily degraded and inactivated by superoxide anion [13]. Further study also showed that EDRF produces relaxation in smooth muscle via activation of soluble guanylate cyclase and elevation of cytosolic cyclic GMP [28]. In 1987, EDRF was identified as nitric oxide (NO), a highly reactive and versatile free radical, able to diffuse through biological membranes from cells where it is synthesized into nearby target cells to directly affect cellular function [25]. Thus, it became clear why EDRF actions on vascular smooth muscle are similar to those of the clinically used vasodilator, nitroglycerin which releases NO as an active metabolite [14, 24]. Following the identification of EDRF as NO, there has been an explosion of scientific research on the role of NO in blood vessels where it functions to regulate, not only vasodilatation, but also platelet aggregation [27], platelet [26] and leukocyte [17] adhesion to the endothelium, endothelin - 1 generation [1], and vascular smooth muscle cell proliferation [29]. Because of the important role of NO in each of these various processes, abnormalities in vascular NO production may contribute significantly to certain vascular disorders such as those of atherosclerosis, diabetes, and hypertension [6].

NO is synthesized in endothelial and other cell types by oxidation of one of the guanidino nitrogens of L-arginine in a reaction catalyzed by the enzyme, NO synthase (NOS). Three distinct NOS isoforms have been identified by cDNA cloning and sequencing. Although none of these enzymes has an absolutely tissue-specific pattern of expression, they are commonly referred to by the names of the tissues from which they were first isolated. Endothelial NOS (eNOS), neuronal NOS (nNOS), and macrophage or inducible NOS (iNOS) all produce NO and L-citrulline via a complex reaction mechanism involving several different cofactors, substrates, and prosthetic groups including L-arginine, NADPH, FAD, FMN, calmodulin (CaM), tetrahydrobiopterin (BH_4), molecular oxygen, and a p450-type iron protoporphyrin IX heme [21]. Each of the three NOS isoforms exists as a homodimer. Individual monomeric subunits possess a bidomain structure consisting of an N-terminal oxygenase domain that contains the heme moiety and BH_4 and binds L-arginine and a C-terminal reductase domain that contains the binding sites for FAD, FMN, and NADPH [31], [12], [3]. Each NOS isoform also has certain unique features. nNOS, for example, contains a 230-amino acid N-terminal extension that is not found in either eNOS or iNOS. This region contains a PDZ domain which targets nNOS to neuronal postsynaptic densities through interaction with the postsynaptic density proteins, PSD-95 and PSD-93 and to the sarcolemma of skeletal muscle cells through interaction with 1-syntrophin in the membrane cytoskeleton dystrophin complex [2]. The nNOS N-terminal extension also interacts with a protein designated PIN for protein inhibitor of NOS [16]. A novel property of iNOS as compared to both nNOS and eNOS is that it is not activated through reversible binding of Ca^{2+}-CaM as occurs with the latter two enzymes. Rather, iNOS is Ca^{2+} - independent and thus tonically active due to irreversible binding of apoCaM during or shortly after translation of the iNOS mRNA, even in cells containing only resting cell Ca^{2+} levels [5]. Finally, eNOS is unique among NOS isoforms in that it is fatty acylated by both myristate and palmitate. These modifications appear to contribute to targeting of eNOS to the plasmalemmal caveolae and golgi membranes of endothelial cells [30], [20].

2. Identification, Characterization, and Comparison of the Calmodulin-Binding Domains of the Endothelial and Inducible Nitric Oxide Synthases

The best-known example of a protein-protein interaction in which eNOS participates is that with Ca^{2+}-CaM, a positive allosteric effector of many different Ca^{2+} - dependent enzymes. Until recently, the CaM-binding domain of eNOS (as well as that of iNOS) was identified solely on the basis of sequence analysis. Identification of CaM-binding domains by sequence analysis involves the use of computer algorithms to search for sequences of appropriate length, charge, hydrophobicity, and helical hydrophobic moment. Prediction of CaM-binding domains solely by sequence analysis, however, can result in misidentification. Therefore, in order to more definitively establish the location of the CaM-binding sequences in eNOS and in iNOS, we prepared synthetic peptides corresponding to the putative CaM-binding domains of the proteins and tested whether the peptides could produce an electrophoretic mobility shift of CaM during polyacrylamide gel electrophoresis in 4 M urea [34]. Depending on the charge and hydrophobicity of the peptide, high affinity binding is detected by this method as a band with increased or decreased mobility relative to the unbound CaM band. In the presence of Ca^{2+}, the electrophoretic mobility of CaM was retarded by a peptide corresponding to bovine eNOS residues 493-512, demonstrating that this sequence contains all of the residues necessary for high affinity binding of Ca^{2+}-CaM by eNOS. This conclusion is also supported by the results of our previous study, in which we found that deletional mutation of residues 493-512 from bovine eNOS results in loss of CaM-binding capacity by the mutant enzyme [33]. A synthetic peptide from iNOS sequence that corresponds to those residues in the murine iNOS sequence (501-523) that are aligned with bovine eNOS residues 493-512 was also tested for its ability to bind CaM. This peptide produced virtually no gel shift of CaM of 4 M urea gels. Thus it appears that high affinity CaM binding by iNOS requires additional residues outside of the sequence that aligns with the complete CaM-binding sequence of eNOS. A longer 501-532 peptide sequence from murine iNOS, however, did produce a gel shift, suggesting that the CaM-binding domain of iNOS may be up to 9 residues longer than that of eNOS.

The CaM-binding domains of eNOS and iNOS were characterized further by using synthetic peptides to inhibit the Ca^{2+}-CaM-dependent activation of nNOS, expressed and purified from a baculovirus expression system. The eNOS 493-512 and iNOS 501-532 peptides were both potent inhibitors of nNOS activity with IC_{50} values of 6 and 2 nM, respectively. The shorter iNOS peptide (501-523) also inhibited nNOS but with a lower potency (IC_{50} = 9 nM). A peptide corresponding to iNOS residues 524-544, which overlaps with the 9 C-terminal residues of the 501-532 sequence was also inhibitory at 100-fold higher concentrations. Thus, iNOS residues 524-532 appear to make important contributions to iNOS CaM binding as these 9 residues by themselves have a low but significant affinity for Ca^{2+}-CaM. The eNOS and iNOS CaM-binding domains were also compared in terms of their dissociation constants for Ca^{2+}-CaM. K_D values for the eNOS 493-512 and iNOS 501-532 peptides were determined to be 4 and 1 nM for the eNOS and iNOS sequences, respectively.

In order to gain additional insight into the molecular basis for differences between eNOS and iNOS with regard to their Ca^{2+}-dependence and reversibility of CaM binding, the two intact proteins plus two different eNOS-iNOS chimeric proteins were

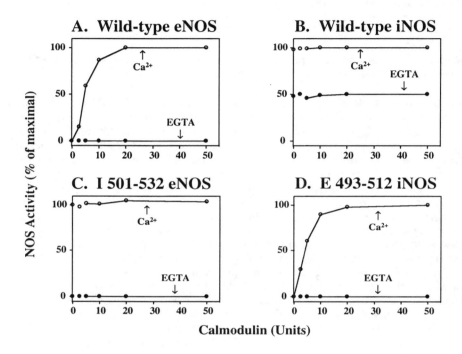

FIGURE 1: Ca^{2+} and CaM dependence of wild-type and chimeric NOS enzymes. Enzymes were expressed in the baculovirus expression system and purified to >90% homogeneity by affinity chromatography on 2', 5'-ADP-Sepharose. Purifications were carried out using buffers containing 2 mM EGTA to remove any CaM bound to the enzymes in a Ca^{2+}-dependent manner. NOS activity of the purified enzymes was determined by monitoring the rate of conversion of L-arginine to L-citrulline. Assays were performed in duplicate in the absence and presence of varying concentrations of exogenously added CaM and in the presence of either 2.5 mM $CaCl_2$ or 10 mM EGTA. Similar results were obtained in three different experiments. A, wild-type eNOS. B, wild-type iNOS. C, I 501-532 eNOS. D, E 493-512 iNOS. (*With permission from* [34]).

characterized after expression and purification from a baculovirus-Sf9 insect cell expression system. Wild-type bovine eNOS and wild-type murine iNOS were each expressed. In addition, a chimeric protein designated as I 501-532 eNOS was expressed in which the wild-type 493-512 sequence in eNOS was replaced by the iNOS 501-532 sequence. A second chimeric protein was expressed in which wild-type 501-523 sequence in iNOS was replaced by the eNOS 493-512 sequence. This protein was designated as E 493-512 iNOS. Each of the four expressed proteins were purified to >90% homogeneity by affinity chromatography on 2', 5' - ADP-Sepharose. Purifications were carried out in buffer containing 2 mM EGTA in order to dissociate during purification any CaM that might bind to the enzymes in a Ca^{2+}-dependent manner. Catalytic activity of the purified enzymes was then measured by the arginine-to-citrulline conversion assay in the presence of various concentrations of exogenously added CaM (Figure 1). Assays were carried out in the presence of Ca^{2+} (2.5 mM) and in the absence of Ca^{2+} (achieved by the addition of 10 mM EGTA). Wild-type eNOS, as expected, was completely dependent on both Ca^{2+} and CaM for activity (Figure 1A). Wild-type iNOS, on the other hand, was completely CaM-independent as well as significantly (although not entirely) Ca^{2+}-independent (Figure 1B). Furthermore, replacement of the CaM-binding sequence of eNOS with the CaM-binding sequence of iNOS in the I 501-532 eNOS chimeric enzyme was sufficient to confer CaM independence on eNOS. Thus, I 501-532 eNOS, like wild-type iNOS, was completely independent of exogenously added CaM (Figure 1C), demonstrating that the iNOS 501-532 sequence has the capacity to bind CaM irreversibly. However, irreversible binding by itself is not sufficient to activate the enzyme in the absence of Ca^{2+}. It appears that bound CaM must be in Ca^{2+}-CaM conformation in order to interact with eNOS in a manner that activates the enzyme because the I 501-532 iNOS chimeric had no activity in the absence of Ca^{2+}. Finally, it also appears that the CaM-binding domain of iNOS is necessary for the Ca^{2+} and CaM independence of this enzyme because the E 493-512 iNOS chimeric enzyme, like the wild-type eNOS enzyme, was completely dependent on both Ca^{2+} and CaM for catalytic activity (Figure 1D).

High affinity CaM-binding domains typically consist of basic, amphiphilic - helices containing 4-5 positively charged residues and 4-5 hydrophobic residues. Typically, several of these residues are important for CaM binding. Therefore, we determined whether specific hydrophobic and basic residues in the eNOS CaM-binding domain contribute to CaM binding by using two different approaches. Synthetic peptides corresponding to bovine eNOS residues 493-512 were prepared in which Phe-498, Val-505, Leu-511, Arg-494, Lys-495, Lys-496, Lys-499, and Lys-506 were each individually replaced by alanine residues. Mutated peptides were then compared to the wild-type peptide for their ability to gel shift CaM on 4 M urea gels as well as for their inhibitory potency for the CaM-mediated activation of nNOS. Peptides that were mutated at either Phe-498, Leu-511, or Lys-499 lost their capacity for high affinity binding of CaM, as assessed by loss of CaM electrophoretic mobility shift on 4 M urea gels. The same three peptides also showed significantly lower potencies for inhibition of nNOS than did the wild-type peptide. The hydrophobic residues, Phe-498 and Leu-511 and the basic residue, Lys-499 thus appear to represent important determinants of the eNOS-CaM interaction. Phe-498 appears to be especially important because mutation of this residue resulted in a 150-fold increase in the IC_{50} of the mutant peptide for inhibition of nNOS.

3. Interactions of Endothelial Nitric Oxide Synthase Monomeric Subunits with Themselves: Comparisons to Inducible Nitric Oxide Synthase

A second type of eNOS protein-protein interaction we have studied is the interaction of eNOS monomeric subunits with themselves in the process of homodimer formation [36]. eNOS, like the other NOS enzymes, is believed to be catalytically active only in dimeric form. Regulation of eNOS subunit interactions could, therefore, provide a mechanism for modulation of enzyme activity *in vivo*. In macrophages, for example, iNOS is 50-75% monomeric under basal conditions and is thus thought to be regulated in part by the binding of L-arginine and BH_4. Interaction with the L-arginine substrate and the BH_4 cofactor promotes dimer assembly. It has not been clear, however, whether eNOS exists in a monomer-dimer equilibrium in endothelial cells. To answer this question we analyzed the quaternary structure of eNOS expressed in bovine aortic endothelial cells

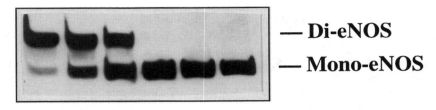

FIGURE 2: Monomer-dimer equilibrium and thermal stability of the eNOS dimer in SDS sample buffer as monitored by LT-PAGE. Bovine aortic endothelial cell lysates were incubated in SDS sample buffer for 30 minutes at the indicated temperatures. Samples were subjected to LT-PAGE and monomeric and dimeric forms of eNOS were visualized by immunoblotting with anti-eNOS antibody. Equivalent results were obtained in four different experiments. (*With permission from [36]*)

(BAEC) using a technique known as LT-PAGE (for low temperature polyacrylamide gel electrophoresis). Because eNOS is an unusually stable dimer it actually migrates in LT-PAGE as a homodimer, even under strongly denaturing conditions. BAEC lysates were suspended in SDS sample buffer (to a final concentration of 3% SDS and 7% 2-mercaptoethanol) and incubated for 30 minutes at 0, 20, 30, 40, 50, and 60°C. Dimeric and monomeric forms of eNOS were then separated by LT-PAGE and visualized by immunoblotting with anti-eNOS antibody. As shown in Figure 2, eNOS migrated in LT-PAGE entirely as a dimer if the samples in SDS sample buffer were not heated prior to running the gel. The critical temperature for subunit dissociation under these denaturing conditions was 30-40°C. These results demonstrate that eNOS in BAEC under basal conditions exists exclusively in dimeric form. It is thus unlikely that cofactor or substrate induction of dimer formation (such as occurs with iNOS) functions as a regulatory mechanism for increasing eNOS activity in endothelial cells.

        To determine whether certain eNOS cofactors or prosthetic groups are required for eNOS dimer assembly we expressed several mutant forms of eNOS in the baculovirus expression system. Expressed proteins were purified by 2', 5'-ADP-Sepharose and analyzed by LT-PAGE. A ΔCaM mutant of bovine eNOS which lacks a CaM-binding domain (residues 493-512 deleted) migrated in LT-PAGE entirely as a dimer suggesting that CaM binding is not a prerequisite for dimer formation. Two additional eNOS mutants were also expressed in the baculovirus system and analyzed by LT-PAGE. A myristoylation-deficient mutant of bovine eNOS, in which glycine 2 has been mutated to an alanine, differs from wild-type eNOS in that it is neither myristoylated nor palmitoylated and, consequently, is not membrane-associated [33]. Like wild-type eNOS, this mutant enzyme migrated in LT-PAGE entirely as a dimer. Neither fatty acylation nor membrane association of eNOS, therefore, appears to required for dimer formation. Another mutant form of eNOS we have studied is a heme-deficient mutant in which the heme-binding cysteine residue of eNOS (residue 186 in the bovine sequence) has been mutated to an alanine. This mutation results in loss of incorporation into eNOS of the heme prosthetic group. This enzyme migrated in LT-PAGE as a monomer. Incorporation of the heme prosthetic group into eNOS, therefore, appears to be a requirement for dimerization of the enzyme.

The iNOS isoform has an absolute dependence on binding of BH_4 for oligomerization. Many investigators, therefore, have assumed that this characteristic of iNOS is also true for eNOS. To determine whether BH_4 is indeed required for eNOS dimer formation we expressed wild-type bovine eNOS in a baculovirus expression system in which Sf9 cells were grown in the presence or absence of 10 mM 2, 4-diamino-6-hydroxypyrimidine (DAHP), a potent inhibitor of GTP cyclohydrolase I, the rate-limiting enzyme in BH_4 biosynthesis. DAHP treatment of cells resulted in the production of a form of the eNOS enzyme which, when purified, was found to be essentially BH_4-free. Analysis of the BH_4-free enzyme in LT-PAGE showed that it was entirely dimeric. Thus, BH_4 binding is not required for eNOS dimer formation. eNOS, therefore, differs significantly from iNOS which has an absolute requirement for BH_4 in order for dimerization to occur.

TABLE I

Interactions between NOS oxygenase and reductase domains in a yeast two-hybrid system

Binding Domain Hybrid	Activation Domain Hybrid	Colony color	β-galactosidase activity
eNOS (1-505)	eNOS (1-505)	Blue	149 ± 30
eNOS (506-1205)	eNOS (506-1205)	Light Blue	38 ± 3
eNOS (1-505)	eNOS (506-1205)	Blue	124 ± 10
eNOS (506-1205)	eNOS (1-505)	Blue	109 ± 7
iNOS (1-498)	iNOS (1-498)	Blue	113 ± 12
iNOS (499-1144)	iNOS (499-1144)	White	4 ± 2
iNOS (1-498)	iNOS (499-1144)	White	2 ± 2
iNOS (499-1144)	iNOS (1-498)	White	3 ± 1

Pairwise combinations of hybrid plasmids were used to cotransform SFY526 yeast cells. Cotransformants were assayed for β-galactosidase activity by the colony lift filter method using X-Gal as substrate and by liquid culture assay with chlorophenolred-β-galactopyranosidase as substrate. β-galactosidase activity is expressed in Miller units. Results shown are mean $\pm$ S.D. from three separate transformations.

Previous studies have also shown that all of the determinants for iNOS dimer formation are contained within the N-terminal oxygenase domain of the enzyme. In order to determine whether similar conclusions can be made about eNOS, we utilized the yeast two-hybrid system developed originally by Fields and Song [9]. The two-hybrid system takes advantage of the modular nature of the yeast GAL4 transcriptional activator. The GAL4 protein contains a site-specific DNA-binding domain that is distinct from the domain responsible for transcriptional activation. Proteins are expressed in the two-hybrid system as fusions with either the GAL4 activation domain or the GAL4 DNA-binding domain. The capacity of the two fusion proteins to interact is detected by cotransformation into a strain of yeast that contains an integrated copy of a LacZ reporter gene. If the two proteins interact, the two domains of GAL4 are brought together in close physical proximity, resulting in reconstitution of GAL4 activity and β-galactosidase reporter gene transcription. GAL4 DNA-binding domain and activation domain fusion plasmids were constructed of the bovine eNOS and murine iNOS oxygenase and reductase domains using the shuttle/expression vectors, pGBT9 and pGAD424. Various pairwise combinations of plasmid constructs were then used to cotransform the yeast strain,

SFY526. Interactions of the fusion proteins were first determined by β-galactosidase activity assay of cotransformants by a colony lift filter assay using X-Gal as substrate. Fusion proteins that interact in the two-hybrid system give a blue signal on filters. Fusion proteins that do not interact give a white signal. The strength of the two-hybrid interaction was then quantitated by a liquid culture assay using chlorophenol red-β-D-galactopyranoside as substrate. As shown in Table I, eNOS oxygenase domain (residues 1-505) fusion proteins interacted strongly in the two-hybrid system in a head to head fashion. Strong head to tail interactions were also detected between either of two different combinations of eNOS oxygenase domain and eNOS reductase domain (residues 506-1205) hybrids. Weaker but significant tail to tail interactions were also detected between eNOS C-terminal reductase domain fusion proteins. However, in marked contrast to the results obtained with the eNOS hybrids, iNOS oxygenase domain (residues 1-498) and reductase domain (residues 499-1144) fusion proteins interacted in the two-hybrid system only through head to head interactions of N-terminal oxygenase domains. No head to tail or tail to tail interactions was detected with the iNOS hybrids. These results provide a potential explanation for the known differences in dimer stability of the eNOS and iNOS isoforms. eNOS dimers are very likely more stable than iNOS dimers due to more extensive interactions between eNOS monomeric subunits.

4. Interactions of Endothelial Nitric Oxide Synthase with Caveolin-1

Plasmalemmal caveolae are small, bulb-shaped invaginations of the plasma membrane that are especially abundant in endothelial cells. These membranes organelles were initially identified because of their function in certain transport processes such as those of endocytosis, potocytosis, and transcytosis. Recently, however, it has been recognized that caveolae also have another important function which is to serve as plasma membrane signal transduction organizing centers that compartmentalize hormone receptors with their downstream effectors. A principal protein component of caveolae is caveolin. Three homologous but distinct isoforms of caveolin are known termed caveolins-1,-2, and -3. The form expressed in endothelial cells is caveolin-1. Full-length caveolin-1 contains three domains: a 101-residue N-terminal cytoplasmic domain, a 33-residue membrane-spanning domain (which is believed to form a hairpin loop within the membrane), and a 44-residue C-terminal cytoplasmic domain. Association of eNOS and caveolin -1 in cultured BAEC and in bovine lung microvascular endothelial cells has been shown previously in coimmunoprecipitation experiments [8,11]. It has not been clear, however, whether eNOS and caveolin-1 interact directly. The interacting domains in the two proteins have also not been identified. Finally, the functional consequences of caveolin-1 interaction on eNOS catalytic activity have not been determined. Each of these questions with regard to the eNOS-caveolin-1 interaction has recently been investigated in our laboratory [15].

      To determine whether eNOS interacts directly with caveolin-1, we expressed full-length bovine caveolin-1 as a glutathione S-transferase (GST)-fusion protein in *E. coli*. In addition, to determine which domains of caveolin-1 are involved in eNOS binding, we also expressed GST-fusion proteins of caveolin-1 residues 1-60, 1-101 (N-terminal cytoplasmic domain), 102-134 (membrane-spanning domain), and 135-178 (C-terminal cytoplasmic domain). The fusion proteins and a GST-nonfusion protein were purified by affinity chromatography on glutathione-Sepharose beads. The GST-caveolin-1 fusion proteins or GST alone prebound to Sepharose beads were then used in *in vitro* binding assays with recombinant bovine eNOS, expressed and purified from a baculovirus system.

Beads were incubated with eNOS at 4°C overnight, washed extensively, and bound proteins were eluted with reduced glutathione. Eluted proteins were separated on SDS polyacrylamide gels, transferred to nitrocellulose, and immunoblotted with anti-eNOS antibody. As shown in Figure 3, eNOS bound specifically to the full-length caveolin-1 (residues 1-178) fusion protein but not to GST alone, demonstrating that eNOS and caveolin-1 interact directly. Furthermore, eNOS bound specifically to GST-fusion proteins that contained only the caveolin-1 N-terminal cytoplasmic domain (residues 1-

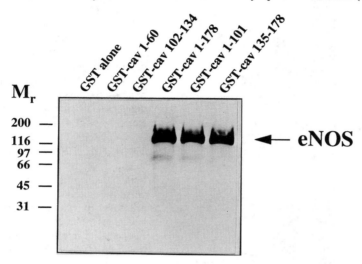

FIGURE 3: *In vitro* binding of eNOS to GST-caveolin-1 fusion proteins. GST-caveolin-1 fusion proteins containing full-length caveolin-1 (GST-cav 1-178), the caveolin-1 N-terminal cytoplasmic domain (GST-cav 1-101), caveolin-1 residues 1-60 (GST-cav 1-60), the caveolin-1 C-terminal cytoplasmic domain (GST-cav 135-178), the caveolin-1 membrane-spanning domain (GST-cav 102-134), plus GST alone were expressed in *E. coli* and purified by affinity binding to glutathione-Sepharose beads. Proteins prebound to beads were incubated with purified baculovirus-expressed recombinant eNOS. Following binding, extensive washing, and elution with reduced glutathione, proteins were separated by SDS polyacrylamide gel electrophoresis, transferred to nitrocellulose, and immunoblotted with anti-eNOS antibody. The result shown is representative of three separate experiments. (*With permission from [15]*)

101) or only the caveolin-1 C-terminal cytoplasmic domain (residues 135-178). In contrast, GST-fusion proteins containing caveolin-1 residues 1-60 or the caveolin-1 membrane-spanning domain (residues 102-134) did not bind eNOS. The eNOS-caveolin-1 interaction, therefore, involves binding of eNOS to both cytoplasmic domains of caveolin-1. Furthermore, either cytoplasmic domain by itself is sufficient to mediate the interaction.

To confirm the conclusions reached based on the *in vitro* binding assays and to determine whether caveolin-1 binds to either the eNOS oxygenase domain or the eNOS reductase domain, or both, we also investigated the eNOS-caveolin-1 interaction in the yeast two-hybrid system. Hybrid cDNA constructs were prepared that encoded full-length bovine caveolin-1 (residues 1-178), the caveolin-1 N-terminal cytoplasmic domain (residues 1-101), the caveolin-1 C-terminal cytoplasmic domain (residues 135-178), the bovine eNOS oxygenase domain (residues 1-505), and the bovine eNOS reductase domain (residues 506-1205) fused to either the GAL4 DNA binding domain or activation domain. Various pairwise combinations of the plasmid constructs were used to cotransform the yeast strain, SFY526. Interactions of the hybrid proteins were assessed by colony lift filter assay of β-galactosidase reporter gene transcription. Both N- and C- terminal cytoplasmic domains of caveolin-1 interacted with eNOS in the two-hybrid system, confirming the conclusions reached based on the GST-fusion protein *in vitro* binding assays. Caveolin-1 interactions were restricted to the eNOS oxygenase domain and did not occur with the eNOS reductase domain. To determine whether the interaction of eNOS with caveolin-1 alters the catalytic activity of the enzyme, we incubated equal quantities of purified, baculovirus-expressed eNOS with equimolar quantities of the GST alone, GST-caveolin 1-60, GST-caveolin 102-134, GST-caveolin 1-178, GST-caveolin 1-101, and GST-caveolin 135-178 fusion proteins. eNOS activity was then determined by arginine-to-citrulline conversion assay in the presence of excess cofactors, Ca^{2+}, and CaM. The full-length caveolin-1 fusion protein inhibited eNOS activity by about 60%. Furthermore, either of the caveolin-1 cytoplasmic domains by itself appears to be sufficient to mediate eNOS inhibition because the GST-caveolin 1-101 and GST-caveolin 135-178 fusion proteins also inhibited enzyme activity by about 60%. In contrast, the GST-caveolin 1-60 and GST-caveolin 102-134 fusion proteins were without effect on activity. Inhibition of eNOS by GST-caveolin 1-101 but not by GST-caveolin 1-60 suggests that the inhibitory region of the N-terminal cytoplasmic of caveolin-1 may correspond to the so-called caveolin-1 scaffolding domain (residues 82-101) shown previously to inhibit other important signaling proteins such as G subunits, Ha-Ras, and the Src family tyrosine kinases [18], [32], [19]. To examine this possibility, we prepared synthetic peptides corresponding to caveolin-1 residues 61-81 and 82-101 and determined what effects, if any, they had on the catalytic activity of purified eNOS. As shown in Figure 4A, the 82-101 peptide potently inhibited eNOS activity with an IC_{50} of about 1 M and complete inhibition at 10 M. A 10 M concentration of the 61-81 peptide, on the other hand, actually increased activity by about 30%. To map the region of the caveolin-1 C-terminal cytoplasmic domain that inhibits eNOS, we prepared two additional synthetic peptides corresponding to caveolin-1 residues 135-156 and 157-178 and tested their effects on eNOS activity. The 135-156

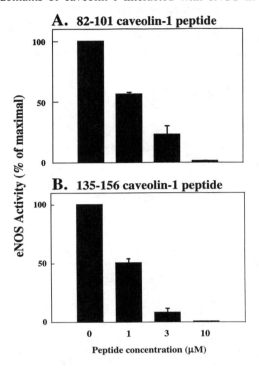

FIGURE 4: Effect of peptides corresponding to caveolin-1 residues 82-101 and 135-156 on eNOS catalytic activity. eNOS activity was determined by arginine-to-citrulline conversion assay in the absence and presence of various concentrations of caveolin-1 peptides. A, caveolin-1 82-101 peptide. B, caveolin-1 135-156 peptide. Results shown are mean ± S.E. of triplicate determinations from three separate experiments. (*With permission from [15]*)

caveolin-1 peptide inhibited eNOS with a potency similar to that of the 82-101 peptide (Figure 4B). In contrast, the 157-178 peptide was without effect on activity.

To determine whether inhibition of eNOS by caveolin-1 is due to an effect of caveolin-1 on the eNOS interaction with Ca^{2+}-CaM, we preincubated purified eNOS with and without the 61-81 and 82-101 caveolin-1 peptides (10 M) and then subjected the enzyme to CaM-Sepharose affinity chromatography. The enzyme was allowed to bind to the column in the presence of 2 mM $CaCl_2$ and was eluted with 2 mM EGTA. The amount of enzyme eluted (and hence bound by CaM-Sepharose) in each condition was

A.

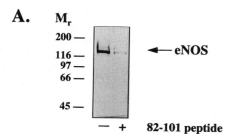

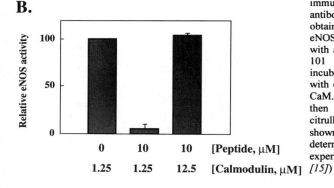

B.

FIGURE 5: Effect of the caveolin-1 82-101 peptide on eNOS binding to CaM-Sepharose and reversal of eNOS inhibition with excess Ca^{2+}-CaM. A, eNOS was incubated in the presence or absence of the caveolin-1 82-101 peptide and then subjected to chromatography on CaM-Sepharose. eNOS was eluted from CaM-Sepharose with 2 mM EGTA. The amount of eNOS eluted in each condition was quantitated by immunoblotting with anti-eNOS antibody. Equivalent results were obtained in three experiments. B, eNOS was incubated for 5 minutes with and without the caveolin-1 82-101 peptide (10 M) and then incubated for an additional 5 minutes with either 1.25 or 12.5 M Ca^{2+}-CaM. eNOS catalytic activity was then determined by arginine-to-citrulline conversion assay. Results shown are mean ± S.E. of triplicate determinations from three separate experiments. (*With permission from* [15])

then quantitated by immunoblotting with anti-eNOS antibody. As shown in Figure 5A, preincubation with the 82-101 peptide almost completely blocked subsequent binding of eNOS to the CaM-Sepharose column. In contrast, the 61-81 peptide had no effect on CaM binding. Furthermore, peptide inhibition was reversible by increasing the molar excess Ca^{2+}-CaM by 10-fold. Purified eNOS was preincubated for 5 minutes at 37 C with the 82-101 peptide (10 M). Enzyme activity was then determined in the presence of the standard concentration of Ca^{2+} (1.25 M) used in the arginine-to-citrulline conversion assay. Activity was confirmed to be completely inhibited in the presence of 10 M peptide and 1.25 M Ca^{2+}-CaM. eNOS was then incubated for an additional 5 minutes at 37 C with 12.5 M of Ca^{2+}-CaM. As shown in Figure 5B, increasing the Ca^{2+}-CaM concentration by 10-fold resulted in a complete reversal of peptide inhibition. Regulation of eNOS activity in endothelial cells, therefore, very likely involves competition between Ca^{2+}-CaM and caveolin-1 for positive and negative interactions, respectively, with the eNOS enzyme. Interactions of NOS enzymes with caveolin proteins are not limited to eNOS and caveolin-1. For example, we have shown recently that nNOS interacts with caveolin-3 in skeletal muscle [37]. Interaction in this case is also mediated by two different membrane-proximal regions of the caveolin-3 N- and C-terminal cytoplasmic domains. These regions correspond to caveolin-1 residues 82-101 and 135-156. Furthermore, we have found that both of these domains are also involved in caveolin inhibition of the c-Src tyrosine kinase. Therefore, we have proposed that caveolin proteins contain both N- and C-terminal scaffolding/inhibitory domains and have suggested that these domains be referred to as scaffolding domains 1 and 2, respectively.

5. Tyrosine Phosphorylation-Dependent Interaction of Endothelial Nitric Oxide Synthase with Other Proteins

Many of the agonists that activate eNOS in endothelial cells also stimulate protein tyrosine phosphorylation. We have, therefore, recently investigated whether eNOS activation is associated with direct tyrosine phosphorylation of the enzyme [35]. BAEC were treated with bradykinin (100 nM) for various times, cells were lysed, and eNOS was immunoprecipitated from lysates with anti-eNOS antibody. Precipitated proteins were separated by gel electrophoresis, transferred to nitrocellulose, and immunoblotted with anti-phosphotyrosine antibody. As shown in Figure 6, neither basal nor bradykinin-stimulated tyrosine phosphorylation of eNOS (130 kDa) was observed in these

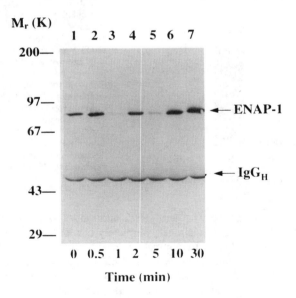

FIGURE 6: Tyrosine phosphorylation of ENAP-1 in response to bradykinin. Cultured bovine aortic endothelial cells ere exposed to bradykinin (100 nM) for 0, 0.5, 1, 2, 5, 10, and 30 minutes. Cells were lysed and eNOS was immunoprecipitated with anti-eNOS antibody. Precipitated proteins were separated by SDS polyacrylamide gel electrophoresis, transferred to nitrocellulose, and immunoblotted with anti-phosphotyrosine antibody. Similar results were obtained in seven separate experiments. (*With permission from* [35])

experiments, consistent with the observations made in other laboratories that eNOS is phosphorylated in endothelial cells exclusively on serine [23, 7]. Tyrosine phosphorylation, however, was detected for a 90 kDa eNOS-associated protein that we have termed ENAP-1 (for eNOS-associated protein 1). ENAP-1 undergoes cycles of tyrosine phosphorylation/dephosphorylation in endothelial cells in response to bradykinin stimulation. As of this writing, the identity of ENAP-1 and the nature of its role in eNOS regulation have not yet been determined. However, in the future we hope to clone the ENAP-1 cDNA (and thus identify the protein) by two-hybrid screening using eNOS as "bait" to screen an endothelial library of candidate interacting proteins.

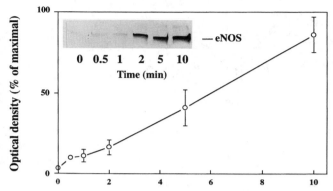

FIGURE 7: Phenylarsine oxide-stimulated eNOS translocation to the cytoskeletal protein fraction. Cultured bovine aortic endothelial cells we treated with phenylarsine oxide (10 M) for 0, 0.5, 1, 2, 5, and 10 minutes. Cells were lysed in buffer containing 1% Triton X-100 and detergent-insoluble, cytoskeletal proteins were pelleted at 10,000 X g. Pelleted proteins were separated by SDS polyacrylamide gel electrophoresis, transferred to nitrocellulose, and immunoblotted with anti-eNOS antibody. Equivalent results were obtained in five separate experiments. (*With permission from [38]*)

eNOS also interacts with detergent-insoluble, cytoskeletal proteins in endothelial cells in a tyrosine phosphorylation-dependent manner. BAEC were treated with bradykinin (100 nM) or the tyrosine phosphatase inhibitor, phenylarsine oxide (10 M) for various times and cells were lysed in buffer containing 1% Triton X-100. Detergent-soluble and detergent-insoluble, cytoskeletal proteins were then separated by centrifugation at 10,000 X g. The amount of eNOS in the detergent-insoluble pellet (and thus presumably associated with cytoskeletal proteins) was then quantitated by immunoblotting with anti-eNOS antibody. Bradykinin stimulated a transient increase in the amount of cytoskeletal-associated eNOS. Furthermore, bradykinin-stimulated eNOS translocation was completely blocked by the tyrosine kinase inhibitor, geldanamycin (1 g/ml). Inhibition of tyrosine dephosphorylation by phenylarsine oxide also resulted in a dramatic increase in the amount of eNOS associated with the detergent-insoluble, cytoskeletal protein compartment (Figure 7). Phenylarsine oxide treatment also produces a dramatic increase in the amount of detergent-insoluble caveolin-1 and in the amount of caveolin-1 associated with eNOS [38]. Treatment with the inhibitor also results in a significant reduction in the eNOS activity of BAEC lysates, possibly due to an increased association of eNOS with its inhibitory protein partner, caveolin-1.

6. Summary and Conclusions

Our studies suggest that eNOS is subject to reciprocal regulation by both Ca^{2+}-CaM and caveolin-1 in endothelial cells (Figure 8). Thus, under basal conditions, eNOS is bound to the plasma membrane, not only due to insertion of myristate and palmitate fatty acyl chains into the hydrophobic membrane interior, but also due to direct protein-protein interactions with caveolin-1. eNOS interacts specifically with two different caveolin-1 membrane-proximal scaffolding domains. These two domains are contained within caveolin-1 amino acid residues 82-101 and 135-156. Interaction of eNOS with these two

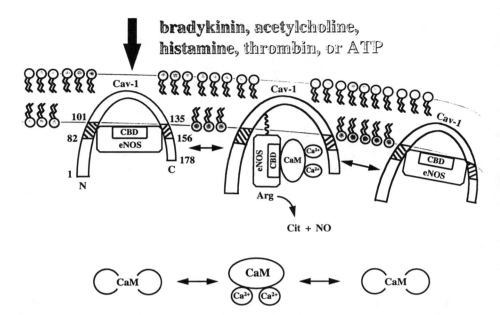

FIGURE 8: Schematic diagram illustrating reciprocal regulation of eNOS in endothelial cells by Ca^{2+}-CaM and caveolin-1

caveolin domains serves to inhibit or suppress enzyme catalytic activity. Following agonist-stimulation of endothelial cells, intracellular Ca^{2+} levels are transiently elevated resulting in conversion of apoCaM to Ca^{2+}-CaM. Ca^{2+}-CaM displaces eNOS from its inhibitory association with caveolin-1 and activates the enzyme. When intracellular Ca^{2+} levels return to basal, Ca^{2+}-CaM reverts to apoCaM and dissociates from eNOS. The enzyme subsequently returns to the state of being inhibited through association with caveolin-1. Furthermore, although it is not yet clear exactly which phosphorylation events are involved, this reciprocal regulation of eNOS by Ca^{2+}-CaM and caveolin-1 appears to be modulated by protein tyrosine phosphorylation. Future study will provide further insight into what these phosphorylation events are and may also lead to the identification of other eNOS-associated proteins. For example, evidence has been presented recently that eNOS may also interact with the CAT1 cationic amino acid transporter in endothelial caveolae. Interaction of eNOS with CAT1 may explain the so-called arginine paradox and provide a mechanism whereby eNOS preferentially utilizes extracellular, rather that intracellular, L-arginine as substrate [22].

References

[1]　　Boulanger, C., and Lüscher, T.F. Release of endothelin from the porcine aorta: inhibition by endothelium-derived nitric oxide. *J.Clin.Invest.* 85:587-590, 1990.

[2]　　Bredt, D.S., Targeting nitric oxide to its targets. *Proc.Soc.Exp., Biol.Med.*211:41-48, 1996.

[3]　　Chen, P.F., Tsai, A.L., Berka, V. And Wu, K.K. Endothelial nitric oxide synthase: evidence for bidomain structure and reconstitution of catalytic activity from two separate domains generated by a baculovirus expression system. *J.Biol.Chem.* 271:14631-14635, 1996.

[4]   Cherry, P.D., Furchgott, R.F., Zawadzki, J.V., and Jothianandan, D.   Role of endothelial cells in relaxation of isolated arteries by bradykinin. *Proc.Natl.Acad.Sci.USA* 79:2106-2110, 1982.

[5]   Cho, H.J., Xie, Z, Calaycay, J., Mumford, R.A., Swiderek, K.M., Lee, T.D., and Nathan, C. Calmodulin is a subunit of nitric oxide synthase from macrophages. *J.Exp.Med.* 176:599-604, 1992.

[6]   Cooke, J.P., and Dzau, V.J. Nitric oxide synthase: role in the genesis of vascular disease. *Annu.Rev.Med.* 48:489-509, 1997.

[7]   Corson, M.A., James, N.L., Latta, S.E., Nerem, R.M., Berk, B.C., and Harrison, D.G. Phosphorylation of endothelial nitric oxide synthase in response to fluid shear stress. *Circ.Res.* 79:984-991, 1996.

[8]   Feron, O., Belhassen, L., Kobzik, L., Smith, T.W., Kelly, R.A., and Michel, T. Endothelial nitric oxide synthase targeting to caveolae: specific interactions with caveolin isoforms in cardiac myocytes and endothelial cells. *J.Biol.Chem.* 271:22810-22814, 1996.

[9]   Fields, S., and Song, O. A novel genetic system to detect protein-protein interactions. *Nature.* 340:245-246, 1989.

[10]   Furchgott, R.F., and Zawadzki, J.V.   The obligatory role of endothelial cells in the relaxation of arterial smooth muscle by acetylcholine. *Nature* 288:373-376, 1980.

[11]   Garc a-Cardeña, G., Fan, R., Stern, D.F., Liu, J., and Sessa, W.C. Endothelial nitric oxide synthase is regulated by tyrosine phosphorylation and interacts with caveolin-1. *J.Biol.Chem.* 271:27237-27240, 1996.

[12]   Ghosh, D.K., and Stuehr, D.J. Macrophage NO synthase: characterization of the isolated oxygenase and reductase domains reveals a head-to-head subunit interaction. *Biochemistry* 34:801-807, 1995.

[13]   Gryglewski, R.J., Palmer, R.M.J., and Moncada, S. Superoxide anion is involved in the breakdown of endothelium-derived vascular relaxing factor. *Nature* 320:454-456. 1986.

[14]   Ignarro, L.J. Biological actions and properties of endothelium-derived nitric oxide formed and released from artery and vein. *Circ.Res.* 65:1-21, 1989.

[15]   Ju, H., Zou, R., Venema, V.J., and Venema, R.C. Direct interaction of endothelial nitric-oxide synthase and caveolin-1 inhibits synthase activity. *J.Biol.Chem.* 272:18522-18525, 1997.

[16]   Jaffrey, S.R., and Snyder, S.H. PIN: An associated protein inhibitor of neuronal nitric oxide synthase. *Science* 274:774-777, 1996.

[17]   Kubes, P., Suzuki, M., and Granger, D.N. Nitric oxide: an endogenous modulator of leukocyte adhesion. *Proc.Natl.Acad.Sci.USA* 88:4651-4655, 1991.

[18]   Li, S., Okamoto, T., Chun, M., Sargiacomo, M., Casanova, J.E., Hansen, S.H., Nishimoto, I., and Lisanti, M.P. Evidence for a regulated interaction between heterotrimeric G proteins and caveolin. *J.Biol.Chem.* 270:15693-15701, 1995.

[19]   Li, S., Couet, J., and Lisanti, M.P. Src tyrosine kinases, G subunits, and Ha-Ras share a common membrane-anchored scaffolding protein, caveolin: caveolin binding negatively regulates the auto-activation of Src tyrosine kinases. *J.Biol.Chem.* 271:29182-29190, 1996.

[20]   Liu, J., Hughes, T.E., and Sessa, W.C. The first 35 amino acids and fatty acylation sites determine the molecular targeting of endothelial nitric oxide synthase into the golgi region of cells: a green florescent protein study. *J.Cell.Biol.* 137:1525-1535, 1997.

[21]   Marletta, M.A. Nitric oxide synthase structure and mechanism. *J.Biol.Chem.* 268:12231-12234, 1993.

[22]   McDonald, K.K., Zharikor, S., Block, E.R., and Kilberg, M.S. A caveolar complex between the cationic amino acid transporter 1 and endothelial nitic-oxide synthase may explain the "arginine paradox". *J.Biol.Chem.* 272:31213-31216, 1997

[23]   Michel, T., Li, G.K., and Busconi, L. Phosphorylation and subcellular translocation of endothelial nitric oxide synthase. *Proc.NaH.Acad.Sci.* USA 90:6252-6256, 1993.

[24]   Moncada, S., Palmer, R.M.J., and Higgs, E.A. Nitric oxide: physiology, pathophysiology, and pharmacology. *Pharmacol.Rev.* 43:109-142, 1991.

[25]   Palmer, R.M.J., Ferrige, A.G., and Moncada, S. Nitric oxide release accounts for the biological activity of endothelium-derived relaxing factor. *Nature* 327:524-526, 1987.

[26]   Radomski, M.W., Palmer, R.M.J., and Moncada, S. The role of nitric oxide and cGMP in platelet adhesion to vascular endothelium. *Biochem.Biophys.Res.Commun.* 148:1482-1489, 1987.

[27]   Radomski, M.W., Palmer, R.M.J., and Moncada, S. An L-arginine: nitric oxide pathway present in human platelets regulates aggregation. *Proc.Natl.Acad.Sci.USA* 87:5193-5197, 1990.

[28]   Rapoport, R.M., and Murad, F. Agonist-induced endothelium-dependent relaxation in rat thoracic aorta may be mediated through cGMP. *Circ.Res.* 52:352-357, 1983.

[29] Scott-Burden, T., Schini, V.B., Elizondo, E., Junquero, D.C., and Vanhoutte, P.M. Platelet-derived growth factor suppresses and fibroblast growth factor enhances cytokine-induced production of nitric oxide by cultured smooth muscle cells: effect on cell proliferation. *Circ.Res.* 71:1088-1100, 1992.

[30] Shaul, P.W., Smart, E.J., Robinson, L.J., German, Z., Yuhanna, I.S., Ying, Y., Anderson, R.G.W., and Michel, T. Acylation targets endothelial nitric-oxide synthase to plasmalemmal caveolae. *J.Biol.Chem.* 271:6518-6522, 1996.

[31] Sheta, E.A, McMillan, K., and Masters, B.S.S. Evidence for a bidomain structure of constitutive cerebellar nitric oxide synthase. *J.Biol.Chem.* 269,15147-15153, 1994.

[32] Song, K.S., Li, S., Okamoto, T., Quilliam, L.A., Sargiocomo, M., and Lisanti, M.P. Co-purification and direct interaction of Ras with caveolin, an integral membrane protein of caveolae microdomains: detergent-free purification of caveolae membranes. *J.Biol.Chem.* 271:9690-9697, 1996.

[33] Venema, R.C. Sayegh, H.S., Arnal, J.-F., and Harrison, D.G. Role of the enzyme calmodulin-binding domain in membrane association and phospholipid inhibition of endothelial nitric oxide synthase. *J.Biol.Chem.* 270:14705-14711, 1995.

[34] Venema, R.C., Sayegh, H.S., Kent, J.D., and Harrison, D.G. Identification, characterization, and comparison of the calmodulin-binding domains of the endothelial and inducible nitric oxide synthases. *J.Biol.Chem.* 271:6435-6440, 1996a.

[35] Venema, V.J., Marrero, M.B., and Venema, R.C. Bradykinin-stimulated protein tyrosine phosphorylation promotes endothelial nitric oxide synthase translocation to the cytoskeleton. *Biochem. Biophys. Res. Commun.* 226:703-710, 1996b.

[36] Venema, R.C., Ju, H., Zou, R., Ryan, J.W., and Venema, V.J. Subunit interactions of endothelial nitric-oxide synthase: comparisons to the neuronal and inducible nitric-oxide synthase isoforms. *J.Biol.Chem.* 270:14705-14711, 1997a.

[37] Venema, V.J., Ju, H., Zou, R., and Venema, R.C. Interaction of neuronal nitric-oxide synthase with caveolin-3 in skeletal muscle: identification of a novel caveolin scaffolding/inhibitory   domain. *J.Biol.Chem.* 272:28187-28190, 1997b.

[38] Venema, V.J., Zou, R., Ju, H., Marrero, M.B., and Venema, R.C. Caveolin-1 detergent solubility and association with endothelial nitric oxide synthase is modulated by tyrosine phosphorylation. *Biochem.Biophys.Res.Commun.* 236:155-161, 1997c

Vascular Endothelium: Mechanisms of Cell Signaling
J.D. Catravas et al. (Eds.)
IOS Press, 1999

REGULATION OF NITRIC OXIDE SYNTHASE BY SUBCELLULAR TARGETING AND PROTEIN-PROTEIN INTERACTIONS

William C. Sessa, Ph.D.
Yale University School of Medicine
Boyer Center for Molecular Medicine
295 Congress Avenue
New Haven, CT 06536, USA

Abstract

Endothelial nitric oxide synthase (eNOS) is a peripheral membrane protein that converts L-arginine to nitric oxide (NO). Our work has focused on understanding the basic cell biology of eNOS as it pertains to the regulation of NO production. eNOS is co-translationally N-myristoylated (at glycine-2) and post-translationally cysteine palmitoylated (at cysteines 15 and 26). These lipid modifications are important for eNOS trafficking into the Golgi region and into cholesterol and glycolipid rich microdomains of the plasma membrane, termed caveolae. Mutations of either site influence eNOS trafficking and block stimulated NO release without influencing eNOS activity in broken cell lysates. Since the compartmentalization of eNOS is critical for optimal NO production, we hypothesized that proper subcellular targeting of the enzyme places eNOS is an environment containing NOS regulatory proteins. Indeed, eNOS interacts with many different proteins based on metabolic labeling experiments including a 22 kDa protein identified as caveolin-1 (CAV-1) and a 90 kDa protein identified as heat shock protein 90 (Hsp90). CAV-1 negatively regulates eNOS signaling while Hsp90 is a positive regulator. This review will outline recent progress in understanding the cell biolgy of eNOS and other NOS isoforms.

1. Introduction

Nitric oxide (NO) is produced by the enzyme family of nitric oxide synthases; neuronal (nNOS or NOS1), inducible (iNOS or NOS 2) and endothelial (eNOS or NOS 3) [1]. NOSs are cytochrome P-450 hemoproteins that utilize L-arginine as the substrate, NADPH and molecular oxygen as co-substrates and calmodulin as a critical regulator. NOSs exhibit approximate 40-50% sequence identity across the family and each isoform is highly homologous across various species (80-94% identity). Based on findings accumulating over the past several years, all NOSs are catalytically competent to produce NO only as homodimers and for iNOS and to lesser extent nNOS and eNOS, tetrahydrobiopterin (BH_4) is an essential co-factor for dimerization in *vitro* and *in vivo* [2-5].

As alluded to above, the production of NO can be regulated by a variety of factors (oxygen, L-arginine, calcium, calmodulin and BH₄) that directly influence the catalytic activity of the enzyme. However, in the past several years a novel concept has emerged suggesting that cell type specific subcellular targeting of the enzyme provides a dynamic mechanism to control NO synthesis.

2. Endothelial Nitric Oxide Synthase

eNOS was originally purified as a 135 kDa membrane protein from both freshly isolated and cultured bovine aortic endothelial cells [6]. eNOS is membrane associated by virtue of co-translational N-myristoylation at glycine 2 and post-translational cysteine palmitoylation at positions 15 and 26 [7-9]. In cultured endothelial cells and intact blood vessels, eNOS is localized on membranes of the Golgi complex and on plamalemma caveolae of endothelial cells [10-12]. Mutation of the N-myristoylation site inhibits the subsequent palmitoylation and prevents Golgi and caveolae targeting [13]. Interestingly, mutation of the palmitoylation sites blocks caveolae targeting suggesting that palmitoylation is a "molecular zip code" for eNOS. In both circumstances, inhibition of proper targeting results in a 50-70% reduction in stimulated NO production demonstrating that cellular compartmentalization is critical for optimal NOS activation. What is the functional consequence of impaired localization? A recent demonstration using a paradigm of memory (long-term potentiation, LTP) in CA1 region neurons of the hippocampus (rich in eNOS) shows that inhibition of eNOS N-myristoylation blocks membrane targeting and attenuates LTP providing support for the concept that compartmentalization is critical for NO production [14]. Thus, it is likely that targeting onto the cytoplasmic face of the Golgi via N-myristoylation and then into the plasma membrane via cysteine palmitoylation are important events necessary for placing eNOS into a milieu rich in NOS substrates (L-arginine, NADPH, oxygen) cofactors (Ca^{2+}, tetrahydrobiopterin and flavins) and NOS regulatory proteins (calmodulin, caveolin and Hsp90).

Palmitoylation of eNOS plays a role in its targeting near to other signaling proteins to form a highly efficient signal transduction cascade in discrete regions of endothelial cells. Interestingly, we and others have showed that eNOS interacts in endothelial cells with caveolin-1 [15, 16], and in cardiac myocytes with caveolin-3 [17]. This interaction is through two cytoplasmic domains of caveolin-1, the scaffolding domain (amino acids 61-101) and the carboxy terminal tail (amino acids 153-178). The scaffolding domain of caveolin is also the docking site for Ha-Ras, c-Src and G-protein α subunits, suggesting that in addition to its role as a structural protein for caveolae, specific protein-protein interactions between caveolin and other resident proteins could regulate signal transduction [18, 19]. Incubation of pure eNOS with peptides derived from the scaffolding domains of caveolin-1 and -3 result in inhibition of eNOS, iNOS and nNOS activities [15]. These results suggest a common mechanism and site of inhibition. The region of eNOS that interacts with caveolin was mapped using a yeast two-hybrid system and GST-fusion proteins to the oxygenase domain between amino acids 310 and 570 [15, 20]. Site directed mutagenesis of the predicted caveolin binding motif within eNOS blocked the ability of caveolin-1 to supress NO release in co-transfection experiments. These results suggests that caveolin negatively regulates NO production and that additional mechanisms of regulation must prevail during stimulation of NO release by shear stress, growth factors and calcium-mobilizing agonists.

Recently, we have identified a novel eNOS regulatory as the protein heat shock protein -90 (Hsp90). The rationale for examining this interaction stems from the observation that eNOS co-precipitates with a 90 kDa protein [21, 22] and Hsp90 may be involved in a variety of signal transduction cascades [23]. A variety of peripheral membrane signaling proteins including Src and its family members, Raf, G-protein βγ subunits and MEK can exist as heterocomplexes with Hsp90. However, the regulation and function of Hsp90 binding to its native cellular substrates in mammalian cells are elusive and not well described.

In cultured bovine lung microvascular endothelial cells and human umbilical vein endothelial cells, Hsp90 coprecipitates with eNOS. The interaction between these proteins is also found in intact blood vessels but does not appear to occur between nNOS and Hsp90 in rat cerebella suggesting a unique interaction in the endothelium. Utilizing in vitro reconstitution assays with purified proteins and co-transfection experiments in COS cells reveal that the binding of Hsp90 to eNOS increases the catalytic eficiency of the enzyme by either a direct allosteric activation or by stabilization the dimeric structure. One interesting finding is the association of eNOS with Hsp90 is stimulus-dependent, i.e. vascular endothelial growth factor, histamine and fluid shear stress all enhance the interaction of eNOS with Hsp90 in a time frame consistent with NO release [24]. Similar results are seen with estrogen and ionomycin suggesting that a variety of activators of NO production interface at the level of Hsp90 prior to NOS activation (unpublished observations).

With caveolin and Hsp90 as negative and postive regulators of eNOS, then how is the production of NO controlled? The model we envision is that when eNOS is in caveolae and bound to caveolin, the recruitment of Hsp90 and/ or calmodulin perhaps via mobilization fo cytoplasmic calcium, can relieve the inhibitory action of caveolin thus promoting NO release. When calcium levels fall, the dissociation of calmodulin from NOS and perhaps Hsp90 will permit caveolin to resume its inhibitory actions on eNOS. When eNOS is not in caveolae or bound to caveolin, which is likely to occur in the Golgi or cytoskeleton, the rate limitng step for eNOS activation may be the recruitment of Hsp90.

3. Subcellular localization and regulation of other NOS Isoforms

3.1. Neuronal Nitric Oxide Synthase

nNOS was purified as 150 kDa protein from cytosolic fractions of rat and porcine cerebellum [25, 26]. In contrast to nNOS purified from brain, human and rat nNOS isolated from skeletal muscle is mostly membrane associated (>80%). nNOS has a unique, 210 amino acid N-terminal extension that contains a PDZ motif , named after the three proteins that contain repeats of this domain, post-synaptic density protein-95 (PSD-95), *Drosophila* disc large protein (Dlg) and zona occludens protein-1 (ZO-1). The PDZ motif permits nNOS to interact biochemically with other PDZ motifs found in PSD-95 and a related protein, PSD-93, in brain extracts [27]. PSD-95 also interacts with other neural signaling proteins such as the NMDA receptor and the Shaker family of K^+ channels via the carboxy terminal amino acid motifs ESDV or ETDV. The precise functional reasons for these molecular interactions of nNOS with PDZ motif containing proteins are not known but likely represents another example of a growing theme in biology; i.e. compartmentalization of signal transduction to defined regions of the cell. In the periphery, PDZ domain interactions also mediate binding of nNOS to the skeletal muscle protein α1-syntrophin, a dystrophin associated protein. This interaction is responsible for the targeting of nNOS to the sarcolemma of fast-twitch fibers of skeletal muscle. Interestingly, *mdx* mice and humans with Duchenne muscular dystrophy (DMD) demonstrate a selective loss of nNOS protein and catalytic activity from muscle membranes, suggesting that aberrant regulation of nNOS may contribute to preferential degeneration of fast-twitch muscle fibers in DMD [28]. In addition, nNOS in sarcolemmal membranes may influence excitation-contraction coupling as evidenced by the ability of NOS inhibitors to increase the amplitude of muscle contraction [29].

3.2. Inducible Nitric Oxide Synthase

iNOS was purified as a 133 kDa protein from the cytosol of activated murine macrophages. In serially passaged murine macrophages, the majority of iNOS is clearly cytosolic. Recently, both in primary cultures of murine macrophages and in activated human neutrophils isolated from patients with ongoing urinary tract infections, a large percentage of the total iNOS activity resides within the particulate fraction [30]. The reasons why iNOS localization varies in different cell lines are not obvious. Based on the cDNA cloning, iNOS does not contain a PDZ motif or is it fatty acylated suggesting a novel mechanism for subcellular targeting into membrane. More importantly, the significance of two pools of iNOS are not clear. In primary cultures of murine macrophages and in neutrophils isolated from patients with urinary tract infections, iNOS localizes in the perinuclear region of the cells. The precise nature of that perinuclear staining remains to be defined, but appears to be regions of the Golgi-complex and in an unidentified vesicle population [31]. As suggested by these authors, perhaps the localization of iNOS in vesicles will facilitate a higher local concentration of NO in the vicinity of a phagocytized pathogen. To date, there are no published experiments reporting the presence of proteins coassociated with iNOS.

4. Summary

In the NOS field, we are viewing the tip of the iceberg studying the importance of subcellular targeting and protein-protein interactions. Clearly, several aspects of complex cell signaling require compartmentalization of proteins for local activation and inactivation of biochemical pathways. All the NOS isoforms display some degree of specific subcellular targeting suggesting that mutiple protein-protein or protein-lipid interactions are yet to be discovered. Elucidation of such interactions will increase our understanding of the molecular mechanisms of NO generation.

References

[1]   Sessa, W. C. 1994. The Nitric Oxide Synthase Family of Proteins. *J. Vasc. Res.* 31:131-143
[2]   Klatt, P., Schmidt, K., Lehner, D., Glatter, O., Bachinger, H. P., et al. 1995. Structural analysis of porcine brain nitric oxide synthase reveals a role for tetrahydrobiopterin and L-arginine in the formation of an SDS-resistant dimer. *Embo J* 14:3687-95
[3]   Lee, C. M., Robinson, L. J., Michel, T. 1995. Oligomerization of endothelial nitric oxide synthase. Evidence for a dominant negative effect of truncation mutants. *J Biol Chem* 270:27403-6
[4]   Nathan, C., Xie, Q. W. 1994. Regulation of biosynthesis of nitric oxide. [Review]. *J Biol Chem* 269:13725-8
[5]   Tzeng, E., Billiar, T. R., Robbins, P. D., Loftus, M., Stuehr, D. J. 1995. Expression of human inducible nitric oxide synthase in a tetrahydrobiopterin (H4B)-deficient cell line: H4B promotes assembly of enzyme subunits into an active dimer. *Proc Natl Acad Sci U S A* 92:11771-5
[6]   Pollock, J. S., Forstermann, U., Mitchell, J. A., Warner, T. D., Schmidt, H. H., et al. 1991. Purification and characterization of particulate endothelium-derived relaxing factor synthase from cultured and native bovine aortic endothelial cells. *Proc Natl Acad Sci U S A* 88:10480-4

[7]   Liu, J., Sessa, W. C. 1994. Identification of covalently bound amino-terminal myristic acid in endothelial nitric oxide synthase. *J Biol Chem* 269:11691-4

[8]   Liu, J., García-Cardeña, G., Sessa, W. C. 1995. Biosynthesis and palmitoylation of endothelial nitric oxide synthase: mutagenesis of palmitoylation sites, cysteines-15 and/or -26, argues against depalmitoylation-induced translocation of the enzyme. *Biochemistry* 34:12333-40

[9]   Liu, J., Garcia-Cardena, G., Sessa, W. C. 1996. Palmitoylation of endothelial nitric oxide synthase is necessary for optimal stimulated release of nitric oxide: Implications for caveolae localization. *Biochemistry* 35:13277-13281

[10] Sessa, W. C., García-Cardeña, G., Liu, J., Keh, A., Pollock, J. S., et al. 1995. The Golgi association of endothelial nitric oxide synthase is necessary for the efficient synthesis of nitric oxide. *J Biol Chem* 270:17641-4

[11] García-Cardeña, G., Oh, P., Liu, J., Schnitzer, J. E., Sessa, W. C. 1996. Targeting of nitric oxide synthase to endothelial cell caveolae via palmitoylation; implications for nitric oxide signaling. *Proc Natl Acad Sci USA* 93:6448-6453

[12] Shaul, P. W., Smart, E. J., Robinson, L. J., German, Z., Yuhanna, I. S., et al. 1996. Acylation targets endothelial nitric-oxide synthase to plasmalemmal caveolae. *J Biol Chem* 271:6518-22

[13] Liu, J., Hughes, T. E., Sessa, W. C. 1997. The First 35 Amino Acids and Fatty Acylation Sites Determine the Molecular Targeting of Endothelial Nitric Oxide Synthase into the Golgi Region of Cells: A Green Fluorescent Protein Study. *J. Cell Biol.* 137:1525-1535

[14] Kantor, D. B., Lanzrein, M., Stary, S. J., Sandoval, G. M., Smith, W. B., et al. 1996. A role for endothelial nitric oxide synthase in LTP revealed by adenovirus-mediated inhibition and rescue. *Science* 274:1744-1748

[15] Garcia-Cardena, G., Martasek, P., Masters, B. S., Skidd, P. M., Couet, J., et al. 1997. Dissecting the interaction between nitric oxide synthase (NOS) and caveolin. Functional significance of the nos caveolin binding domain in vivo. *J Biol Chem* 272:25437-40

[16] Feron, O., Belhassen, L., Kobzik, L., Smith, T. W., Kelly, R. A., et al. 1996. Endothelial nitric oxide synthase targeting to caveolae. Specific interactions with caveolin isoforms in cardiac myocytes and endothelial cells. *J Biol Chem* 271:22810-4

[17] Feron, O., Smith, T. W., Michel, T., Kelly, R. A., Feron, O., et al. 1997. Dynamic targeting of the agonist-stimulated m2 muscarinic acetylcholine receptor to caveolae in cardiac myocytes Endothelial nitric oxide synthase targeting to caveolae. Specific interactions with caveolin isoforms in cardiac myocytes and endothelial cells. *J Biol Chem* 272:17744-8

[18] Li, S., Couet, J., Lisanti, M. P. 1996. Src tyrosine kinases, Galpha subunits, and H-Ras share a common membrane-anchored scaffolding protein, caveolin. Caveolin binding negatively regulates the auto-activation of Src tyrosine kinases. *J Biol Chem* 271:29182-90

[19] Song, K. S., Li, S., Okamoto, T., Quilliam, L. A., Sargiacomo, M., et al. 1996. Co-purification and direct interaction of Ras with caveolin, an integral membrane protein of caveolae microdomains. *Journal of Biological Chemistry* 271:9690-7

[20] Ju, H., Zou, R., Venema, V. J., Venema, R. C. 1997. Direct interaction of endothelial nitric-oxide synthase and caveolin-1 inhibits synthase activity. *J Biol Chem* 272:18522-5

[21] Venema, V. J., Marrero, M. B., Venema, R. C. 1996. Bradykinin-stimulated protein tyrosine phosphorylation promotes endothelial nitric oxide synthase translocation to the cytoskeleton. *Biochem Biophys Res Commun* 226:703-10

[22] Garcia-Cardena, G., Fan, R., Stern, D. F., Liu, J., Sessa, W. C. 1996. Endothelial nitric oxide synthase is regulated by tyrosine phosphorylation and interacts with caveolin-1. *J Biol Chem* 271:27237-27240

[23] Pratt, W. B. 1997. The Role of the Hsp90-Based Chaperone System in Signal Transduction by Nuclear Receptors and Receptors Signaling via MAP Kinase. *Annu. Rev. Pharmacol. Toxicol.* 37:297-326

[24] Garcia-Cardena, G., Fan, R., Shah, V., Sorrentino, R., Cirino, G., et al. 1998. Dynamic activation of endothelial nitric oxide synthase by Hsp90. *Nature* 392:821-824

[25] Schmidt, H. H. H. W., Pollock, J. S., Nakane, M., Gorsky, L. D., Forstermann, U., et al. 1991. Purification of a soluble isoform of guanylyl cyclase-activating-factor synthase. *Proc. Natl. Acad. Sci.* 99:365-369

[26] Bredt, D. S., Snyder, S. H. 1990. Isolation of nitric oxide synthetase, a calmodulin-requiring enzyme. *Proc Natl Acad Sci U S A* 87:682-5

[27] Brenman, J. E., Chao, D. S., Gee, S. H., McGee, A. W., Craven, S. E., et al. 1996. Interaction of nitric oxide synthase with the postsynaptic density protein PSD-95 and α1-syntrophin mediated by PDZ domains. *Cell* 84:757-67

[28] Brenman, J. E., Chao, D. S., Xia, H., Aldape, K., Bredt, D. S. 1995. Nitric oxide synthase complexed with dystrophin and absent from skeletal muscle sarcolemma in Duchenne muscular dystrophy. *Cell* 82:743-52

[29] Kobzik, L., Reid, M. B., Bredt, D. S., Stamler, J. S. 1994. Nitric oxide in skeletal muscle [see comments]. *Nature* 372:546-8

[30] Wheeler, M. A., Smith, S. D., Garcia-Cardena, G., Nathan, C., Weiss, R. M., et al. 1997. Bacterial infection induces nitric oxide synthase in human neutrophils. *J Clin Invest* 99:110-116

[31] Vodovotz, Y., Russell, D., Xie, Q.-w., Bogdan, C., Nathan, C. 1995. Vesicle membrane association of nitric oxide synthase in primary mouse macrophages. *J Immunology* 154:2914-2925

Part V

Thrombosis

Vascular Endothelium: Mechanisms of Cell Signaling
J.D. Catravas et al. (Eds.)
IOS Press, 1999

ENDOTHELIAL AND SMOOTH MUSCLE PLASMINOGEN ACTIVATORS IN FIBRINOLYSIS, CELL MIGRATION AND REPAIR-ASSOCIATED ANGIOGENESIS

Victor W.M. van Hinsbergh, Pieter Koolwijk, Annemie Collen, Marielle Kroon,
Roeland Hanemaaijer, Jan H.Verheijen, Paul H.A. Quax
Gaubius Laboratory TNO-PG, Leiden
And Institute of Cardiovascular Research, Vrije Universiteit
Amsterdam, The Netherlands

1. Introduction

Fibrin is a temporary matrix, which is formed after wounding of a blood vessel and when plasma leaks from blood vessels forming a fibrous exudate, often seen in areas of inflammation and in tumors [38]. The fibrin matrix not only acts as a barrier preventing further blood loss, but also provides a structure in which new microvessels can infiltrate during wound healing. Proper timing of the outgrowth of microvessels as well as the subsequent (partial) disappearance of these vessels is essential to ensure adequate wound healing and to prevent the formation of scar tissue. It is generally believed that plasminogen activators play an important role in the migration and invasion of leukocytes and endothelial cells, and in the dissolution of the fibrin matrix [82, 106, 81, 148]. Plasminogen activators are serine proteases, which enzymatically convert the zymogen plasminogen into the active protease plasmin, the prime protease that degrades fibrin. The production of plasminogen activators by endothelial cells not only contributes to the proteolytic events related to the formation of microvessels in a wound, but also plays a crucial role in the prevention of thrombosis. If fibrin becomes deposited within the lumen of a blood vessel, cessation of the blood flow may occur accompanied by ischemia and eventually death of the distal tissues. The endothelium contributes considerably to the maintenance of blood fluidity by exposing anticoagulant molecules, by providing factors that interfere with platelet aggregation, and by its ability to stimulate fibrinolysis. Lysis of intravascularly generated fibrin must occur rapidly. However, it should be limited to a local area, because a general elevation of fibrinolysis upon wounding would result in recurrent bleeding. Hence, endothelial cells apply plasminogen activators for initial events in angiogenesis, for the degradation of the temporary fibrin matrix during wound healing, and for the immediate dissolution of a fibrinous thrombus originating within a blood vessel [143]. These cells are able to execute all these processes adequately by orchestrating in time and space the synthesis and action of two types of plasminogen activators as well as that of specific inhibitors and cellular receptors for plasminogen activators and plasminogen.

2. Components of the Plasmin/Plasminogen Activator System

Figure 1 summarizes the proteases and the inhibitors involved in fibrinolysis. Fibrin degradation and probably also activation of several matrix metalloproteinases is accomplished by the serine protease plasmin, which is formed from its zymogen plasminogen by plasminogen activators (PAs). The actual activities of plasmin and the PAs are regulated not only by their concentration and activation, but also by their interaction with inhibitors, cellular receptors, and matrix proteins.

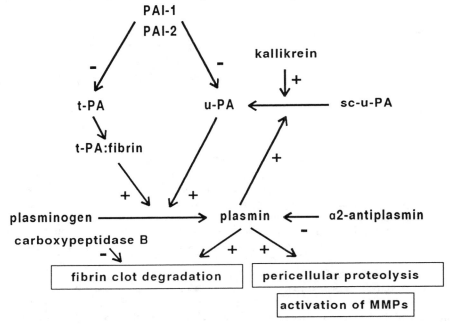

Figure 1. Schematic representation of the plasminogen activation system. +: activation; -: inhibition. Inhibitors are indicated in italics. PA: plasminogen activator; t-PA: tissue-type PA; u-PA: urokinase type PA; sc-u-PA: single-chain u-PA; PAI: PA inhibitor.

2.1. Proteases

Plasmin is formed from its zymogen plasminogen by proteolytic activation by PAs. Two types of mammalian PAs are presently known: tissue-type plasminogen activator (t-PA) and urokinase-type plasminogen activator (u-PA). The three serine proteases, plasminogen, t-PA and u-PA, are synthesized as single polypeptide chains, and each of them is converted by specific proteolytic cleavage to a molecule with two polypeptide chains connected by a disulphide bond. The carboxy-terminal part of the molecule (the so called B-chain) contains the proteolytically active site, whereas the amino-terminal part of the molecule (the A-chain) is built up of domains that determine the interaction of the proteases with matrix proteins and cellular receptors. The proteolytic cleavage of plasminogen and single-chain u-PA to their respective two-chain forms is necessary to disclose the proteolytically active site and to activate the molecule. In contrast, t-PA activity markedly increases by interaction of t-PA with fibrin. Once bound to this substrate, both the single-chain and two-chain form of t-PA are active. The interaction of plasminogen with fibrin or the cell surface occurs predominantly via binding sites in the kringle structures, which recognize lysine residues of proteins, in particular carboxy-terminal lysines. Because B-type carboxypeptidases remove carboxy-terminal lysine residues from potential binding sites for plasminogen in fibrin or on the cell surface, they can act as negative regulators of the fibrinolytic system [123].

2.2. Inhibitors

The activities of the proteases of the fibrinolytic system are controled by potent inhibitors, which are members of the serine protease inhibitor (serpin) superfamily [45]. Plasmin, if not bound to fibrin, is instantaneously inhibited by α_2-antiplasmin [71]. Because this interaction is facilitated by the lysine binding domain of plasmin, it is attenuated when plasmin is bound to fibrin. The predominant regulators of t-PA and u-PA activities are PAI-1 and PAI-2 [47, 3]. PAI-1 is a 50 kD glycoprotein present in blood platelets and synthesized by endothelial cells, smooth muscle cells and many other cell types in culture [134, 89]. PAI activity in human plasma is normally exclusively PAI-1. PAI-1 binds to vitronectin, which stabilizes its inhibitory activity. PAI-1 is the main if not the sole inhibitor of PAs synthesized by endothelial cells, vascular smooth muscle cells and hepatocytes. PAI-2 is produced by monocytes/macrophages, placental trophoblasts and certain tumor cell lines [3]. It can be found as a glycosylated secreted molecule and as an non-glycosylated molecule intracellularly [153].

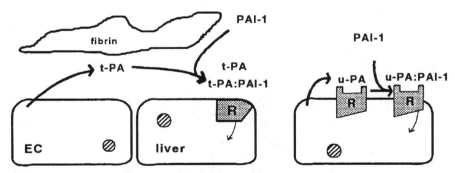

Figure 2. Schematic presentation of the synthesis and cellular uptake of plasminogen activators (PAs). Left: fibrinolysis; right: pericellular proteolysis. After secretion the PA binds to a matrix or cellular receptor (R) where it becomes active and performs its proteolytic activity until it is inhibited by its inhibitor PAI-1. The PA:PAI-1 complex is subsequently internalized by the same or another cell. PAs that do not interact with a suitable matrix or receptor are cleared by the liver. EC: endothelial cell; uPAR: u-PA receptor. (From [148], with permission).

2.3. Receptors

Regulation of fibrinolytic activity also occurs by cellular receptors. These receptors direct the action of PAs and plasmin to focal areas on the cell surface, or are involved in the clearance of the PAs (Figure 2). The presently available knowledge indicates that t-PA acts predominantly in the blood and body cavities. It is produced by endothelial and mesothelial cells and taken up rather rapidly by the liver or mesothelium. If t-PA encounters fibrin after being released from cells, it binds and activates plasminogen. The other plasminogen activator, u-PA, acts mainly in direct association with the membrane of the cell by which it is produced, and by which it is taken up after activation and complexation with the inhibitor PAI-1. Hence, cellular receptors are important for activation on the cell surface and for clearance of PAs and their inhibitor complexes.

High affinity binding sites for plasminogen [93,113, 97, 60], t-PA [59, 60] and u-PA [149, 8, 33] are found on various types of cells including endothelial cells. Endothelial cells in vitro bind plasminogen with a moderate affinity (120 to 340 nM depending on whether the Lys- or Glu-form of plasminogen is used) but with a high capacity (3.9 to 14 x 10^5 molecules per cell) [61, 113]. This binding, which is also observed with many other cell types, is mediated by the lysine binding sites of kringles 1-3 of the plasmin (ogen) molecule. Because these lysine binding sites are also involved in the interaction of plasmin with $α_2$-antiplasmin, occupation of lysine binding sites protects plasmin from instantaneous inhibition by $α_2$-antiplasmin not only when plasmin is bound to fibrin (see above) but also when it is bound to the cellular receptors. The nature of the plasminogen receptors is not fully resolved. In addition to gangliosides, which directly or indirectly contribute to the plasminogen binding [95], at least eight proteins have been reported to be involved in plasminogen binding. Among them are members of the low density lipoprotein receptor family, such as gp330 and LRP; annexin II; a not yet identified 45 kD protein; GbIIb/IIIa and α-enolase (see [60] for review). In neural cells plasminogen binding to amphoterin was found. Lipoprotein Lp(a), which has strong structural homology with a large part of the plasminogen molecule, can compete for plasminogen binding to endothelial cells [94, 97]. This competition also involves lysine binding sites.

Specific binding of t-PA to human endothelial cells has been reported [67, 6, 4]. t-PA binds via its growth factor domain with high affinity to annexin II on human endothelial cells in culture [64]. Different epitopes of the annexin II molecule are involved in plasminogen and t-PA binding. It is conceivable that annexin II, like fibrin, forms a ternary complex with t-PA and plasminogen on the endothelial cell surface [60]. In addition, t-PA interacts with matrix-bound PAI-1 [4].

Binding of u-PA with the cell surface limits plasminogen activation to focal areas such as the focal attachment sites and cellular protrusions involved in cell migration and invasion. Furthermore, u-PA interaction with its cellular receptor evokes signal transduction and phosphorylation of several proteins [24, 36, 12, 9]. A specific u-PA receptor has been identified and cloned [149, 33, 8]. It is present on many cell types, including endothelial cells [5]. It is a glycosyl phosphatidyl inositol- (GPI-) anchored glycoprotein, which binds both single-chain u-PA and two-chain u-PA via their growth factor domain [33]. The u-PA receptor is heavily glycosylated. It belongs to the cysteine-rich cell surface proteins. After synthesis it is proteolytically processed at its carboxyl-terminus and subsequently anchored in the plasma membrane by a GPI-group [112]. It comprises three domains, which are structurally homologous to snake venom α-toxins [33]. The u-PA receptor has been found in focal attachment sites, where integrin-matrix interactions occur, and in cell-cell contact areas [114, 31]. Human endothelial cells in vitro contain about 140,000 u-PA receptors per cell [58]. The expression of the u-PA receptor is enhanced by angiogenic growth factors including basic and acidic fibroblast growth factor (bFGF, aFGF) and vascular endothelial growth factor (VEGF) [92, 91, 81]. The number of u-PA receptors on human and bovine endothelial cells is also enhanced by activation of protein kinase C and by elevation of the cellular cAMP concentration [83, 143].

The u-PA receptor both acts as a site for focal pericellular proteolysis by u-PA and in involved in the clearance of the u-PA:PAI-1 complex. Upon secretion, single-chain u-PA binds to the u-PA receptor and is subsequently converted to the proteolytically active two-chain u-PA. Since the endothelial cell also contains plasmin(ogen) receptors, an interplay between receptor-bound u-PA and receptor-bound plasmin(ogen), and plasmin formation is likely to happen. The generated plasmin can degrade a number of matrix proteins. In addition, a direct plasmin-independent proteolytic action of u-PA on matrix proteins may also occur [120]. Like free u-PA activity, receptor-bound two-chain u-PA is subject to inhibition by PAI-1. As a consequence u-PA is only active over a short period of time. In contrast to receptor-bound single-chain or non-inhibited two-chain u-PA, the u-PA:PAI-1 complex is rapidly internalized together with the u-PA receptor [102], followed by degradation of the u-PA:PAI-1 complex and return of the empty u-PA receptor to the plasma membrane. Internalization of the GPI-linked u-PA receptor occurs probably after interaction with (an)other receptor(s), such as the α_2-macroglobulin/low density lipoprotein receptor-related protein (LRP) [100] or the VLDL-receptor [69]. VLDL-receptors were demonstrated on capillary and arteriolar endothelial cells in vivo [155]. The u-PA receptor may have additional roles [24]. The u-PA receptor can also form complexes with integrins. In leukocytes u-PA receptor forms complexes with β_2-integrins [9] and can interfere with β_1-integrin ligation [156]. In addition, vitronectin directly interacts with the u-PA receptor. This binding occurs to the second domain of the u-PA receptor and is influenced by u-PA binding to its receptor, which occurrs to the first domain [150, 72, 25]. By this interaction with vitronectin, u-PA receptor may function additionally in cell adherence and cell migration.

The LRP and LRP-like proteins on liver hepatocytes are involved in the clearance of plasmin- 2-antiplasmin, PA:PAI-1 complexes [103, 15, 14] and probably free PAs from the circulation. In addition, t-PA can also be cleared by mannose receptors present on macrophages and liver endothelial cells [104] and by α-fucose receptors on hepatocytes [62].

3. Synthesis, Storage And Release Of T-Pa: Role In The Prevention Of Intravascular Fibrin Deposition

The fibrinolytic activity in blood is largely determined by the concentration of t-PA, which is synthesized by the endothelium [124, 154]. After release into the blood stream, t-PA resides only for a short period in the blood, unless it encounters a specific binding site, in particular fibrin. This is due to the short half life time of t-PA in the circulation, which is 5 to 10 minutes in man. This rapid clearance, which occurs in the liver, and the ability of endothelial cells to release a relatively large amount of t-PA immediately after exposure to vasoactive agents make that the plasma concentration of t-PA can change rapidly [40, 43].

Endothelial cells contain a storage pool of t-PA, which can be rapidly released after exposure of the cells to vasoactive substances, such as bradykinin, platelet activating factor and thrombin [141, 43, 44]. Intracellularly stored t-PA has been demonstrated in small vesicles [44], which are different from the Weibel-Palade bodies, the storage organelles for von Willebrand factor and P-selectin. The t-PA storage granules are part of a system by which endothelial cells can meet acute needs that are required as soon as they become exposed to the initiation of coagulation or to vasoactive agents (Table 1). The acute t-PA release mechanism enables an enhanced t-PA concentration, exclusively at those sites of the vascular system where fibrin deposition is pending or occurs. Hence, it contributes to the local protection against an emerging unwanted thrombus. If a generalized stimulation of the endothelium occurs, for example by catecholamines or after dDAVP infusion, the acute release mechanism causes a rapid temporary increase in the systemic blood t-PA concentration. Recent studies have demonstrated that under the proper experimental conditions, acute t-PA release can also be demonstrated in cultured endothelial cells (Figure 3) [131, 141, 44].

Table 1. ACUTE RELEASE OF PRODUCTS FROM ENDOTHELIAL CELLS.

From Weibel Palade bodies:
       von Willebrand factor
       P-glycoprotein
       Multimerin
From storage vesicles:
       tissue-type plasminogen activator (t-PA)
       tissue factor pathway inhibitor (TFPI-1)
       protein S
       endothelin-1
By enzymatic activity:
       Nitric oxide (NO)
       Prostacyclin, prostaglandin E2
       Platelet activating factor (PAF)

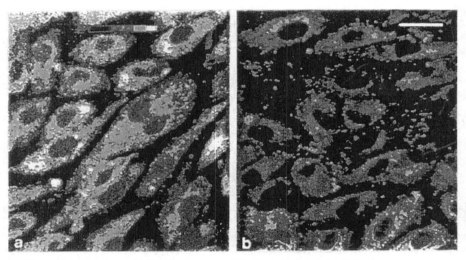

Figure 3. Acute release of t-PA from human umbilical vein endothelial cells in vitro. Immunohistochemical staining for t-PA in first passage human umbilical vein endothelial cells before (A) and 3 min after stimulation of the cells with thrombin (B). Bar: 25 μm. (From Emeis et al, 1997, with permission).

The size of the intracellular t-PA pool depends on the rate of t-PA synthesis [141]. Hence, influencing t-PA synthesis can influence both constitutive t-PA production and the amounts of acutely released t-PA. The t-PA synthesis rate is different in various types of blood vessels, e.g. veins produce more t-PA than arteries. Furthermore, t-PA synthesis can be enhanced pharmacologically or physiologically by various mediators [79]. Insight has been gained regarding the regulation of the synthesis of t-PA in endothelial cells in vitro. Activation of protein kinase C has been implicated in the regulation of transcription of the t-PA gene and t-PA synthesis in human endothelial cells. The stimulation of t-PA synthesis by histamine and thrombin is caused by this process. The induction of t-PA by protein kinase C activation is potentiated by a simultaneous increase of the cellular cAMP concentration [87, 76]. It has been suggested that the proto-oncogenes c-fos and c-jun, which can form homo- (jun-jun) or heterodimers (jun-fos) called AP1, are involved in the regulation of the t-PA gene in endothelial cells by interacting with one or more AP1-binding site(s) of the t-PA promoter [76]. In favour of the involvement of AP-1 is an experiment of nature, in which a single mutation in an AP-1 binding site of the t-PA promoter (-TGACATCA-) alters this PMA-responsive element in a cAMP-responsive element (-TGACGTCA-) [48]. In contrast to human and mouse cells, rat endothelial cells enhance their t-PA synthesis markedly upon stimulation of the cAMP generation alone, whereas rat t-PA synthesis does not respond to the sole addition of PMA [42].

Other - pharmacologically interesting - agents that can enhance t-PA synthesis are retinoids [77, 137] and certain benzodiazepines [78]. Retinoic acid and vitamin A have been demonstrated also to enhance t-PA synthesis in the rat, an elevation which is still present after a feeding period of six weeks [140]. As these components have little effect on the production of PAI-1, vitamin A derivatives are interesting candidates for pharmacological enhancement of t-PA synthesis. They act via specific nuclear receptors in the endothelial cell [80, 84]. Furthermore, exposure of endothelial cells to high shear forces causes an increase the production of t-PA by these cells [35, 90].

4. Effect of Inflammatory Mediators on the Regulation of Plasminogen Activation and Pericellular Proteolysis.

The primary cytokines interleukin-1 (IL-1) and tumor necrosis factor-a (TNFa) exert many effects on the vascular endothelium. Their most prominent feature is the induction or increase of the transcription of many genes. These genes include amongst others the leukocyte adhesion molecules E-selectin, VCAM-1 and ICAM-1, cyclooxygenase-2, and a number proteases and protease inhibitors. It was early recognized that TNFa and IL-1, as well as bacterial lipopolysaccharide (LPS), markedly increase the production of PAI-1 in endothelial cells in vitro [29, 41, 130, 144]. This induction was also demonstrated at the transcriptional level, and was largely inhibited by the isoflavone compound genistein [147]. In vivo, administration of TNFa, IL-1 or LPS causes an increase in PAI-1 concentration in the circulation. After infusion of LPS in animals, PAI-1 mRNA increased in vascularized tissues and PAI-1 mRNA was elevated in the endothelium of various organs [117, 74]. Administration of LPS or TNFa to tumor patients or healthy volunteers caused after about 2 hours a large increase in blood PAI-1 levels, which was preceded by a rapid and sustained increase in t-PA concentration [135, 146, 142]. An increase in t-PA gene transcription after TNFa exposure was demonstrated in human umbilical vein endothelial cells [147], but an increase in t-PA synthesis was only found in microvascular endothelial cells [144, 81], but not in those of umbilical vein [130, 144, 47]. The mechanism underlying the stimulation of t-PA synthesis in vivo by LPS or TNFa is probably bimodal. The rapid initial increase in t-PA level is most likely due to indirect stimulation of the acute release of t-PA. The continuously increased concentration of t-PA in the plasma is caused by an increase in t-PA synthesis. Simultaneously, a large increase in PAI-1 production observed two hours after TNFa - or LPS-administration, which far exceeds that of t-PA [135, 146, 142]. This may result - after an initial rise in fibrinolytic activity - in a prolonged attenuation of the fibrinolysis process. It is generally believed that induction of PAI-1 by inflammatory mediators may contribute to the thrombotic complications in endotoxemia and sepsis. Nevertheless, during infusion of TNFa the fibrinolytic system acted still to such extent that all fibrin formed was immediately converted into fibrin degradation products, also during the period that a large excess of circulating PAI-1 was detected [146].

The inflammatory mediators TNFα, IL-1 and LPS elicit also another effect on the regulation of plasminogen activator production in endothelial cells. Simultaneous with the increase in PAI-1 and t-PA, these inflammatory mediators induce the synthesis of u-PA in human endothelial cells in vitro [145]. Whereas u-PA is normally not found in endothelial cells in vivo, association of u-PA with the endothelium was observed in acute appendicitis [56] and in rheumatoid arthritis [151]. Induction of endothelial u-PA by TNFα in vitro is associated by an increased degradation of matrix [98]. The enhanced secretion of u-PA occurs entirely towards the basolateral side of the cell, whereas the secretion of t-PA and PAI-1 proceeds equally to the luminal and basolateral sides of the [145]. The polar secretion of u-PA suggests that u-PA may be involved in local remodeling of the basal membrane of the cell. u-PA activity is controled in space by interaction of u-PA with its cellular receptor and by the inhibitor PAI-1. The increase of PAI-1 induced by inflammatory mediators may represent, in addition to a role in the modulation of fibrinolysis, a protective mechanism of the cell against uncontroled u-PA activity.

In line with a putative role of TNFα and IL-1 in inflammation-induced local pericellular proteolysis is the observation that TNF also increases the production of matrix-degrading metalloproteinases (MMPs) by endothelial cells. In human microvascular and vein endothelial cells, TNFα increases the mRNA levels and the synthesis of interstitial collagenase (MMP-1), neutrophil collagenase (MMP-8), stromelysin-1 (MMP-3) and - if protein kinase C is also activated - gelatinase-B (MMP-9), whereas the mRNAs levels and synthesis of their physiological inhibitors TIMP-1 and TIMP-2 are not changed [66, 67, 32]. Furthermore, activation of gelatinase A (MMP-2) was observed after exposure of the cells to TNFα [66]. Recently, it has been shown that activation of gelatinase A depends on the activity of membrane-type MMP (MT-MMP) [126, 50], and that MMP-2 interacts with $\alpha_v \beta_3$ integrin [13]. Interestingly, secretion of gelatinases by bovine endothelial cells occurs predominantly towards the basolateral side of the cells [139] similar to the TNFα -induced production of uPA [145]. A role of MMPs in endothelial cell-matrix remodeling has indeed been shown in a three dimensional collagen matrix in vitro [49, 108]. Furthermore, MMPs have been detected in vivo in proliferating endothelial cells during development [75] and in endothelial cells present in atherosclerotic plaques and growing tumors [55, 99, 122].

The plasmin-plasminogen activator system and the matrix metalloproteinases cooperate in the degradation of extracellular matrix proteins [88]. Figure 4 depicts the interaction between the two systems. It should be noted, however, that this schematic picture is based on in vitro data and that it still uncertain whether all the depicted steps also act in vivo. Nevertheless, u-PA and MMP expression frequently coincide in time and location in pathological tissues. Taken these data together, it will be clear that activation of endothelial cells by TNF affects multiple sites in the proteolytic cascades involved in the degradation of matrix proteins such that it markedly enhances the breakdown and remodeling of the endothelial cell basal membrane.

5. Involvement of u-PA and u-PA Receptor in Cell Migration and Realignment of Endothelial Cells and Smooth Muscle Cells

Concentration of u-PA activity at the cellular protrusions of migrating or invading cells has been frequently observed. [7] Suggested that a continuous activation and removal of u-

PA bound to the receptor could contribute to the formation and detachment of focal attachment sites and hence to locomotion of the cell. Indeed, migrating and invading cells,

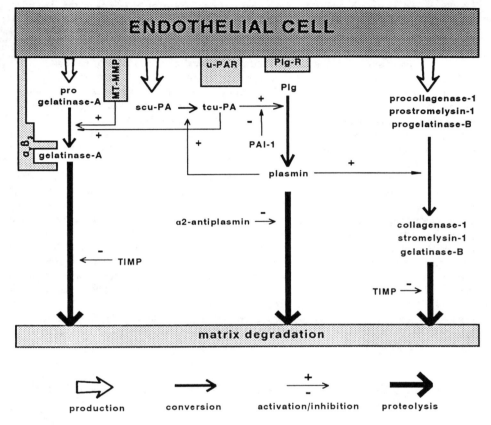

Figure 4. Schematic representation of the interaction between the u-PA-plasmin system and the presumed activation of matrix degrading metalloproteinases (MMPs). Abbreviations: PA: plasminogen activator; u-PA urokinase-type PA; sc-u-PA: single-chain u-PA; tc-u-PA: two-chain u-PA; u-PAR: u-PA receptor; Plg: plasminogen; Plg-R: Plg receptor; PAI-1: PA inhibitor-1; MT-MMP: membrane-bound MMP; TIMP: tissue inhibitor of MMP. +: stimulation; -: inhibition.

such as monocytes and tumor cells, express u-PA activity bound to u-PA receptors on their cellular protrusions [46] and on focal attachment sites [114, 68]. Receptor-bound u-PA activity is also thought to be involved in smooth muscle and endothelial cell migration and in the formation of new blood vessels (angiogenesis). Inhibition of plasminogen activation interferes with smooth muscle cell migration in vitro [129; 118, 152] and affects smooth muscle migration and proliferation in vivo [27]. In mice lacking u-PA intimal hyperplasia of injured arteries is less pronounced than in wild-type or t-PA-deficient mice [20]. Moreover, PAI-1-deficient mice show an exacerbated intimal proliferation [20]. Animals made deficient for plasminogen show comparable pathological features as those with a combined deficiency for u-PA and t-PA [111, 17]. These data suggest a role of u-PA and plasminogen in cell recruitment.

    An involvement of u-PA and the u-PA receptor in the migration of bovine endothelial cells has been demonstrated by several investigators [105, 108, 128]. After wounding of a monolayer of these endothelial cells, the cells that migrate into the wounded area express u-PA activity [105] bound to the u-PA receptor [108]. The migration and expression of u-PA depended on the release of bFGF from the wounded area [128]. bFGF is a potent inducer of plasminogen activator activity, in particular u-PA, in bovine endothelial cells [125, 57], but not in human endothelial cells [81]. In both species bFGF increases the number of u-PA receptors on endothelial cells [92, 108, 81].

Receptor-bound u-PA was demonstrated in focal adhesion sites of fibroblasts [68] and endothelial cells [31]. It may act proteolytically on these structures and hence influence cell-matrix interactions and cell migration. This was suggested for smooth muscle cells by the plasminogen dependency of cell migration [129, 152]. Additional mechanisms are also possible, as it has been suggested that u-PA can act on cell migration without involvement of its proteolytic activity [101], either by u-PA receptor-dependent signal transduction [36, 121] or by interaction of the occupied u-PA receptor with vitronectin [150].

In a group of experiments we have evaluated the inhibition of the cell-bound u-PA/plasmin activities on smooth muscle cell migration in explants of human saphenous vein. A recombinant adenovirus (Ad.ATF.BPTI) encoding a hybrid protein consiting of the receptor binding aminoterminal fragment of u-PA (ATF) linked to the mature protein of bovine pancreas trysin inhibitor (BPTI) [119]. BPTI, also known as aprotinin, is a potent plasmin inhibitor. When pieces of sapenous vein are maintained in culture they develop a pseudoneointima by invasion of cells from the cut edges of the vessel [133]. This neointima has a morphology similar to that observed in early coronary artery by-pass vein grafts that failed within one or two weeks. Infection of these grafts with Ad.ATF.BPTI prior to culture reduced neointima formation strongly, while in control segments transfected with an adenovirus encoding β-galactosidase neointima was not inhibited [119]. This further underlines the importance of cell-bound u-PA and plasmin in smooth muscle migration.

6. Role of the Plasmin/Plasminogen Activator System in the Formation of Endothelial Tubes in A Fibrin Matrix

The outgrowth of new blood vessels from existing ones, angiogenesis, is an essential process during development, but normally stops when the body becomes adult. The half life of endothelial cells in the adult body varies between 100 to 10,000 days in normal tissues, whereas it is reduced to several days in placenta and tumors [70]. With the exception of the female reproductive system, angiogenesis in the adult is associated with tissue repair after injury by wounding or inflammation. Repair-associated angiogenesis in the adult is usually accompanied by the presence of fibrin and inflammatory cells or mediators, in contrast to developmental angiogenesis in the embryo. The temporary repair matrix, fibrin, acts on the one hand as a barrier preventing further blood loss, and provides on the other hand a structure in which new microvessels can infiltrate during wound healing. A proper timing of the outgrowth of microvessels as well as the subsequent (partial) disappearance of these vessels is essential to ensure adequate wound healing and to prevent the formation of scar tissue. Although essential for the formation of granulation tissue and tissue repair, angiogenesis, once under control of pathological stimuli, can contribute to a number of pathological conditions, such as tumor neovascularisation, pannus formation in rheumatoid arthritis, and diabetic retinopathy. Understanding the mechanisms involved in angiogenesis may provide clues to prevent pathological angiogenesis without seriously impairing tissue repair. A number of studies and reviews have focused on angiogenic factors and the formation of capillary-like structures [51, 18, 96, 1, 52, 132, 127, 39]. Among them, [37] and [30] have pointed to the importance of fibrin in angiogenesis. Furthermore, work of Polverini and colleagues have demonstrated the involvement of monocytes and their products in the induction of angiogenesis [115, 86, 53, 75]. Because of the specific roles of fibrin and inflammatory cells and mediators in pathological angiogenesis in the adult, we have focused our studies on the invasion of human endothelial cells into three-dimensional fibrin matrices and the role of endothelial plasminogen activators in this process (Figure 5). This model resembles recanalization of a fibrin clot by invading endothelial cells. This invasion is usually preceded by infiltration of inflammatory cells, which interact with the vascular structures from which subsequently endothelial cells migrate into the fibrin clot [82].

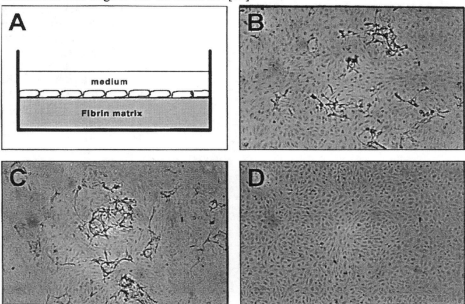

Figure 5. Formation of capillary-like tubular structures in a three dimensional fibrin matrix by human endothelial cells. Human microvascular endothelial cells grown under control conditions on top of a three-dimensional fibrin matrix (A). Model (B-D): Formation of tubular structures is induced by the simultaneous addition of b-FGF (50 ng/mL) and TNF (20 ng/mL) (B), or VEGF (100 ng/mL) and TNF (20 ng/mL) (C). When b-FGF, VEGF or TNF were added solely, no tubular structures were induced (D).

Previous studies by Pepper and Montesano using a similar model demonstrated a direct correlation between the expression of PA activity and the formation of capillary sprouts by bovine microvascular endothelial cells in vitro [106, 96]. The outgrowth of tubular structures was increased by bFGF, which increases both u-PA activity and u-PA receptor in bovine endothelial cells. Interestingly, the extent of tube formation and the diameter of the formed tubes were reduced by simultaneous presence of TGF-β [106]. The latter is a growth factor, which amongst others exerts a strong enhancement of PAI-1 synthesis in cultured endothelial cells, and thus inhibits PA activity [125]. In addition to bFGF, VEGF can also stimulate bovine endothelial cells to form tubular structures. It acts cooperatively with bFGF in this induction [107].

Studies in human endothelial cells showed that no tubular structures are formed when a quiescent monolayer of human microvascular endothelial cells grown on a fibrin matrix is exposed to bFGF or VEGF. However, when bFGF or VEGF are added simultaneously with TNF, a large number of capillary-like tubular structures are formed (Figure 5) [81]. The outgrowth of tubular structures requires u-PA activity and is completely reduced by anti-u-PA immunoglobulins but not by anti-t-PA antibodies and is paralleled by an increased degradation of fibrin (Figure 6). It is also reduced by inhibiting the interaction of u-PA with its receptor. Furthermore, proteolytic activation of plasminogen appears to be involved, because the plasmin inhibitor aprotinin largely inhibits the formation of tubular structures. Expression of both u-PA and u-PA receptor was localized at the invading tips of the tubular structures, while they were almost absent in the endothelial cells covering the fibrin matrix. These data agree with the data on bovine endothelial cells, except that in human endothelial cells a second mediator is required to induce u-PA synthesis. Many factors influence the formation of tubular structures in a fibrin matrix, including several nuclear hormone receptors. When human foreskin microvascular cells are used, dexamethasone and testosteron and to a minor extent 17 β-estradiol and the metabolite 2-methoxy-estradiol inhibited angiogenesis in vitro, while this process was enhanced by all-trans retinoic acid and 9-cis retinoic acid (Figure 7) [85]. Such studies have to be extended with studies on female microvascular endothelial cells.

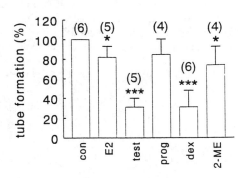

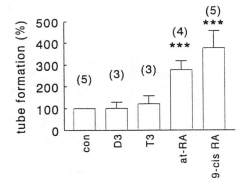

Figure 6. Effect of various inhibitors on the formation of tubular structures and fibrin degradation by human microvascular endothelial cells in a three-dimensional fibrin matrix in vitro (from Collen et al, 1998, with permission).

Not only the proteolytic activities of u-PA and plasmin determine the extent of outgrowth of capillary-like tubular structures, but also the fibrin structure per se is an important determinant in the formation and maintenance of these structures [28]. When fibrin gels were prepared at a pH of 7.0 they consisted of malleable gels with thick fibrin fibers, which were very sensitive to fibrinolysis. On the other hand when these fibrin matrices were prepared at pH 7.8, they were rigid, finely dispersed and more resistant to fibrinolysis. When these gels were equilbrated to a pH of 7.4 and subsequently covered by endothelial cells that became exposed to angiogenic growth factor (bFGF or VEGF) and TNF the cells formed much easier and faster tubular structures on the fibrin matrix originally prepared at pH 7.0, but the stability of these structures was less than in the fibrin gels prepared at pH 7.4 or 7.8, because of excessive fibrinolysis. This indicates that the structure of fibrin also is an important determinant for angiogensis.

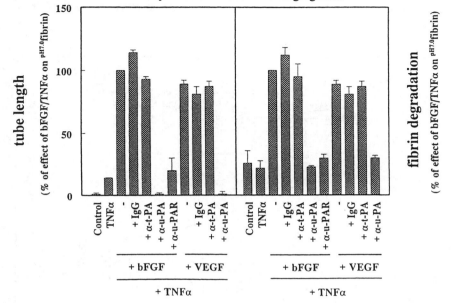

Figure 7. Effect of sex hormones and other hormones acting via nuclear hormone receptors on the formation of tubular structures by human microvascular endothelial cells cultures on a three-dimensional fibrin matrix. Con: control (βFGF- and TNFα -stimulated): E2 17 -estadiol; test: testosterone, prog: progesterone; dex: dexamethasone; 2-ME: 2-methyloxyestradial; D3: 1,25 dihydroxyvitamin D3; T3: thyroid hormone; at-RA: all-trans retinoic acid: 9-cis RA: 9-cis retinoic acid (all tested at 1 μmol/L). (from [85] with permission).

Proteolysis of the basement membrane of endothelial cells and invasion of endothelial cells into the underlying matrix are prerequisites for angiogenesis [2]. However, not only proteolysis, but also the formation of new cell attachment sites are important for the formation of tubular structures. It should be noted that fibrin contains cell binding domains for endothelial cells: a RGD sequence in its γ-chains which binds to the vitronectin receptor, i.e. the α_v β_3 integrin [34; 136] and another site in the γ-chain. [11, 12] and [65] have shown that inhibition of the α_v β_3 integrin reduces angiogenesis in several in vivo models. [54] Reported that both α_v β_3 and α_v β_5 integrin are involved in growth factor-stimulated angiogenesis in the rabbit cornea, but via distinct mechanisms. It is of interest that these authors showed that bFGF- and TNFα -induced angiogenesis is inhibited by an antibody against the α_v β_3 integrin, whereas angiogenesis induced by VEGF or by a protein kinase C activating phorbol ester required α_v β_5 integrin. It remains to be established whether both α_v β_3- and α_v β_5-dependent mechanisms are active in the invasion of endothelial cells into a fibrin matrix. The involvement of α_v β_3-integrin interaction with the fibrin matrix is likely [23], while a role of α_v β_5 integrin, which more selectively interacts with vitronectin, has to be evaluated. Irrespective of the exact role of fibrin in stimulating angiogenesis, the fibrin structure has important consequences for wound healing, and proteolytic modification of fibrin, e.g. by leukocyte elastase, or interaction of fibrin with other matrix proteins, such as vitronectin and fibronectin, may affect cell invasion and angiogenesis and the success of wound healing. Furthermore, the recent observation that MMP-2 (gelatinase-A) binds to $\alpha_v \beta_3$ [13] further points to the complexity of interactions that the $\alpha_v \beta_3$ integrin may play in fibrinous exudates, in which the matrix consists of a mixture of fibrin, collagens and other extracellular matrix components.

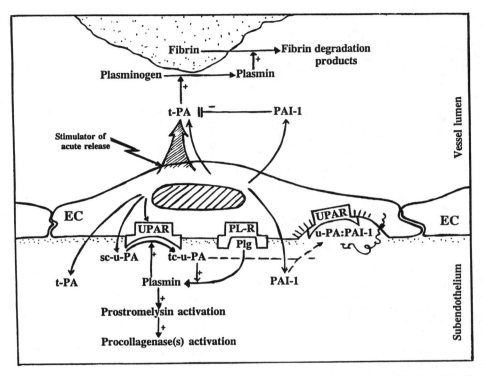

Figure 8. Schematic representation of postulated aspects of the involvement of endothelial cell plasminogen activators in fibrinolysis and local proteolysis. Abbreviations: PA: plasminogen activator; t-PA: tissue-type PA; u-PA urokinase-type PA; sc-u-PA: single-chain u-PA; tc-u-PA: two-chain u-PA; Plg: plasminogen; UPAR: u-PA receptor; Pl-R: plasminogen receptor; PAI-1: PA inhibitor-1; EC: endothelial cell. +: stimulation; -: inhibition.

7. Summary

The endothelial cell uses PAs for several functions (Figure 8). The endothelium is able to respond to emerging fibrin deposits in the blood stream by regulating the production of t-PA, the main fibrinolysis regulator in blood. In addition it can fine-tune fibrinolytic activity by the simultaneous production of PAI-1, so that re-bleeding of a wound is prevented. On the other side of the coin, the endothelium uses PAs, in particular u-PA, for proteolytically changing its interaction with its underlying matrix and for remodelling of its basement membrane, processes which are necessary for cell migration and angiogenesis. This process is limited in space and time by interaction of u-PA with its specific receptor and by the presence of PAI-1. Locally generated u-PA and plasmin activities interact with those of matrix metalloproteinases, which degrade another spectrum of extracellular matrix proteins. The expression of u-PA, u-PA receptor and many matrix metalloproteinases in endothelial cells is under the control of the monocyte-derived cytokines TNFα and IL-1 and by angiogenic growth factors. Cell migration and invasion require not only proteolytic activity but also the formation of new cell-matrix contacts needed for the cell to pull itself ahead. Smooth muscle migration and the formation of capillary-like tubular structures by human microvascular endothelial cells into a three-dimensional fibrin matrix are controled by cell-bound u-PA and plasmin. In addition the structure of the fibrin matrix itself is an important determinant in the extent of formation and maintenance of capillary-like tubular structures. These data point to a close interaction of proteins involved in cell-matrix interaction and cell surface-bound pericellular proteolysis.

Acknowledgement

The financial support by the Netherlands Heart Foundation (grants M93.001, 93.154 and 95.193), the Dutch Cancer Society (grants TNOP 97-1511 and 94.748) and the Praeventiefonds (grants 28-2621 and 28-2622) is gratefully acknowledged.

References

[1] Aiello, L.P., Avery, R.L., Arrigg, P.G., Keyt, B.A., Jampel, H.D., Shah, S.T., Pasquale, L.R. et al. (1994) Vascular endothelial cell growth factor in ocular fluid of patients with diabetic retinopathy and other retinal disorders. N. Engl. J. Med. 331:1480-1487.

[2] Ausprunk, D. and Folkman, J. (1977) Migration and proliferation of endothelial cells in preformed and newly formed blood vessels during tumor angiogenesis. Microvasc. Res. 14: 52-65.

[3] Bachmann, F. (1995) The enigma PAI-2. Gene expression, evolutionary and functional aspects. Thromb. Haemostas. 74: 172-179.

[4] Barnathan, E.S., Kuo, A., Van der Keyl, H., McCrae, K.R., Larsen, G.R. and Cines, D.B. (1988) Tissue-type plasminogen activator binding to human endothelial cells. Evidence for two distinct sites. J. Biol. Chem. 263: 7792-7799.

[5] Barnathan, E. S. (1992) Characterization and regulation of the urokinase receptor of human endothelial cells. Fibrinolysis, 6: 1-9.

[6] Beebe, D. P. (1987) Binding of tissue plasminogen activators to human umbilical vein endothelial cells. Thromb. Res., 46: 241-254.

[7] Blasi, F. (1993) Urokinase and urokinase receptor - A paracrine/autocrine system regulating cell migration and invasiveness. Bioessays, 15: 105-111.

[8] Blasi, F., Conese, M., Møller, L. B., Pedersen, N., Cavallaro, U., Cubellis, M., Fazioli, F., Hernandez-Marrero, L., Limongi, P., Munoz-Canoves, P., Resnati, M., Riittinen, L., Sidenius, N., Soravia, E., Soria, M., Stoppelli, M., Talarico, D., Teesalu, T., and Valcamonica, S. (1994) The urokinase receptor: Structure, regulation and inhibitor- mediated internalization. Fibrinolysis, 8: 182-188.

[9] Bohuslav, J., Horejsi, V., Hansmann, C., Stöckl, J., Weidle, U.H., Majdic, O., Bartke, I., Knapp, W., Stockinger, H. (1995) Urokinase plasminogen activator receptor, β$_2$-integrins, and src-kinases within a single receptor complex of human monocytes. J. Exp. Med. 181: 1381-1390.

[10] Broadley, K.N., Aquino, A.M., Woodward, S.C., Buckley-Sturrock, A., Sato, Y., Rifkin, D. and Davidson, J.M. (1989) Monospecific antibodies implicate basic fibroblast growth factor in normal wound repair. Lab. Invest. 61: 571-575.

[11] Brooks, P.C., Clark, R.A. and Cheresh, D.A. (1994a) Requirement of vascular integrin α$_v$ β$_3$ for angiogenesis. Science 264: 569-571.

[12] Brooks, P.C., Montgomery, A.M., Rosenfeld, M., Reisfeld, R.A., Hu, T., Klier, G and Cheresh, D.A. (1994b) Intergrin α$_v$ β$_3$ antagonists promote tumor regression by inducing apoptosis of angiogenic blood vessels. Cell 79: 1157-1164.

[13] Brooks, P.C., Strömblad, S., Sanders, L.C., von Schalscha, T.L., Aimes, R.T., Stetler-Stevenson, W.G., Quigley, J.P., and Cheresh, D.A., 1996, Localization of matrix metalloproteinase MMP-2 to the surface of invasive cells by interaction with integrin α$_v$ β$_3$. Cell 85: 683-693.

[14] Bu, G., Warshawsky, I., and Schwartz, A. L. (1994) Cellular receptors for the plasminogen activators. Blood, 83: 3427-3436.

[15] Bu, G., Williams, S., Strickland, D.K. and Schwartz, A.L. (1992) Low density lipoprotein receptor-related protein/ α_2-macroglobulin receptor is an hepatic receptor for tissue-type plasminogen activator, Proc. Natl. Acad. Sci. U.S.A. 89: 7427-7431.

[16] Bugge, T.H., Suh, T.T., Flick, M.J., Daugherty, C.C., Rømer, J., Solberg, H., Ellis, V., Danø, K. and Degen, J.J., 1995a, The receptor for urokinase-type plasminogen activator is not essential for mouse development or fertility. J.Biol. Chem. 270: 16886-16894.

[17] Bugge, T.H., Flick, M.J., Daugherty, C.C., and Degen, J.L., 1995b, Plasminogen deficiency causes severe thrombosis but is compatible with development and reproduction. Genes & Development 9: 794-807.

[18] Burgess, W.H., and Maciag, T., 1989 The heparin-binding (fibroblast) growth factor family of proteins. Annu. Rev. Biochem. 58:575-606.

[19] Carmeliet, P., Schoonjans, L., Kieckens, L., Ream, B., Degen, J., Bronson, R., De Vos, R., Van den Oord, J. J., Collen, D., and Mulligan, R. C. (1994) Physiological consequences of loss of plasminogen activator gene function in mice. Nature, 368: 419-424.

[20] Carmeliet, P. and Collen, D. (1994) Evaluation of the plasminogen/plasmin system in transgenic mice. Fibrinolysis 8: 269-276.

[21] Carmeliet, P., Stassen, J. M., Schoonjans, L., Ream, B., Van den Oord, J. J., De Mol, M., Mulligan, R. C., and Collen, D. (1993) Plasminogen activator inhibitor-1 gene-deficient mice. II. Effects on hemostasis, thrombosis, and thrombolysis. J. Clin. Invest., 92: 2756-2760.

[22] Carmeliet, P., Kieckens, L., Schoonjans, L., Ream, B., Van Nuffelen, A., Prendergast, G., Cole, M., Bronson, R., Collen, D., and Mulligan, R. C. (1994) Plasminogen activator inhibitor-1 gene-deficient mice. I. Generation by homologues recombination and characterization. J. Clin. Invest., 92: 2746-2755.

[23] Chang, M-C., Wang, B-R. and Huang T-F. (1995) Characterization of endothelial cell differential attachment to fibrin and fibrinogen and its inhibition by Arg-Gly-Asp-containing peptides. Thromb. Haemostas. 74:764-769.

[24] Chapman, H.A. (1997) Plasminogen activators, integrins, and the coordinated regulation of cell adhesion and migration. Curr. Opinion Cell Biol. 9: 714-724.

[25] Chavakis, T., Kanse, S.M., Yutzy, B., Lijnen, H.R., and Preissner, K.T. (1998) Vitronectin concentrates proteolytic activity on the cell surface and extracellular matrix by trapping soluble urokinase receptor-urokinase complexes. Blood 91: 2305-2312.

[26] Ciambrone, G. J., and McKeown-Longo, P. J. (1992) Vitronectin regulates the synthesis and localization of urokinase-type plasminogen activator in HT-1080 cells. J. Biol. Chem., 267: 13617-13622.

[27] Clowes, A.W., Clowes, M.M., Au, Y.P.T., Reidy, M.A. and Belin, D. (1990) Smooth muscle cells express urokinase during mitogenesis and tissue-type plasminogen activator during migration in injured rat carotid artery. Circ. Res. 67: 61-67.

[28] Collen, A., Koolwijk, P., Kroon, M., and van Hinsbergh, V.W.M. (1998) Influence of fibrin structure on the formation and maintenance of capillary-like tubules by human microvascular endothelial cells. Angiogenesis 2: 153-165.

[29] Colucci, M., Paramo, J.A., and Collen, D., 1985, Generation in plasma of a fast-acting inhibitor of plasminogen activator in response to endotoxin stimulation. J. Clin. Invest. 75: 818-824.

[30] Colvin R.B. (1986) Wound Healing Processes in Hemostasis and Thrombosis. in: "Vascular Endothelium in Hemostasis and Thrombosis," M.A. Gimbrone Jr., ed., pp. 220-241, Churchill Livingstone, Edinburgh.

[31] Conforti, G., Dominguez-Jimenez, C., Rønne, E., Høyer-Hansen, G., and Dejana, E. (1994) Cell-surface plasminogen activation causes a retraction of in vitro cultured human umbilical vein endothelial cell monolayer. Blood, 83: 994-1005.

[32] Cornelius, L. A., Nehring, L. C., Roby, J. D., Parks, W. C., and Welgus, H. G. (1995) Human dermal microvascular endothelial cells produce matrix metalloproteinases in response to angiogenic factors and migration. J. Invest. Dermatol., 105: 170-176.

[33] Danø, K., Behrendt, N., Brünner, N., Ellis, V., Ploug, M., and Pyke, C. (1994) The urokinase receptor Protein structure and role in plasminogen activation and cancer invasion. Fibrinolysis, 8: 189-203.

[34] Dejana E., Lampugnani, M.G., Giorgi, M., Gaboli, M., and Marchisio, P.C., 1990, Fibrinogen induces endothelial cell adhesion and spreading via the release of endogenous matrix proteins and the recruitment of more than one integrin receptor. Blood 75: 1509-1517.

[35] Diamond, S.L., Eskin, S.G., and McIntire, L.V. (1989) Fluid flow stimulates tissue plasminogen activator secretion by cultured human endothelial cells. Science 243: 1483- 1485.

[36] Dumler, I., Petri, T., and Schleuning, W-D. (1993) Interaction of urokinase-type plasminogen activator (u-PA) with its cellular receptor (u-PAR) induces phosphorylation on tyrosine of a 38 kDa protein. FEBS Letters, 322: 37-40.

[37] Dvorak, H.F. (1986) Tumors: wounds that do not heal: similarities between tumor stroma generation and wound healing. N. Engl. J. Med. 315: 1650-1659.

[38] Dvorak, H. F., Nagy, J. A., Berse, B., Brown, L. F., Yeo, K-T., Yeo, T-K., Dvorak, A. M, Van De Water, L., Sioussat, T. M, and Senger, D. R. (1992) Vascular permeability factor, fibrin, and the pathogenesis of tumor stroma formation. Ann. N. Y. Acad. Sci., 667: 101-111.

[39] Dvorak, H. F, Brown, L. F., Detmar, M., and Dvorak, A. M. (1995) Vascular permeability factor/vascular endothelial growth factor, microvascular hyperpermeability, and angiogenesis. Am. J. Pathol., 146: 1029-1039.

[40] Emeis, J. J. (1992) Regulation of the acute release of tissue-type plasminogen activator from the endothelium by coagulation activation products. Ann. N. Y. Acad. Sci., 667: 249-258.

[41] Emeis, J.J., and Kooistra, T., 1986, Interleukin-1 and lipopolysaccharide induce a fast-acting inhibitor od tissue-type plasminogen activator in vivo and in cultured endothelial cells. J. Exp. Med. 163: 1260-1266.

[42] Emeis, J.J., and Kooistra, T. (1993) Animal models and experimental procedures to study the synthesis and acute release of tissue-type plasminogen activator, Fibrinolysis 7, Suppl.1: 31-32.

[43] Emeis, J.J., van den Eijnden-Schrauwen, Y., and Kooistra, T., 1996, Tissue-type plasminogen activator and the vessel wall: synthesis, storage and secretion. in: "Vascular Control of Hemostasis", V.W.M. van Hinsbergh ed., pp. 187-206, Harwood Acad. Publ., Amsterdam.

[44] Emeis, J.J., van den Eijnden-Schrauwen, Y., van den Hoogen, C.M., de Priester, W., Westmunckett, A., and Lupu, F. (1997) J. Cell Biol. 139: 245-256.

[45] Emeis, J.J., Verheijen, J.H., Ronday, H.K., De Maat M.P.M., Brakman, P. (1997a). Progress in clinical fibrinolysis. Fibrinolysis and proteolysis 11: 67-84.

[46] Estreicher, A., Mühlhauser, J., Carpentier, J-L., Orci, L., and Vassalli, J-D. (1990) The receptor for urokinase type plasminogen activator polarizes expression of the protease to the leading edge of migrating monocytes and promotes degradation of enzyme inhibitor complexes. J. Cell Biol., 111: 783-792.

[47] Fearns, C., Samad, F., and Loskutoff, D.J., 1996, Synthesis and localization of PAI-1 in the vessel wall. in: "Vascular Control of Hemostasis", V.W.M. van Hinsbergh ed., pp. 207-226, Harwood Acad. Publ., Amsterdam.

[48] Feng, P., Ohlsson, M., and Ny, T. (1990) The structure of the TATA-less rat tissue-type plasminogen activator gene. Species-specific sequence divergences in the promoter predict differences in regulation of gene expression, J. Biol. Chem. 265: 2022- 2027.

[49] Fisher, C., Gilbertsonbeadling, S., Powers, E.A., Petzold, G., Poorman, R., and Mitchell, M.A., 1994, Interstitial collagenase is required for angiogenesis in vitro. Dev. Biol. 162: 499-510.

[50] Foda, H.D., George, S., Conner, C., Drews, M., Tomkins, D.C., Zucker, S., 1996, Activation of human umbilical vein endothelial cell progelatinase A by phorbol myristate: a protein kinase C-dependent mechanism involving a membrane-type matrix metalloproteinase. Lab. Invest. 74: 538-545.

[51] Folkman, J., 1995, Tumor angiogenesis. in: "The Molecular Basis of Cancer", J. Mendelsohn, P.M. Howley, M.A. Israel, and L.A. Liotta, eds., pp. 206-232, W.B. Saunders Comp., Philadelphia.

[52] Fong, G-H., Rossant, J., Gertsenstein, M. and Breitman, M.L. (1995) Role of the flt-1 receptor tyrosine kinase in regulating the assembly of vascular endothelium. Nature 376: 66-70.

[53] Fràter-Schröder, M., Risau, W., Hallman, R., Gautschi, P., and Böhlen, P. (1987) Tumor necrosis factor type α, a potent inhibitor of endothelial cell growth in vitro, is angiogenic in vivo. Proc. Natl. Acad. Sci. USA, 84: 5277-5281.

[54] Friedlander, M., Brooks, P.C., Shaffer, R.W., Kincais, C.M., Varner, J.A. and Cheresh, D.A. (1995) Definition of two angiogenic pathways by distinct α_v integrins. Science 270: 1500-1502.

[55] Galis Z.S., Sukhova, G.K., Lark, M.W., and Libby, P., 1994, Increased expression of matrix metalloproteinases and matrix degrading activity in vulnerable regions of human atherosclerotic plaques. J. Clin. Invest. 94: 2493-2503.

[56] Grøndahl-Hansen, J., Kirkeby, L., Ralfkiær, Kristensen, P., Lund, L.R., Danø, K., 1989, Urokinase-type plasminogen activator in endothelial cells during acute inflammtion of the appendix. Am. J. Pathol. 135: 631-636.

[57] Gualandris, A., and Presta, M. (1995) Transcriptional and posttranscriptional regulation of urokinase-type plasminogen activator expression in endothelial cells by basic fibroblast growth factor. J. Cell. Physiol., 162: 400-409.

[58] Haddock, R. C., Spell, M. L., Baker III, C. D., Grammer, J. R, Parks, J. M., Speidel, M., and Booyse, F. M. (1991) Urokinase binding and receptor identification in cultured endothelial cells. J. Biol. Chem., 266: 21466-21473.

[59] Hajjar, K.A. (1991) The endothelial cell tissue plasminogen activator receptor. Specific interaction with plasminogen, J. Biol. Chem. 266: 21962-21970.

[60] Hajjar, K. A. (1995) Cellular receptors in the regulation of plasmin generation. Thromb. Haemostas., 74: 294-301.

[61] Hajjar, K.A. and Nachman, R.L. (1988) Endothelial cell-mediated conversion of Glu-plasminogen to Lys-plasminogen. Further evidence for assembly of of the fibrinolytic system on the endothelial cell surface. J. Clin. Invest. 82: 1769-1778.

[62] Hajjar, K. A., and Reynolds, C. (1994) α-Fucose-mediated binding and degradation of tissue-type plasminogen activator by HepG2 cells. J. Clin. Invest., 93: 703-710.

[63] Hajjar, K. A., Hamel, N. M., Harpel, P. C., and Nachman, R. L. (1987) Binding of tissue plasminogen activator to cultured human endothelial cells. J. Clin. Invest., 80: 1712-1719.

[64] Hajjar, K., Jacovina, A. and Chacko, J. (1994) An endothelial cell receptor for plasminogen tissue plasminogen activator 1 identity with annexin II. J. Biol. Chem. 269: 21191-21197.

[65] Hammes, H.P., Brownlee, M., Jonczyk, A., Sutter, A., and Preissner, K., 1996, Subcutaneous injection of a cyclic peptide antagonist of vitronectin receptor-type integrins inhibits retinal neovascularization. Nature Medicine 2: 529-533.

[66] Hanemaaijer, R., Koolwijk, P., Leclercq, L., De Vree, W. J. A., and Van Hinsbergh, V. W. M. (1993) Regulation of matrix metalloproteinase expression in human vein and microvascular endothelial cells - Effects of tumour necrosis factor-α, interleukin-1 and phorbol ester. Biochem. J., 296: 803-809.

[67] Hanemaaijer, R., Sorsa, T., Konttinen, Y.T., Ding, Y., Sutinen, M., Visser, H., van Hinsbergh, V.W.M., Helaakoski, T., Kainulainen, T., Rönkä, H., Tschesche, H., Salo, T. (1997) Matrix metalloproteinase-8 is expressed in rheumatoid synovial fibroblasts and endothelial cells. Regulation by tumor necrosis factor-α and doxycycline. J. Biol. Chem. 272: 31504-31509.

[68] Hébert, C. A., and Baker, J. B. (1988) Linkage of extracellular plasminogen activator to fibroblast cytoskeleton: Colocalization of cell surface urokinase with vinculin. J. Cell Biol., 105: 1241-1247.

[69] Heegaard, C.W., Wiborg Simonsen, A.C., Oka, K., Kjøller, L., Christensen, A., Madsen, B., Ellgaard, L., Chan, L., and Andreasen, P.A., 1995, Very low density lipoprotein receptor binds and mediates endocytosis of urokinase-type plasminogen activator-type-1 plasminogen activator inhibitor complex. J. Biol. Chem. 270: 20855-20861.

[70] Hobson B. and Denekamp J. (1984) Endothelial proliferation in tumours and normal tissues: Continuous labelling studies. Br. J. Cancer 49: 405-413.

[71] Holmes, W.E., Nelles, L., Lijnen, H.R. and Collen, D. (1987) Primary structure of human α2-antiplasmin, a serine protease inhibitor (Serpin), J. Biol. Chem. 262: 1659-1664.

[72] Kanse, S.M., Kost, C., Wilhelm, O.G., Andreasen, P.A., and Preissner, K.T. (1996) Exp. Cell Res. 224: 344-353.

[73] Karelina, T.V., Goldberg, G.I., and Eisen, A.Z., 1995, Matrix metalloproteinases in blood vessel development in human fetal skin and in cutaneous tumors. J. Invest. Dermatol. 105: 411-417.

[74] Keeton, M., Eguchi, Y., Swadey, M., Ahn, C. and Loskutoff, D. (1993) Cellular localization of type 1 plasminogen activator inhibitor messenger RNA and protein in murine renal tissue, Am. J. Pathol. 142: 59-70.

[75] Koch, A.E. Polverini, P.J., Kunkel, S.L., Harlow, L.A., DiPietro, L.A., Elner, V.M., Elner S.G., and Strieter, R.M., 1991, Interleukin-8 as a macrophage-derived mediator of angiogenesis. Science 258: 1798-1801.

[76] Kooistra, T., Bosma, P.J., Toet, K., Cohen, L.H., Griffioen, M., Van den Berg, E., Le Clercq, L., and Van Hinsbergh, V.W.M., 1991a, Role of protein kinase C and cyclic adenosine monophosphate in the regulation of tissue-type plasminogen activator, plasminogen activator inhibitor-1, and platelet-derived growth factor mRNA levels in human endothelial cells. Possible involvement of proto-oncogenes c-jun and c-fos. Arterioscler. Thrombos. 11: 1042-1052.

[77] Kooistra, T., Opdenberg, J.P., Toet, K., Hendriks, H.F.J., Van den Hoogen, R.M., and Emeis, J.J., 1991b, Stimulation of tissue-type plasminogen activators synthesis by retinoids in cultured human endothelial cells and rat tissues in vivo, Thromb. Haemostas. 65: 565-572.

[78] Kooistra, T., Toet, K., Kluft, C., Von Voigtlander, P.F., Ennis, M.D., Aiken, J.W., Boadt, J.A. and Erickson, L.A., 1993, Triazolobenzodiazepines: a new class of stimulators of tissue-type plasminogen activator synthesis in human endothelial cells, Biochem. Pharmacol. 46: 61-67.

[79] Kooistra, T., Schrauwen, Y., and Emeis, J. J. (1994) regulation of endothelial cell t-PA synthesis and release. Int. J. Hematol., 59: 233-255.

[80] Kooistra, T., Lansink, M., Arts, J., Sitter, T., and Toet, K., 1995, Involvement of retinoic acid receptor in the stimulation of tissue-type plasminogen activator gene expression in human endothelial cells. Eur. J.Biochem 232: 425-432.

[81] Koolwijk, P., van Erck, M.G.M., de Vree, W.J.A., Vermeer, M.A., Weich, H.A., Hanemaaijer, R. and van Hinsbergh, V.W.M., 1996, Cooperative effect of TNF, bFGF and VEGF on the formation of tubular structures of human microvascular endothelial cells in a fibrin matrix. Role of urokinase activity. J. Cell Biol. 132: 1177-1188

[82] Kwaan, H.C. 1966, Tissue fibrinolytic activity studied by a histochemical method, Fed. Proc. 25:52-56.

[83] Langer, D. J., Kuo, A., Kariko, K., Ahuja, M., Klugherz, B. D., Ivanics, K. M, Hoxie, J. A., Williams, W. V., Liang, B. T., Cines, D. B., and Barnathan, E. S., 1993, Regulation of the endothelial cell urokinase-type plasminogen activator receptor - Evidence for cyclic AMP-dependent and protein kinase-C dependent pathways. Circ. Res., 72: 330-340.

[84] Lansink, M., and Kooistra, T., (1996) Stimulation of tissue-type plasminogen activator expression by retinoic acid in human endothelial cells requires retinoic receptor 2 induction. Blood 88: 531-541.

[85] Lansink, M., Koolwijk, P., van Hinsbergh, V. and Kooistra T. (1998) Effect of steroid hormones and retinoids on the formation of capillary-like structures of human microvascular endothelial cells in fibrin matrices is related to urokinase expression. Blood 92: 927-938.

[86] Leibovich S.J., Polverini, P.J., Shepard, H.M., Wiseman, D.M., Shively, V. and Nuseir, N. (1987) Macrophage-induced angiogenesis is mediated by tumour necrosis factor-α. Nature 329: 630-632.

[87] Levin, E.G., Marotti, K.R., and Santell, L., (1989) Protein kinase C and the stimulation of tissue plasminogen activator release from human endothelial cells. Dependence on the elevation of messenger RNA, J. Biol. Chem. 264: 16030-16036.

[88] Liotta, L.A., Steeg, P.S., and Stetler-Stevenson, W.G. (1991) Cancer metastasis and angiogenesis - An imbalance of positive and negative regulation. Cell, 64: 327-336.

[89] Loskutoff, D.J. (1991) Regulation of PAI-1 gene expression, Fibrinolysis 5: 197-206.

[90] Malek, A.M., Jackman, R., Rosenberg, R.D., Izumo, S. (1994) Endothelial expression of thrombomodulin is reversibly regulated by fluid shear stress. Circ. Res. 74: 852-860.

[91] Mandriota, S., Seghezzi, G., Vassalli, J-D., Ferrara, N., Wasi, S., Mazzieri, R., Mignatti, P. and Pepper, M. (1995) Vascular endothelial growth factor increases urokinase receptor expression in vascular endothelial cells. J. Biol. Chem. 270: 9709-9716.

[92] Mignatti, P., Mazzieri, R., and Rifkin, D. B., 1991, Expression of the urokinase receptor in vascular endothelial cells is stimulated by basic fibroblast growth factor. J. Cell Biol., 113: 1193-1201.

[93] Miles, L.A., Levin, E.G., Plescia, J., Collen, D. and Plow, E.F., 1988, Plasminogen receptors, urokinase receptors, and their modulation on human endothelial cells, Blood 72: 628-635.

[94] Miles, L. A., Fless, G. M., Levin, E. G., Scanu, A. M., and Plow, E. F., 1989a, A potential basis for the thrombotic risks associated with lipoprotein(a). Nature, 399: 301-303.

[95] Miles, L. A., Dahlberg, C. M., Levin, E. G., and Plow, E. F., 1989b, Gangliosides interact directly with plasminogen and urokinase and may mediate binding of these fibrinolytic components to cells. Biochem., 28: 9337-9343.

[96] Montesano, R. (1992) Regulation of angiogenesis in vitro. Eur. J. Clin. Invest., 22: 504-515.

[97] Nachman, R.L. (1992) Thrombosis and atherogenesis: molecular connections. Blood 79: 1897-1906.

[98] Niedbala, M. J., and Stein-Picarella, M. (1992) Tumor necrosis factor induction of endothelial cell urokinase-type plasminogen activator mediated proteolysis of extracellular matrix and its antagonism by γ-interferon. Blood, 79: 678-687.

[99] Nikkari S.T., O'Brien, K.D., Ferguson, M., Hatsukami, T., Welgus, H.G., Alpers, C.E., and Clowes, A.W., 1995, Interstitial collagenase (MMP-1) expression in human carotid atherosclerosis. Circulation 92: 1393-1398.

[100] Nykjær, A., Petersen, C. M., Møller, B., Jensen, P. H., Moestrup, S. K., Holtet, T. L., Etzerodt, M., Thogersen, H. C., Munch, M., Andreasen, P. A., and Gliemann, J. (1992). Purified α2-macroglobulin receptor/LDL receptor-related protein binds urokinase activator inhibitor type-1 complex - Evidence that the 2-macroglobulin receptor mediates cellular degradation of urokinase receptor-bound complexes. J. Biol. Chem., 267: 14543-14546.

[101] Odekon, L. E., Sato, Y., and Rifkin, D. B. (1992) Urokinase-type plasminogen activator mediates basic fibroblast growth factor-induced bovine endothelial cell migration independent of its proteolytic activity. J. Cell. Physiol., 150: 258-263.

[102] Olson, D., Pöllänen, J., Høyer-Hansen, G., Rønne, E., Sakaguchi, K., Wun, T-C., Appella, E., Danø, K. and Blasi, F. (1992) Internalization of the urokinase-plasminogen activator inhibitor type-1 complex is mediated by the urokinase receptor, J. Biol. Chem. 267: 9129-9133.

[103] Orth, K., Madison, E. L., Gething, M-J., Sambrook, J. F., and Herz, J. (1992) Complexes of tissue-type plasminogen activator and its serpin inhibitor plasminogen-activator inhibitor type-1 are internalized by means of the low density lipoprotein receptor- related protein/ 2-macroglobulin receptor. Proc. Natl. Acad. Sci. USA, 89: 7422-7426.

[104] Otter, M., Barrett-Bergshoef, M.M. and Rijken, D.C. (1991) Binding of tissue-type plasminogen activator by the mannose receptor. J. Biol. Chem. 266:13931-13935.

[105] Pepper, M. S., Vassalli, J-D., Montesano, R., and Orci, L. (1987) Urokinase-type plasminogen activator is induced in migrating capillary endothelial cells. J. Cell Biol., 105: 2535-2541.

[106] Pepper, M. S., Belin, D., Montesano, R., Orci, L., and Vassalli, J. (1990) Transforming growth factor-ß-1 modulates basic fibroblast growth factor induced proteolytic and angiogenic properties of endothelial cells in vitro. J. Cell Biol., 111: 743-755.

[107] Pepper, M. S., Ferrara, N., Orci, L., and Montesano, R. (1992) Potent synergism between vascular endothelial growth factor and basic fibroblast growth factor in the induction of angiogenesis in vitro. Biochem. Biophys. Res. Commun., 189: 824-831.

[108] Pepper, M. S, Sappino, A-P., Stocklin, R., Montesano, R., Orci, L., and Vassalli, J-D. (1993) Upregulation of urokinase receptor expression on migrating endothelial cells. J. Cell Biol., 122: 673-684.

[109] Pepper, M. S., Vassalli, J-D., Wilks, J. W., Schweigerer, L., Orci, L., and Montesano, R. (1994) Modulation of bovine microvascular endothelial cell proteolytic properties of inhibitors of angiogenesis. J. Cell. Biochem., 55: 419-434.

[110] Pepper, M.S., Mandiota, S.J., Jeltsch, M., Kumar, V. And Alitalo, K. (1998) Vascular endothelial growth factor (VREGF)-C synergizes with basic fibroblast growth factor and VEGF in the induction of angiogenesis in vitro, and alters endothelial extracellular proteolytic activity. J. Cell. Physiol. In press.

[111] Ploplis, V.A., Carmeliet, P., Vazirzadeh, S., Van Vlaenderen, I., Moons, L., Plow, e.f., and Collen, D., 1995, Effects of disruption of the plasminogen gene on thrombosis, growth, and health in mice. Circulation 92:2585-2593.

[112] Ploug, M., Behrendt, N., Lober, D., and Danø, K. (1991) Protein structure and membrane anchorage of the cellular receptor for urokinase-type plasminogen activator. Seminars in Thromb. Haemostas. 17: 183-193.

[113] Plow, E.F., Felez, J. and Miles, L.A. (1991) Cellular regulation of fibrinolysis. Thromb. Haemostas. 66: 32-36.

[114] Pöllänen, J., Hedman, K., Nielsen, L. S., Danø, K., and Vaheri, A. (1988) Ultrastructural localization of plasma membrane-associated urokinase-type plasminogen activator at focal contacts. J. Cell Biol., 106: 87-95.

[115] Polverini, P. (1989) Macrophage-induced angiogenesis - A review. Macrophage-Derived Cell Regulatory Factors, 1: 54-73.

[116] Presta, M., Maier, J. A. M., and Ragnotti, G. (1989) The mitogenic signalling pathway but not the plasminogen activator-inducing pathway of basic fibroblast growth factor is mediated through protein kinase C in fetal bovine aortic endothelial cells. J. Cell Biol., 109: 1877-1884.

[117] Quax, P. H. A., Van den Hoogen, C. R., Verheijen, J. H., Padro, T., Zeheb, R., Gelehrter, T. D., van Berkel, T. J. C., Kuiper, J., and Emeis, J. J. (1990) Endotoxin induction of plasminogen activator and plasminogen activator inhibitor type 1 mRNA in rat tissues in vivo. J. Biol Chem., 265: 15560-15563.

[118] Quax, P.H.A., Koolwijk, P., Verheijen, J.H.M., and Van Hinsbergh, V.W.M., 1996, The role of plasminogen activators in vascular pericellular proteolysis. in "Vascular Control of Hemostasis", V.W.M. van Hinsbergh, ed., pp. 227-245, Harwood Academic Publishers, Amsterdam.

[119] Quax PHA, Lamfers MLM, Grimbergen JG, Verheijen JH, van Hinsbergh VWM (1997) Inhibition of neointima formation in cultured human saphenous vein segments by an adenovirus expressing an urokinase receptor binding plasmin inhibitor. Circulation 96: I-699.

[120] Quigley, J. P., Gold, L. I., Schwimmer, R., and Sullivan, L. M. (1987) Limited cleavage of cellular fibronectin by plasmin activator purified from transformed cells. Proc. Natl. Acad. Sci. USA, 84: 2776-2780.

[121] Rao, N. K., Shi, G-P., and Chapman, H. A. (1995) Urokinase receptor is a multifunctional protein: Influence of receptor occupancy on macrophage gene expression. J. Clin. Invest., 96: 465-474.

[122] Rao, J.S., Yamamoto, M., Mohaman, S., Gokaslan, Z.L., Stetler-Stevenson, W.G., Roa, V.H., Liotta, L.A., Nicolson, G.l.,and Sawaya, R.E., 1996, Expression and localization of 92 kD type IV collagenase genatinase B (MMP-9) in human gliomas. Clin. Exp. Metastasis 14: 12-18.

[123] Redlitz, A., Tan, A. K., Eaton, D. L., and Plow, E. F. (1995) Plasma carboxypeptidases as regulators of plasminogen system. J. Clin. Invest., 96: 2534-2538.

[124] Rijken, D. D., Wijngaards, G., and Welbergen, J. (1980) Relationship between tissue plasminogen activator and the activators in blood and vascular wall. Thromb. Res., 18: 815-830.

[125] Saksela, O.D., Moscatelli, D. and Rifkin, D. (1987) The opposing effects of basic fibroblast growth factor and transforming growth factor beta on the regulation of plasminogen activator activity in capillary endothelial cells. J.Cell. Biol. 105: 957-963.

[126] Sato, H., Takin, T., Okada, Y., Cao, J., Shinagawa,A., Yamamoto, E., and Seiki, M., 1994, A matrix metalloproteinase expressed in the surface of invasive tunour cells. Nature 370: 61-65.

[127] Sato, T.N., Tozawa, Y., Deutsch, U., Wolburg-Buchholz, K., Fujiwara, Y., Gendron-Maguire, M., Gridley, T., Wolburg, H., Risau, W. and Qin, Y. (1995) Distinct roles of the receptor tyrosine kinases tie-1 and tie-2 in blood vessel formation. Nature 376: 70-74.

[128] Sato, Y., and Rifkin, D. B. (1988) Autocrine activities of basic fibroblast growth factor : Regulation of endothelial cell movement, plasminogen activator synthesis, and DNA synthesis. J. Cell Biol., 107: 1199-1205.

[129] Schleef, R. R., and Birdwell, C. R. (1982) The effect of proteases on endothelial cell migration in vitro. Exp. Cell Res., 141: 503-508.

[130] Schleef, R. R., Bevilacqua, M. J., Sawdey, M., Gimbrone, M. A., and Loskutoff, D. J. (1988) Cytokine activation of vascular endothelium Effect on tissue-type plasminogen activator and type 1 plasminogen activator inhibitor. J. Biol. Chem., 263: 5797-5803.

[131] Schrauwen, Y., de Vries, R.E.M., Kooistra T. and Emeis, J.J. (1994) Acute release of tissue-type plasminogen activator (t-PA) from the endothelium; regulatory mechanisms and therapeutic target. Fibrinolysis 8 (suppl.2): 8-12.

[132] Shalaby, F., Rossant, J., Yamaguchi, T.P., Gertsenstein, M., Wu, X-F., Breitman, M.L. and Schuh, A.C. (1995) Failure of blood-island formation and vasculogenesis in flk-1-deficient mice. Nature 376: 62-66.

[133] Slomp, J., Gittenberger-de Groot, A.C., van Munsteren, J.C., Huysmans, H.A., van Bockel, J.H., van Hinsbergh, V.W.M. and Poelmann, R.E. (1996) Nature and origin of the neointima in whole vessel wall organ culture of the human saphenous vein. Virchows Arch. 428: 59-67.

[134] Sprengers, E.D. and Kluft, C. (1987) Plasminogen activator inhibitors, Blood 69: 381-387.

[135] Suffredini, A.F., Harpel, P.C. and Parrillo, J.E. (1989) Promotion and subsequent inhibition of plasminogen activation after administration of intravenous endotoxin to normal subjects, N. Engl. J. Med. 320: 1165-1172.

[136] Thiagarajan, P., Rippon, A.J., and Farrell, D.H., 1996, Alternative adhesion sites in human fibrinogen for vascular endothelial cells. Biochemistry 35: 4169-4175.

[137] Thompson, E.A., Nelles, L., and Collen, D., 1991, Effect of retinoic acid on the synthesis of tissue-type plasminogen activator and plasminogen activator inhibitor-1 in human endothelial cells, Eur. J. Biochem. 201: 627-632.

[138] Thompson, J.A., Anderson, K.D., DiPietro, J.M., Zwiebel, J.A., Zametta, M., Anderson, W.F. and Maciag, T., 1988, Site-directed neovessel formation in vivo. Science 241: 1349-1352.

[139] Unemori, E.N., Bouhana, K.S. and Werb, Z. (1990) Vectorial secretion of extracellular matrix proteins, matrix-degrading proteinases, and tissue inhibitor of metalloproteinases by endothelial cells. J. Biol Chem. 265: 445-451.

[140] Van Bennekum, A.M., Emeis, J.J., Kooistra, T., and Hendriks, H.F.J., 1993, Modulation of tissue-type plasminogen activator by retinoids in rat plasma and tissues, Am. J. Physiol. 264: R931-R937.

[141] Van den Eijnden-Schrauwen, Y., Kooistra, T., De Vries, R. E. M., and Emeis, J. J. (1995) Studies on the acute release of tissue-type plasminogen activator from human endothelial cells in vitro and in rats in vivo: Evidence for a dynamic storage pool. Blood, 85: 3510-3517.

[142] Van Deventer, S.J.H., Büller, H.R., Ten Cate, J.W., Aarden, L.A., Hack, E. and Sturk, A. (1990) Experimental endotoxemia in humans: analysis of cytokine release and coagulation, fibrinolytic, and complement pathways, Blood 76: 2520-2526.

[143] Van Hinsbergh, V. W. M. (1992) Impact of endothelial activation on fibrinolysis and local proteolysis in tissue repair. Ann. N. Y. Acad. Sci., 667: 151-162.

[144] Van Hinsbergh, V.W.M., Kooistra, T., Van den Berg, E.A., Princen, H.M.G., Fiers, W. and Emeis, J.J. (1988) Tumor necrosis factor increases the production of plasminogen activator inhibitor in human endothelial cells in vitro and in rats in vivo. Blood 72: 1467-1473.

[145] Van Hinsbergh, V. W. M., van den Berg, E. A., Fiers, W., and Dooijewaard, G. (1990a) Tumor necrosis factor induces the production of urokinase-type plasminogen activator by human endothelial cells. Blood, 75: 1991-1998.

[146] Van Hinsbergh, V. W. M., Bauer, K. A., Kooistra, T., Kluft, C., Dooijewaard, G., Sherman, M. L., and Nieuwenhuizen, W. (1990b) Progress of fibrinolysis during tumor necrosis factor infusions in humans Concomitant increase in tissue-type plasminogen activator, plasminogen activator inhibitor type-I, and fibrin(ogen) degradation products. Blood, 76: 2284-2289.

[147] Van Hinsbergh, V.W.M., Vermeer, M., Koolwijk, P., Grimbergen, J., and Kooistra, T. (1994) Genistein reduces tumor necrosis factor α -induced plasminogen activator inhibitor-1 transcription but not urokinase expression in human endothelial cells. Blood 84: 2984-2991.

[148] Van Hinsbergh, V.W.M., Koolwijk, P., and Hanemaaijer, R. (1997) Role of fibrin and plasminogen activators in repair-associated angiogenesis: In vitro studies with human endothelial cells., in: "Regulation of Angiogenesis", I.D.Goldberg and E.M. Rosen, eds., pp.391-411, Birkhauser Verlag, Basel.

[149] Vassalli, J-D. (1994) The urokinase receptor. Fibrinolysis, 8: 172-181.

[150] Wei, Y., Waltz, D., Rao, N., Drummond, R., Rosenberg, S., and Chapman, H. (1994) Identification of the urokinase receptor as cell adhesion receptor for vitronectin. J. Biol. Chem., 269: 32380-32388.

[151] Weinberg, J.B., Pippen, A.M.M and Greenberg, C.S. (1991) Extravascular fibrin formation and dissolution in synovial tissue of patients with osteoarthitis and rheumatoid arthritis. Arthitis Rheum. 34: 996-1005.

[152] Wijnberg, M.J., Quax, P.H.A., Nieuwenbroek, N.M.E., Verheijen, J.H. (1997). The migration of human smooth muscle cells in vitro is mediated by plasminogen activation and can be inhibited by alpha-2-macroglobulin receptor associated protein. Thromb. Haemostas. 78: 880-886.

[153] Wohlwend, A., Belin, D. and Vassalli, J-D. (1987) Plasminogen activator-specific inhibitors produced by human monocytes/macrophages, J. Exp. Med. 165: 320-339 (1987).

[154] Wun, T-C. and Capuano, A. (1985) Spontaneous fibrinolysis in whole human plasma. Identification of tissue activator-related protein as the major plasminogen activator causing spontaneous activity in vitro, J. Biol. Chem. 260: 5061-5066.

[155] Wyne, K.L., Pathak, R.K., Seabra, M.C., and Hobbs, H.H. (1996) Expression of the VLDL receptor in endothelial cells. Arterioscl. Thromb. Vasc. Biol. 16: 407-415.

[156] Wei, Y., Lukashev, M., Simon, D.I., Bodary, S.C., Rosenberg, S., Doyle, M.V. and Chapman, H.A. (1996) Regulation of integrin function by the urokinase receptor. Science 273:1551-1555.

Vascular Endothelium: Mechanisms of Cell Signaling
J.D. Catravas et al. (Eds.)
IOS Press, 1999

ENDOTHELIAL CELL MATRIX INTERACTIONS

Philip G. de Groot & Inge W.G. Bobbink

Department of Haematology, University Medical Centre Utrecht
PO Box 85500
3508 GA Utrecht, The Netherlands

Abstract

Maintenance of the integrity of the vessel wall is one of the most important functions of the vascular endothelium. The subendothelium, a protein rich matrix underneath the endothelial cells, is crucial in the preservation of the optimal endothelial cell functioning. The matrix contributes to the maintenance of an intact endothelial cell layer by the interaction between specific receptors on the endothelial cell membrane and specific matrix ligands in the substratum. These interactions are responsible not only for keeping up the polarity of the cells and the maintenance of an non-permeable barrier for a number of blood components, they are also involved in the regulation of cell spreading and cell proliferation. In this overview the interactions between matrix and endothelial cells is discussed on the basis of vascular complications present in diabetes mellitus.

1. Introduction

The maintenance of the integrity of the vascular wall is essential in the prevention of the process of atherosclerosis. The integrity of the vascular wall is predominantly determined by the presence of an intact and healthy endothelial layer covering the luminal side of the vessel. The interaction between endothelial cells and their substratum, the endothelial cell matrix, is an important determinant of the delicate pro-and antithrombotic balance accomplished by the endothelium, in maintaining the polarity of the cells, preserving the permeability layer between blood and tissue and for the re-endothelization after injury.

The extracellular matrix produced by cultured endothelial cells has been shown to contain a large series of adhesive proteins such as fibronectin, vitronectin, thrombospondin, laminin, von Willebrand factor and various types of collagen. Besides proteins the matrix also contains a number of proteoglycans. The adhesive proteins present in the matrix directly interact via specific receptors with the covering endothelial cells, thereby influencing the function of the cells. One of the endothelial cell functions is to prevent the direct contact between the flowing blood and the underlying subendothelium. The process of vascular subendothelial biosynthesis, assembly and the regulation in vivo is poorly understood. Almost all studies on the assembly of the subendothelium are performed in vitro. In vitro cultures of endothelial cells have the disadvantage that the studies are performed with proliferating endothelial cells or cells that have recently been proliferating. In vivo almost all the endothelial cells are of a non-proliferating phenotype. A growing cell produces a completely different matrix compared to a quiescent cell. Results of in vitro experiments could not be translated easily into the in vivo situation.

While the endothelial cells express a large number of anti-thrombotic properties, the underlying subendothelium is highly thrombogenic. In this review the influence of the matrix composition on endothelial cell function is discussed on the basis of vascular complications present in diabetes mellitus. The influence of endothelial cells on matrix composition is discussed with von Willebrand factor as example. Von Willebrand factor in the matrix plays an important role in the interaction of blood platelets with the vessel wall. Finally some general remarks will be made on the mechanism by which platelets interact with the vessel wall.

2. The Influence Of The Composition of the Matrix on Endothelial Cell Adhesion, Shape and Proliferation

Vascular disease involving both the micro-and macrovasculature is one of the main complications of diabetes mellitus. Morbidity and mortality in diabetes mellitus are mainly caused by its vascular complications. Hyperglycation is known to be an important factor in the development of the vascular complications [1]. One of the main mechanisms proposed to explain the effects of hyperglycaemia on vascular cell damage is the non-enzymatic glycation of proteins. Non-enzymatic glycation of proteins is the chemical reaction between a reducing sugar and a protein. Glycation begins with the covalent attachment of glucose to reactive free amino groups from lysine residues in proteins. The reactivity of a particular sugar depends on the fraction of the sugar in the aldehyde form. The product of this step is a Schiff base that can undergo Amadori rearrangements to form the more stable Amadori-type early glycosylation products. This reaction is reversible and the rate at which the early glycation products are formed is proportional to the glucose concentration and time. These early glycation products slowly undergo a series of complex irreversible chemical rearrangements resulting in a heterologous group of compounds, known as advanced glycated end products (AGEs) [2]. AGE formation is irreversible and it primarily affects macromolecules with long half lives, such as haemoglobin and extracellular matrix components. These matrix components are therefor subject to accumulation of glycated products. Adhesive proteins present in the matrix exert a regulatory function on the overlying cells and changes in the structure of these proteins or composition of the matrix may therefor influence cellular properties. Therefore we investigated the effect of glycation of the extracellular matrix of endothelial cell function.

In vitro incubation of endothelial cell matrices with glucose or glucose-6-phosphate resulted in a time and concentration dependent degree of glycation of the matrix. Endothelial cell adhesion to these glycated endothelial cell matrices was significantly reduced compared to non-glycated matrices. Additionally, mean cell size of adhered cells was reduced up to 40% at the highest level of matrix glycation, indicating a severe impaired endothelial cell spreading. Proliferation of endothelial cells on glycated matrices was retarded compared to non-glycated matrices. Analysis of cell-cycle progression revealed that endothelial cell entrance into S-phase was impaired. Experiments with purified glycated matrix proteins (fibronectin, vitronectin, von Willebrand factor, laminin and collagen) indicate that the decrease in endothelial cell adhesion, spreading and proliferation may result from glycation of vitronectin [3].

The effects of glycated adhesive proteins on EC biology may be induced by an altered interaction of glycated adhesive proteins in the matrix with their specific transmembrane receptors on the EC-surface. The matrix is known to be an important regulator of cell shape [4]. Adhesion of cells to the matrix induces changes in cytoskeletal organization, involving polymerization and changes in actin filament distribution. Since the cytoskeleton is the major determinant of cell shape [5], the cytoskeleton rearrangements will affect the cell shape. The link between matrix and the cytoskeleton is provided among others by integrins on the cell surface which mediate outside-in as well as inside-out signalling. Interaction of endothelial cell integrins with their specific adhesive proteins in the matrix could be profoundly impaired by glycation of these proteins. Glycation induced changes in protein structure as a consequence of modification of lysines in the cell attachment site or flanking regions in the molecule may impair integrin interaction by a hampered recognition of the RGD-sequence as a consequence of sterical hindrance. Furthermore, non-integrin-dependent cell adhesion is mediated by heparin-binding domains in matrix proteins that often contain many lysine residues. Thus both in integrin dependent and non integrin-dependent cell adhesion, glycation may lead to a decrease in density of cell-matrix contacts and rounding up of the cells.

Endothelial cell attachment to vitronectin is mediated by both the RGD-sequence in vitronectin and a heparin binding domain at position 371-383 of the vitronectin sequence. Inhibition of endothelial cell adhesion to vitronectin with RGD-containing peptides resulted not only in decreased number of attached endothelial cells but also in a strongly decreased cell spreading. Inhibition with peptides which comprises the heparin binding site only results in less adhering cells not in a decreased cell spreading [6]. Most likely glycation of vitronectin results in a decreased interaction with the endothelial cell vitronectin receptor $\alpha_v\beta_3$. The decreased spreading of the cells may also explain the increased endothelial cell permeability associated with vascular dysfunction in diabetes.

Alterations in cytoskeleton organization are not only involved in determination of cellular shape, but also influence other cellular properties. A matrix-integrin action that reorganizes the cytoskeleton is necessary for the progression of cells through the cell-cycle. The enzymes that mediate cell-cycle progression through G1-phase are cyclin-dependent kinases. In anchorage-dependent cells, the induction of these cyclins is strongly dependent on signals from the matrix [7]. Since cell spreading is affected by glycation of the matrix, impaired integrin signalling can explain the impaired endothelial cell proliferation.

Cell adhesion to a substratum is not a static event, instead there is a continuous movement of cells along their substratum. This means that adhesive interactions of cells with the matrix have to be modulated continuously by proteolysis. This pericellular proteolysis, i.e. loosening of the cell-matrix interactions by partially degrading structural proteins in the matrix, is accomplished by the fibrinolytic system [8]. The activation of plasminogen to plasmin requires the presence of a macro molecular surface acting as a template that brings the enzyme (plasminogen activator) and substrate (plasminogen) in close proximity. This provides a well-designed mechanism for matrix proteins to localize pericellular proteolysis.

Vitronectin is not only an important adhesive extracellular matrix protein, it also plays a role in the plasminogen activating system. The plasminogen activating system is an enzyme cascade in which plasminogen is activated to plasmin by either tissue plasminogen activator (t-PA) or urokinase (u-PA). The efficiency of the system is strongly enhanced when the enzymes are immobilized on a macromolecular surface. The most well known template is fibrin. Vitronectin can also fulfil the template function for plasminogen activation, it binds both plasminogen and plasminogen activators [9]. Both plasminogen and plasminogen activator bind with much higher affinity to glycated vitronectin compared to non-glycated vitronectin. This leads to an increased generation of plasmin on glycated vitronectin compared to non-glycated vitronectin. Increased plasmin formation may lead to increased degradation of matrix proteins. Whether this increased matrix remodeling plays a role in the altered endothelial cellular functions remains to be established.

3. The Influence of the Cells on the Deposition of Matrix Proteins

Two different types of endothelial cell activation can be distinguished. Short-term activation by substances such as thrombin and histamine induce release of von Willebrand factor from endothelial cells which can bind to the matrix of the cells. A different type of activation is seen after stimulation of endothelial cells with tumor necrosis factor (TNF) or interleukin-1 [10]. Stimulation of endothelial cells with IL-1 or TNF resulted in a decreased amount of von Willebrand factor in the extracellular matrix after 2 to 3 days. IL-1 and TNF have little effect on the total level of synthesis of von Willebrand factor by endothelial cells. The decrease in von Willebrand factor in the matrix is due to an altered routing of the newly synthesized von Willebrand factor. Most of the newly synthesized von Willebrand factor is released to the medium or stored inside the Weibel-Palade bodies. After activation hardly any von Willebrand factor is deposited in the extracellular matrix. This makes the subendothelium less reactive for platelets.

In diabetic patients the plasma levels of von Willebrand factor are increased, just like a large number of other plasma markers for endothelial cell injury. In a study with 40 diabetic patients we found also increased plasma levels of ED-1 fibronectin (Fijnheer & de Groot, unpublished observations). ED-1 fibronectin is a cellular fibronectin which is synthesized by endothelial cells and fibroblast and which contains an extra type II connecting segment not present in plasma fibronectin [11]. Increased levels of ED-1 fibronectin indicate an increased metabolism of the subendothelium. Interestingly, there was a very high correlation between plasma levels of ED-1 fibronectin and von Willebrand factor in individual patients. When an individual patient has a high level of plasma von Willebrand he also has a high level of ED-1 fibronectin. The same correlation was not found between the plasma levels of E-selectin or thrombomodulin and von Willebrand factor in the same individual patients. This indicates that the increased level of plasma von Willebrand factor found in plasmas of diabetic patients may be the result of an altered endothelial cell matrix metabolism, von Willebrand factor and fibronectin synthesize by the cells and normally deposited in the matrix are (partly) released to the plasma under diabetic conditions.

Cultured endothelial cells and their extracellular matrix are often used as a model to study the interaction between blood platelets and the vessel wall. However, the culture conditions strongly influence the amount of von Willebrand factor in the matrix [12]. Not only the presence of growth factors but also passage number and time of confluence influence the amount of von Willebrand factor in the matrix. Keeping human umbilical vein endothelial cells confluent for two weeks in a 50% reduction of the amount of von Willebrand factor in the matrix. The observations suggest that growing cells synthesize more von Willebrand factor compared to quiescent cells and that a part of the extra von Willebrand factor synthesized by the proliferating cells is deposited in the matrix. It is understandable that growing cells produce more matrix proteins because there is a need for a new matrix on which the growing cells can optimally adhere. The matrix of cultured cells is thus a matrix of proliferating cells with other characteristics of quiescent cells.

The amount of von Willebrand factor in the matrix is one of the primary factors determining the reactivity of the matrix for platelets. The amount of von Willebrand factor correlated with the number of platelets adhering to the matrix. Thus when the matrix of endothelial cells is used for studies on platelet reactivity, standardized conditions regarding time in culture and culture conditions are essential.

4. The Matrix Composition and the Interaction of the Matrix with Blood Cells.

Platelet adhesion to a damaged vessel wall is the first step in haemostasis and thrombosis. Plug formation only occurs when platelets first adhere to subendothelial or connective tissue components. Platelet adhesion is also the first step in the development of a thrombus when subendothelial structures are exposed to the circulation after superficial injury of the vessel wall. Platelet adhesion is strongly dependent on the flow rate of the blood. Shear has a dominating effect on platelets adhesion by regulating the transport of the platelets to the vessel wall. Shear forces also act on an attached platelet and the affinity of a receptor on the platelet membrane must be high enough to withstand the shear forces. Up till recently it was thought that the interaction between platelet GPIb and von Willebrand factor was strong enough to prevent the withdrawn of platelets by the shear forces. Recently the view on the function of von Willebrand factor was changed from a adhesive protein with high affinity for platelets to a protein responsible for rolling of platelet on a surface. The slowing down of platelets is probably necessary to allow other receptors to interact with other matrix compounds. An improved mechanism of how platelets interact with subendothelial structures under conditions of flow is given.

After exposure of subendothelial cell structures to flowing blood the first event that occurs is the binding of plasma von Willebrand factor to collagen type I and III present in the subendothelium. Subsequently, platelets will adhere to von Willebrand factor via glycoprotein Ib. The interaction of a platelet via GPIb with von Willebrand factor is transient, it allows the platelet to roll over von Willebrand factor in the direction of flow. The rolling stops when the platelet interacts with collagen probably via VLA-2 ($\alpha_2\beta_1$, GPIaIIa). This interaction activates the platelet enough to allow enough to allow spreading of the platelet over the surface. The spreading of the platelet is stabilized via the interaction of GPIIbIIIa ($\alpha_{IIb}\beta_3$) on the platelet membrane and fibronectin present in the matrix. The affinity of a spread platelet for the matrix is high enough to withstand the shear forces of the blood and allows the building of a thrombus on this spread platelet. After spreading the platelet membrane receptor GPVI interacts with collagen and the platelet is activated. The adhered and activated platelet can bind fibrinogen via GPIIbIIa and von Willebrand factor via GPIb. Circulating platelets will bind to the platelet bound fibrinogen and von Willebrand factor and a thrombus is formed.

At lower shear rates of the blood platelets can adhere directly to matrix proteins such as fibronectin, laminin or thrombospondin. The next step then is the binding of plasma von Willebrand factor to the platelet membrane GPIb and the spreading of the platelet via the already mentioned mechanism. Besides activation of platelets by collagen via GPVI, platelets can also activated by thrombin via the thrombin receptor.

References

[1]   M. Brownlee. Nonenzymatic glycation of macromolecules. Prospects of pharmacologic modulation. *Ann. Rev. Med.* **46** (1995) 223-234
[2]   G. Means and M.Chang. Nonenzymatic glycation of proteins. Structure and function changes. *Diabetes* **31** (1982) 1-4

[3]   W.G. Bobbink, H.C. de Boer, W.L.H. Tekelenburg, J.D. Banga and Ph.G. de Groot.   Effect of
      extracellular matrix glycation on endothelial cell adhesion and spreading. *Diabetes* **46** (1997) 87-93
[4]   D. Gospodarowicz, G. Greenburg and C.R. Birdwell.   Determination of cellular shape by the
      extracellular matrix and its correlation with the control of cellular growth. *Cancer Res.* **38** (1978)
      4155-4171
[5]   A. Wang and D.A. Ingber.   Control of cytoskeletal mechanics by extracellular matrix, cell shape and
      mechanical tension. *Biophys. J.* **66** (1994) 2181-2189
[6]   H.C. de Boer, K.T. Preissner, B.N. Bouma and Ph.G. de Groot.   Internalization of vitronectin-
      trhombin-antithrombin III complexes by endothelial cells leads to deposition of the complex into the
      subendothelial matrix. *J. Biol. Chem.* **270** (1995) 30733-30740
[7]   R.K. Assoian. Anchorage-dependent cell cycle progression. *J Cell Biol.* **136** 1997) 1-4
[8]   C.S. He, S.M. Wilhelm, A.P. Pentland, B.L. Marmer, G.A. Grant, A.Z. Eisen and G.I. Goldberg.
      Tissue cooperation in the proteolytic cascade activating human interstitial collagenase. *Proc. Nat.*
      Acad. Sci. USA **86** (1989) 2623-2636
[9]   M.S. Stack, M. Gonzalez-Gronow and S.V. Pizzo.   Regulation of plasminogen activation by
      components of the extracellular matrix. *Biochemistry* **307** (1990) 4966-4970
[10] Ph.G. de Groot, J.H. reinders and J.J. Sixma. Perturbation of human endothelial cells by thrombin or
      PMA changes the reactivity of these extracellular matrix towards platelets.   *J. Cell. Biol.* **104** (1987)
      697-704
[11] A.R. Kornblihtt, K. Umezawa, K. Vibe-Petersen and E.E. Baralle.   Primary structure of human
      fibronectin: different spkicing may generate at least 10 polypeptides from a single gene. *EMBO J.* **4**
      (1985) 1755-1762
[12] Y.P. Wu, J.J. Sixma and Ph.G. de Groot. Cultured endothelial cells regulate platelet adhesion to their
      extracellular matrix by regulation its von Willebrand factor content. *Thromb. Haemostas.* **73** 91995)
      713-718

Vascular Endothelium: Mechanisms of Cell Signaling
J.D. Catravas et al. (Eds.)
IOS Press, 1999

ENDOTHELIAL CELL CONTROL OF PLATELET ACTIVATION: REGULATION OF SYNTHESIS AND SECRETION OF PROSTACYCLIN, NITRIC OXIDE AND VON WILLEBRAND FACTOR

Jeremy D. Pearson

Professor of Vascular Biology, King's College London, Campden Hill Road, London W8 7AH, U.K.

Abstract

Following vessel damage, endothelial cell properties are rapidly modulated to ensure that platelet activation and haemostatic plug formation occur efficiently at the site of the injury but do not lead to intravascular thrombosis. The main endothelium-derived mediators are von Willebrand Factor (vWF), prostacyclin (PGI_2) and nitric oxide (NO). Early studies demonstrated the importance of raised cytosolic Ca^{2+}, $[Ca^{2+}]_i$, in the signal transduction pathways leading to secretion of vWF, PGI_2 and NO in response to agonists such as thrombin. More recently, it has been shown that NO synthesis can occur due to influx of external Ca^{2+} in the absence of detectable elevations of $[Ca^{2+}]_i$. We have now shown that rapid activation of the p42 MAP kinase pathway occurs when endothelial cells are stimulated by thrombin or histamine, and that this pathway in conjunction with raised $[Ca^{2+}]_i$ is needed for PGI_2 synthesis, but not for NO synthesis. In contrast, sustained NO production in response to physical forces can be maintained in the absence of extracellular Ca^{2+} and apparently involves tyrosine phosphorylation signalling events in a manner that is not yet fully understood. Although thrombin and histamine are effective vWF secretagogues, other Ca^{2+}-mobilising agonists are not, indicating the existence of other as yet undefined signalling pathways, and recent reports suggest these can include activation of adenylyl cyclase. Thus despite substantial recent progress, the picture of receptor-linked and mechanically transduced mediator secretion by endothelial cells is not complete.

1. Introduction

Endothelial cells normally present a non-thrombogenic and anticoagulant surface to flowing blood. However, following vessel damage, their properties are rapidly modulated to ensure that platelet activation and haemostatic plug formation occur efficiently at the site of the injury but are strictly limited, and do not lead to intravascular thrombosis. The main endothelial mediators of platelet function are von Willebrand factor (vWF), prostacyclin (PGI$_2$), and nitric oxide (NO). vWF, a highly multimeric glycoprotein, is the primary cofactor for platelet adhesion to exposed collagen under flow conditions [1]. It is secreted by exocytosis from granular stores, notably in response to thrombin [2]. PGI$_2$ and NO are labile, synergistic, powerful inhibitors of platelet aggregation synthesised in response to stimuli that include platelet release products such as ATP, ADP and serotonin [3]. In addition to secreting modulators of platelet activation, the luminal plasma membrane of the endothelial cells constitutively expresses several integral membrane proteins that are important regulators of platelet activation and blood coagulation, including thrombomodulin [4] and ectonucleotidase enzymes [5]. The latter dephosphorylate ATP and ADP and contribute significantly to the antiplatelet actions of endothelium by inactivating the pro-aggregatory ADP [6].

2. Prostacyclin

Although it was the first described endothelium-derived inhibitor of platelet function [7] and powerful vasodilator [8], PGI$_2$ has been (perhaps unfairly) somewhat neglected since the discovery that NO is usually the major endothelium-derived relaxing factor (see below) and also potently inhibits platelet activation. The two mediators are often secreted concomitantly from endothelial cells in response to stimuli and are synergistic in their antiplatelet activity [9]. Direct elevation of intracellular Ca^{2+} concentration, $[Ca^{2+}]_i$, using a calcium ionophore, or increasing $[Ca^{2+}]_i$ in response to G protein-coupled agonists above a threshold value at least 5-fold higher than resting levels, triggers PGI$_2$ release. It was demonstrated that this rise in $[Ca^{2+}]_i$ was necessary and sufficient to explain PGI$_2$ production in response to agonists [10,11], and together with evidence that synthesis of PGI$_2$ from exogenous arachidonic acid did not involve a rise in $[Ca^{2+}]_i$ it was concluded that activation of phospholipase (PL) A$_2$ by Ca^{2+} was the sole signalling pathway controlling PGI$_2$ synthesis. There are two components to the rise in $[Ca^{2+}]_i$ due to agonists: a short-lived peak caused by release of Ca^{2+} from internal stores and a consequential entry of Ca^{2+} across the plasma membrane that is longer-lived in the continuing presence of the agonist. PGI$_2$ release is short-lived and relatively insensitive to removal of extracellular Ca^{2+}, showing that store release is the important component.

   The possibility that other second messenger systems may be involved in controlling PGI$_2$ synthesis was first raised by finding that deliberate activation of protein kinase (PK) C with phorbol esters was capable of enhancing agonist-driven PGI$_2$ production despite a concomitant reduction in Ca^{2+} mobilisation [12]. Indeed, prolonged treatment with phorbol ester alone causes gradual PGI$_2$ release in the absence of any detectable change in $[Ca^{2+}]_i$. These results strongly suggest that phosphorylation events alter the Ca^{2+}-dependence of PLA$_2$. However, PKC activation is unlikely to contribute to the extent of agonist-induced PGI$_2$ synthesis, since PKC inhibitors have no effect.

   More recent experiments, however, have implicated the p42 mitogen activated protein kinase (MAPK) as an equally critical signal as elevated $[Ca^{2+}]_i$ in PGI$_2$ production. We found that tyrosine protein kinase inhibitors could block agonist-stimulated PGI$_2$ release without inhibiting Ca^{2+} mobilisation [13]. By immunoblotting several major bands were noted to be rapidly and transiently phosphorylated in response to agonists such as thrombin or histamine, including one of 42 kDa which was identified as p42 MAPK. Inhibiting phosphorylation and activation of p42 MAPK by selective inhibition of the upstream kinase (MEK) with PD98059 inhibited phosphorylation of PLA$_2$ and reduced PGI$_2$ synthesis in parallel [14]. Similar results were concurrently reported by another group [15], and at the same time it was shown that endothelial p42 MAPK activation caused the phosphorylation of PLA_2, while the agonist-stimulated rise in $[Ca^{2+}]_i$ caused translocation of PLA_2 from cytosol to membranes (primarily the nuclear membrane) [16]. Thus, the translocation and activation of PLA_2, allowing the production of arachidonate from membrane phospholipids as the rate-limiting step in eicosanoid synthesis, is under the dual control of cytosolic $[Ca^{2+}]$ and phosphorylation of p42 MAPK. Activation of MAPK alone is insufficient to trigger substantial PGI_2 synthesis, since cytokines such as IL-1 and TNF efficiently phosphorylate p42 MAPK [17] but do not elevate $[Ca^{2+}]_i$ and cause only slow and weak production of PGI_2 (R. Houliston, C. Wheeler-Jones & J.D. Pearson; unpublished data).

3. Nitric Oxide

Nitric oxide, first described as EDRF [18], is synthesised in endothelial cells from arginine by a Ca^{2+}/calmodulin-dependent isoform of NO synthase [19,20]. It is produced, like PGI_2, in response to Ca^{2+}-mobilising agonists, and as noted above, can act synergistically with PGI_2 [9]. However, endothelial NO synthase is fully activated by $[Ca^{2+}]_i$ that are perhaps only 3-fold above resting levels [21], i.e. levels that are alone too low to induce PGI_2 release. As a consequence, NO production can be prolonged by comparison with PGI_2 synthesis, since $[Ca^{2+}]_i$ elevation due to entry across the plasma membrane is sufficient; indeed agonist-induced NO production, unlike PGI_2 synthesis, is abolished in the absence of external Ca^{2+} [22]. Recently, Lantoine et al have extended these findings to demonstrate that agonist-induced release of Ca^{2+} from internal stores does not cause NO release, while entry of Ca^{2+} across the plasma membrane directly controls NO synthesis [23]. These authors therefore favour a model in which NO synthase is in a local microenvironment just beneath the plasma membrane and preferentially utilises Ca^{2+} that crosses the plasma membrane rather than Ca^{2+} from the bulk cytosolic pool. As discussed elsewhere in this volume (see chapters by Schnitzer, Sessa and Venema) there is now considerable evidence that endothelial caveolae form the appropriate microenvironment, where arginine transporters and NO synthase are colocalised, consistent with our original finding that agonist-induced NO release is accompanied by a transient increase in arginine uptake despite the presence of sufficient cytosolic arginine to saturate NO synthase [24].

There is also increasing interest in how NO production can be modulated by protein phosphorylation events. A major physiological regulator of endothelium-dependent vasodilatation is altered shear stress, and several groups have now reported that induction of NO release by shear stress occurs independently of a sustained elevation in $[Ca^{2+}]_i$ and is sensitive to modulators of tyrosine phosphorylation [25-27]. Although a variety of specific novel protein-protein interactions that can affect NO synthase localisation and activity have recently been described [e.g. 28-31], and longer-term serine phosphorylation of NO synthase has been demonstrated in response to shear [32], the direct basis for Ca^{2+}-insensitive maintenance of NO synthesis remains to be elucidated. A plausible explanation is that altered interactions with other proteins leads to much tighter binding of Ca^{2+}/calmodulin to NO synthase, rendering the enzyme insensitive to external Ca^{2+} by the same mechanism as in the inducible NO synthase isoform, though this has not been demonstrated.

4. Von Willebrand Factor

Plasma vWF, which is responsible for carrying coagulation Factor VIII, is derived from endothelial cells, and circulating levels are maintained primarily by constitutive secretion, which can be modulated in response to agents such as cytokines [2]. In contrast, highly multimerised vWF, stored in endothelial granules (Weibel-Palade bodies) and released by triggered exocytosis, is required for adequate local control of haemostasis. Like PGI_2 synthesis, vWF exocytosis can be induced by calcium ionophores, and requires elevation of $[Ca^{2+}]_i$; it additionally requires extracellular Ca^{2+} [33-35]. Raised $[Ca^{2+}]_i$ alone does not seem to be sufficient to activate exocytosis, because while certain Ca^{2+}-mobilising agonists (thrombin, histamine, peptido-leukotrienes) are potent and effective, others (bradykinin, ATP) are weak or inactive vWF secretagogues [36,37].

We therefore sought evidence of other signal transduction pathways that contribute to agonist-induced vWF secretion. Activation of protein kinase C with phorbol esters induces vWF release [38], and the response is synergistically enhanced by elevation of $[Ca^{2+}]_i$. However, selective inhibition of protein kinase C does not reduce agonist-induced vWF secretion [36]. Similarly, protein tyrosine kinase inhibitors are inactive [14]. Thus these two signalling pathways do not appear to play a role.

Recently, it has been shown that several agonists capable of raising $[cAMP]_i$, or cell-permeable cAMP analogues, induce vWF secretion, albeit relatively weakly, and can potentiate the secretory response to other agonists [39-42]. It is therefore likely that protein kinase A activation contributes to the physiological control of vWF exocytosis, though there is no evidence that this pathway is activated by thrombin or histamine.

In attempts to investigate the control of vWF secretion more directly, we and other groups have used permeabilised endothelial cells [43-45]. In an electropermeabilised cell system, where the plasma membrane was rendered freely permeable to molecules of molecular mass up to about 1 kDa, we found similar dose response curves for Ca^{2+}-driven PGI_2 synthesis and vWF secretion, which were in the same range as agonist-induced $[Ca^{2+}]_i$ changes in intact cells [44]. Considerable vWF secretion occurred in the absence of ATP, but it was further enhanced when ATP was repleted [44], suggesting that a fraction of secretion took place from granules already primed for exocytosis or docked at the plasma membrane [46]. To study the expected involvement of small GTP-binding proteins in exocytosis, we added the stable GTP analog GTPγS. This, surprisingly, did enhance Ca^{2+}-drive PGI_2 synthesis, but did not affect vWF secretion [44]. More recently, Fayos and Wattenberg [45], using digitonin-permeabilised cells, noted that GTPγS could stimulate vWF secretion in the absence of added Ca^{2+} , though the effect was not apparent in the presence of Ca^{2+}. They also found that secretion was dependent on a thiol-sensitive cytosolic component, consistent with known vesicular transport mechanisms. Our experiments with permeabilised cells also support the possible involvement of protein kinase A, since addition of a cAMP analogue in the place of ATP enhanced Ca^{2+}-driven secretion (J. Frearson & J.D. Pearson; unpublished results).

5. Conclusions

Thrombin, generated as blood coagulation is initiated, and products secreted in high local concentrations from granular stores in activated platelets (ATP, ADP, serotonin) each act at G protein-coupled receptors on the endothelial surface to cause, as a primary intracellular signal, mobilisation of cytosolic Ca^{2+} from intracellular stores, and the consequent capacitative entry of Ca^{2+} across the plasma membrane. The importance of Ca^{2+} signalling in the control of PGI_2 and NO synthesis and vWF secretion was recognised rapidly, but the involvement of additional or alternative signal transduction pathways is still being explored. Rapid activation of the p42 MAPK pathway by G protein-coupled agonists has only been described in the last five years, and it is now apparent that this is an integral component, probably acting in parallel with elevated $[Ca^{2+}]_i$, of the acute control of PLA_2 activity and hence PGI_2 synthesis in endothelium. Other functions of the transient activation of p42 MAPK are less obvious: while it may contribute to the reported mitogenic effects of agonists such as thrombin, it is apparently not involved in NO synthesis or vWF secretion.

The hydrolysis of arachidonate from phospholipids, the rate-limiting step in eicosanoid synthesis, occurs when PLA_2 is translocated from cytosol primarily to intracellular membranes. By contrast, although a fraction of endothelial NO synthase is detectable in the Golgi compartment, there is good evidence that NO production mainly occurs close to plasma membrane. This is consistent with the relative importance of Ca^{2+} influx as a primary regulator of NO production. The ability of shear stress to convert endothelial NO synthase into a Ca^{2+}-insensitive enzyme is intriguing, and has recently been mimicked by the use of phenylarsine oxide, a tyrosine phosphatase inhibitor [27], but remains poorly understood despite the increasing number of potentially regulatory protein-protein interactions with NO synthase that have been described. Whatever the mechanism may be, it must be rapidly reversible.

Acute vWF secretion has apparently an absolute requirement for elevated $[Ca^{2+}]_i$ and for external Ca^{2+}, which is in common with exocytic secretion in other cell types. However, unless there is an as yet unrecognised spatial or quantitative difference between the capacity of different phospholipase Cß-coupled agonists to mobilise Ca^{2+}, other signalling pathways must be important to account for the selective secretagogue ability of thrombin and histamine. Pathways involving protein kinase C (at least the conventional isoforms) or tyrosine protein kinases seem to be irrelevant. The ability of agonists such as epinephrine to stimulate vWF secretion, albeit weakly, implicates protein kinase A, but thrombin does not raise intracellular cAMP levels [42], indicating the likely involvement of a further signalling pathways. In experiments with wortmannin, we found no evidence for a role for PI-3-kinase (C. Wheeler-Jones & J.D. Pearson; unpublished results).

In summary, the signal transduction events leading to the rapid secretion of a series of powerful haemostatic mediators from endothelial cells in response to local vessel damage and platelet activation overlap, particularly in their requirement for Ca^{2+}. However, they each additionally involve distinct pathways that are not yet fully delineated, but are the focus of current research. This research is likely to yield results with wider cell biological impact, relating for example to the importance of spatially compartmentalised reaction sequences in biochemical control (NO synthesis) and to the mechanisms regulating exocytosis (vWF secretion).

References

[1]   P.G. De Groot and J.J. Sixma. Platelet-vessel wall interactions. *Vascular Medicine Review 1993; 4: 145-155.*

[2]   E.M. Paleolog, M.A. Carew, J.A. Frearson, C.P.D. Wheeler-Jones and J.D. Pearson. Modulation of secretion of von Willebrand factor from endothelial cells. *Chapter 7 in "Modern Visualisation of the Endothelium" ed. J. Polak, Harwood, 1998, pp. 151-161.*

[3]   J.D. Pearson and C.P.D. Wheeler-Jones.   Platelet - endothelial cell interactions: regulation of prostacyclin and von Willebrand factor secretion. *In "New horizons in vascular endothelium: physiology, pathology and therapeutic opportunities"*, eds. G.V.R. Born and C.J. Schwartz, Schattauer, 1997, pp. 157-166.

[4]   C.T. Esmon.   Thrombomodulin as a model for molecular mechanisms that modulate protease specificity and function at the vessel surface. *FASEB Journal 1995, 9: 956-955.*

[5]   H. Zimmermann and J.D. Pearson.   Extracellular metabolism of nucleotides and adenosine in the cardiovascular system. *In "Cardiovascular biology of purines"* eds. G. Burnstock , J.C. Dobson, B.T. Liang and J. Linden, Kluwer, 1998, in press.

[6]   A.J. Marcus, L.B. Safier, K.A. Hajjar, H.L. Ullman, N. Islam, M.J. Broekman and A.M. Eiroa. Inhibition of platelet-function by an aspirin-insensitive endothelial-cell ADPase - Thromboregulation by endothelial cells. *Journal of Clinical Investigation 1991; 88: 1690-1696.*

[7]   D.E. MacIntyre, J.D. Pearson and J.L. Gordon.   Localisation and stimulation of prostacyclin production in vascular cells. *Nature 1978; 271: 549-551.*

[8]   S. Moncada, R.J. Gryglewski, S. Bunting and J.R. Vane. An enzyme isolated from arteries transforms prostaglandin endoperoxides to an unstable substance that inhibits platelet aggregation. *Nature 1976; 263: 633-635.*

[9]   M.W. Radomski, R.M.J. Palmer and S. Moncada.   Comparative pharmacology of endothelium-derived relaxing factor, nitric oxide and prostacyclin in platelets. *British Journal of Pharmacology 1987; 92: 181-187.*

[10]   T.J. Hallam, J.D. Pearson and L.A. Needham.   Thrombin-stimulated elevation of human endothelial cell cytoplasmic free calcium concentration causes prostacyclin production. *Biochemical Journal 1988; 251: 243-249.*

[11]   E.A. Jaffe, J. Grulich, B.B. Weksler, G. Hampel and K. Watanabe.   Correlation between thrombin-induced prostacyclin production and inositol trisphosphate and cytosolic free calcium levels in cultured human endothelial cells. *Journal of Biological Chemistry 1987; 262: 8557-8565*

[12]   T.D. Carter, T.J. Hallam and J.D. Pearson.   Protein kinase C activation alters the sensitivity of agonist-stimulated endothelial cell prostacyclin production to intracellular Ca^{2+}. *Biochemical Journal 1989; 262:431-437.*

[13]   C.P.D. Wheeler-Jones, M.J. May, A.J. Morgan and J.D. Pearson.   Protein tyrosine kinases regulate agonist-stimulated prostacyclin release but not von Willebrand factor secretion from human umbilical vein endothelial cells. *Biochemical Journal 1996; 315: 407-416.*

[14]   C.P.D. Wheeler-Jones , R. Houliston, M.J. May and J.D. Pearson.   Inhibition of MAP kinase kinase (MEK) blocks endothelial PGI_2 release but has no effect on von Willebrand factor secretion or E-selectin expression. *FEBS Letters 1996; 388: 180-184.*

[15]   V. Patel, C. Brown, A. Goodwin, N. Wilkie and M.R. Boarder.   Phosphorylation and activation of p42 and p44 mitogen-activated protein-kinase are required for the P2 purinoceptor stimulation of endothelial prostacyclin production. *Biochemical Journal 1996; 320: 221-226.*

[16]   H. Kan, Y. Ruan and K.U. Malik.   Involvement of mitogen-activated protein-kinase and translocation of cytosolic phospholipase A(2) to the nuclear-envelope in acetylcholine-induced prostacyclin synthesis in rabbit coronary endothelial cells. *Molecular Pharmacology 1996; 50: 1139-1147.*

[17]   M.J. May, C.P.D. Wheeler-Jones, R. Houliston and J.D. Pearson.   Activation of p42[mapk] in human umbilical vein endothelial cells by interleukin-1α and tumour necrosis factor -α. *American Journal of Physiology 1998; 274: C789-C798.*

[18]   R.F. Furchgott and J.V. Zawadzki.   The obligatory role of endothelial cells in the relaxation of arterial smooth muscle by acetylcholine. *Nature 1980; 288: 373-376.*

[19]   R.M.J. Palmer, D.S. Ashton and S. Moncada.   Vascular endothelial cells synthesise nitric oxide from L-arginine. *Nature 1998; 333: 664-666.*

[20]   I. Fleming, J. Bauersachs and R. Busse.   Calcium-dependent and calcium-independent activation of the endothelial NO synthase. *Journal of Vascular Research 19097; 34: 165-174.*

[21]   A. Mülsch, E. Bassenge and R. Busse.   Nitric oxide synthesis in endothelial cytosol: evidence for a calcium-dependent and a calcium-independent mechanism. *Naunyn Schmiedebergs Archives of Pharmacology 1989; 340: 767-770.*

[22]   C.J. Long and T.W. Stone.   The release of endothelium-derived relaxant factor is calcium-dependent. *Blood Vessels 1985; 22: 205-208.*

[23]   F. Lantoine, L. Iouzalen, M-A. Devynck, E. Millanvoye-van Brussel and M. David-Dufilho.   Nitric oxide production in human endothelial cells stimulated by histamine requires Ca^{2+} influx. *Biochemical Journal 1998; 330: 695-699.*

[24] R.G. Bogle, S.B. Coade, S. Moncada, J.D. Pearson and G.E. Mann. Bradykinin and ATP stimulate L-arginine uptake and nitric oxide release in vascular endothelial cells. *Biochemical and Biophysical Research Communications 1991; 180: 926-932.*

[25] W.C. O'Neill. Flow-mediated NO release from endothelial cells is independent of K+ channel activation or intracellular Ca^{2+}. *American Journal of Physiology 1995; 269: C863-C869.*

[26] K. Ayajiki, M. Kindermann, M. Hecker, I. Fleming and R. Busse. Intracellular pH and tyrosine phosphorylation but not calcium determine shear stress-induced nitric oxide production in native endothelial cells. *Circulation Research 1996; 78: 750-758.*

[27] I. Fleming, J Bauersachs, B Fisslthaler and R Busse. Ca^{2+}-independent activation of the endothelial nitric oxide synthase in response to tyrosine phosphatase inhibitors and fluid shear stress. *Circulation Research 1998; 82: 686-695.*

[28] V.J. Venema, M.B. Marrero and R.C. Venema. Bradykinin-stimulated protein tyrosine phosphorylation promotes endothelial nitric oxide synthase translocation to the cytoskeleton. *Biochemical and Biophysical Research Communications 1996; 226: 703-710.*

[29] H. Ju, R. Zou, V.J. Venema and R.C. Venema. Direct association of endothelial nitric oxide synthase and caveolin-1 inhibits synthase activity. *Journal of Biological Chemistry 1997; 272: 18522-18525.*

[30] G. Garcia-Cardena, R. Fan, D.F. Stern, J. Liu and W.C. Sessa. Endothelial nitric oxide synthase is regulated by tyrosine phosphorylation and interacts with caveolin-1. *Journal of Biological Chemistry 1996; 271: 27237-27240.*

[31] G. Garcia-Cardena, R. Fan, V. Shah, R. Sorrention, G. Cirino, A. Papapetropoulos and W.C. Sessa. Dynamic activation of endothelial nitric oxide synthase by Hsp90. *Nature 1998; 392: 821-824.*

[32] M.A. Corson, N.L. James, S.E. Latta, R.M. Nerem, B.C. Berk and D.G. Harrison. Phosphorylation of endothelial nitric oxide synthase in response to fluid shear stress. *Circulation Research 1996; 79: 975-972.*

[33] C. Loesberg, M.D. Gonsalves, J. Zandbergen, C. Nillems, W.G. van Aken, H. Stel, J.A. van Mourik and P.G. de Groot. The effect of calcium on the secretion of factor VIII-related antigen by cultured human endothelial cells. *Biochimica et Biophysica Acta 1983; 763: 160-168.*

[34] L.A. Sporn, V.J. Marder and D.D. Wagner. Inducible secretion of large biologically potent von Willebrand factor multimers. *Cell 1986; 46: 185-190.*

[35] K.K. Hamilton and P.J. Sims. Changes in cytosolic Ca^{2+} associated with von Willebrand factor release in human endothelial cells exposed to histamine. *Journal of Clinical Investigation 1987; 79: 600-608.*

[36] M.A. Carew, E.M. Paleolog and J.D. Pearson. The roles of protein kinase C and intracellular Ca^{2+} in the secretion of von Willebrand factor from human vascular endothelial cells. *Biochemical Journal 1992; 286: 631-635.*

[37] Y.H. Datta, M. Romano, B.C. Jacobson, D.E. Golan, C.N. Serhan and B.M. Ewenstein. Peptido-leukotrienes are potent agonists of von Willebrand factor secretion and P-selectin surface expression in human umbilical vein endothelial cells. *Circulation 1995; 92: 3304-3311.*

[38] J.H. Reindeers, R.C. Vervoorn, C.L. Verweij, J.A. van Mourik and P.G. de Groot. Perturbation of cultured human vascular endothelial cells by phorbol ester on thrombin alters the cellular von Willebrand factor distribution. *Journal of Cellular Physiology 1987; 133: 79-81.*

[39] U.M. Vischer and C.B. Wollheim. Epinephrine induces von Willebrand factor release from cultured endothelial cells: Involvement of cyclic AMP-dependent signalling in exocytosis. *Thrombosis and Haemostasis 1997; 77: 1182-1188.*

[40] U.M. Vischer, U. Lang and C.B. Wollheim. Autocrine regulation of endothelial exocytosis: von Willebrand factor release is induced by prostacyclin in cultured endothelial cells. *FEBS Letters 1998; 424: 211-215.*

[41] U.M. Vischer and C.B. Wollheim. Purine nucleotides induce regulated secretion of von Willebrand factor: Involvement of cytosolic Ca^{2+} and cyclic adenosine monophosphate-dependent signalling in endothelial exocytosis. *Blood 1998; 91: 118-127.*

[42] R.J. Gegeman, Y. van den Eijnden-Schrauwen and J.J. Emeis. Adenosine 3':5'-cyclic monophosphate induces regulated secretion of tissue-type plasminogen activator and von Willebrand factor from cultured human endothelial cells. *Thrombosis and Haemostasis 1998; 79: 853-858.*

[43] K.A. Birch, J.S. Pober, G.B. Zavoico, A.R. Means and B.M. Ewenstein. Calcium/calmodulin transduces thrombin-stimulated secretion: studies in intact and minimally permeabilised human umbilical vein endothelial cells. *Journal of Cell Biology 1992; 118: 1501-1510.*

[44] .A. Frearson, P. Harrison, M.C. Scrutton and J.D. Pearson. Differential regulation of von Willebrand factor exocytosis and prostacyclin synthesis in electropermeabilised endothelial cell monolayers. *Biochemical Journal 1995; 309: 473-479.*

[45] B.E. Fayos and B.W. Wattenberg. Regulated exocytosis in vascular endothelial cells can be triggered by intracellular guanine nucleotides and requires a hydrophobic, thiol-sensitive component. Studies of regulated von Willebrand factor secretion from digitonin permeabilised endothelial cells. *Endothelium 1997; 5: 339-350.*

[46] J.C. Hay and T.F.J. Martin. Resolution of regulated secretion into sequential MgATP-dependent and calcium-dependent stages mediated by distinct cytosolic proteins. *Journal of Cell Biology 1992; 119: 39-151.*

Part VI

Angiogenesis/Metastases

Vascular Endothelium: Mechanisms of Cell Signaling
J.D. Catravas et al. (Eds.)
IOS Press, 1999

THROMBIN AS AN ANGIOGENIC FACTOR: PATHOPHYSIOLOGICAL IMPLICATIONS

Michael E. Maragoudakis and Nikos Tsopanoglou

Department of Pharmacology, Medical School, University of Patras
261 10 Rio Patras, Greece

Abstract

The original observation made by Trousseau in 1872 that there is an association between thrombosis and cancer has been confirmed by numerous clinical, laboratory, histopathological and pharmacological studies. These data can provide the basis for the molecular mechanisms and an explanation for the hypercoagulability observed in cancer patients. However, the mechanism by which blood coagulation promotes tumor growth and metastasis remains unknown. A plausible explanation might be our finding that thrombin is a potent promoter of angiogenesis, a process essential in solid tumor growth and metastasis. The angiogenic action of thrombin is specific, independent of fibrin formation and requires the active catalytic site of thrombin. A synthetic peptide (TRAP) that mimics many of the actions of the activated thrombin receptor is also angiogenic. Thrombin has a multitude of effects on a variety of cell types including endothelial cells, which are mediated through activation of thrombin receptor, and may contribute to the angiogenesis-promoting effect of thrombin. These effects of thrombin are discussed along with the transduction mechanisms involved. Speculations on the possible pathophysiological implications and potential therapeutic applications are suggested not only for tumor growth and metastasis but also for inflammation, wound healing, restenosis of vascular grafts etc.

1. Introduction

Numerous clinical, laboratory, histopathological and pharmacological studies have confirmed the original observations by Trousseau (1872), that there is an association between thrombosis and cancer [13]. These data provide an explanation for the molecular mechanisms involved for the hypercoagulability which is observed very frequently in cancer patients. For example it has been shown that many tumor cells elicit procoagulant activity directly or through interactions with platelets leukocytes and endothelial cells [14]. Using an immunohistochemical technique [20] have shown localisation of thrombin in tumor cells from small cell carcinoma of the lung, renal cell carcinomas, melanomas and also in macrophages of adenosarcoma and squamous cell sarcoma.

The generation of thrombin by tumors may also influence tumor progression and metastasis. Indeed, it has been shown that in animals tumor models thrombin dramatically increases lung colonies of B16 melanoma cells [10]. Pre-treatment of these cells with thrombin increased 156 fold the number of pulmonary metastasis. These results prompted the use of anticoagulants for antitumor effects and the success of experiments with animals led to clinical trials with warfarin on small cell lung carcinomas [16].

More recently in a large epidemiological study [15] have shown that there is an increase in the risk of a diagnosis of cancer after primary thromboembolism. Standardised increase ratio for cancer was three times higher in patients with thromboembolism for the first six months period.

Although the molecular mechanism by which cancer can lead to hypercoagulability has been studied, the mechanisms by which blood coagulation can promote tumor growth and metastasis remains unknown. A plausible explanation might be our finding that thrombin is a potent promoter of angiogenesis [19].

2. Promotion of Angiogenesis by Thrombin

In the chick chorioallantoic membrane (CAM) system of angiogenesis it has been shown that thrombin promotes angiogenesis by a mechanism which is independent of fibrin formation. [19]. Gamma-thrombin, which has the catalytic site but not the anion binding exocite of α-thrombin and consequently can not cleave fibrinogen to fibrin, has the same effect as α-thrombin on angiogenesis. These angiogenic effects of α- and γ-thrombin are specific, since it can be completely abolished by heparin and hirudin. The catalytic site of thrombin is essential for this effect, because PPACK-thrombin, which has the active site chemically inactivated, is without effect. For the angiogenic action of thrombin, the activation of thrombin receptor is essential. In fact the synthetic 14peptide TRAP, which represents the amino-terminal peptide of the activated thrombin receptor, that mimics many of the actions of thrombin, is also angiogenic [9].

[Dimitropoulou et al. 1998] were able to make corrosion casts from CAM in the presence and absence of thrombin and demonstrate the increase in the vascular density obtained with thrombin. Both the vascular plexus density and thickness were increased and the small capillaries (first order vessels) arising from the plexus increased in number, length and diameter. The effects of thrombin on larger capillaries (second and third order vessels) were less pronounced. This is a direct demonstration of the impressive changes that thrombin is causing in the vascular development of this system.

In another in vivo system of angiogenesis, the Matrigel plug assay in mice, [7] have shown that in the absence of thrombin or other angiogenic factors the Matrigel plug remain clear with no visible blood vessels going into it. However, when plugs contained 0.3-3.0 IU of thrombin/ml Matrigel were appeared pink with a large number of vessels infiltrating into the Matrigel plugs. Histological evaluation revealed a 15-20 fold increase in the area of cells that have infiltrated into the Matrigel plug containing thrombin.

3. Cellular Mechanisms for the Angiogenic Action of Thrombin

The aforementioned results suggested a novel action of thrombin on angiogenesis. The activated thrombin receptor is involved but the detailed cellular events and transduction mechanisms have not been elucidated.

Thrombin in addition to its pivotal role in blood coagulation has many other actions on a variety of cell types, which may be related to its angiogenesis-promoting effect. For example, thrombin has many cellular actions on smooth muscle cells, platelets, macrophages, fibroblasts and endothelial cells (for review see [8]), which may play a role in activating the angiogenic cascade. On smooth muscle cells thrombin stimulates growth and proliferation, which is mediated at least in part via the induction of synthesis of autocrine growth factors such as basic fibroblast growth factor (bFGF) and platelet derived growth factor (PDGF). Similarly, fibroblasts express thrombin receptors and their activation leads to mitogenic effects. On platelets thrombin is a potent activator and causes shape changes, granule release and secretion, activation of phospholipase C and mobilisation of Ca^{++}. On monocytes and macrophages thrombin synergizes and potentiates the mitogenic effect of colony stimulating factor I and induces recruitment and proliferation of these inflammatory cells. This action of thrombin on inflammatory cells may be of importance in relation to angiogenesis in tumors, wound healing and inflammatory diseases.

Particularly on endothelial cells, which are the prime player in angiogenesis, thrombin has many effects that could play a role in activating angiogenesis:

- Thrombin causes changes in the endothelial cell burrier function [4] and increases permeability, which is associated with changes in cell to cell junction organization [12].
- Thrombin causes increase of endothelial cell proliferation, migration and changes in cell shape. Exposure of endothelial cells to thrombin lead to increased synthesis of platelets activating factor, PDGF, prostacyclin, thrombomodulin, synthesis and cell surface expression of tissue factor, tissue plasminogen activator and its inhibitor (for review see [8]).
- Thrombin also activates gelatinase [21] and increases the vectorial secretion of extracellular matrix proteins [11]. These events are of particular importance in the initial and final steps of the angiogenic cascade respectively.

Recently, we have shown that brief exposure of human umbilical vein endothelial cells (HUVECs) to thrombin caused a marked dose-dependent inhibition of adhesion [18]. One IU/ml of thrombin caused 50% inhibition even after 5 minutes of exposure of HUVECs to thrombin. This effect was reversible since reincubation of thrombin-treated HUVECs with fresh growth medium for 15 minutes restored their ability for attachment.

This short term inhibitory effect of thrombin on the adhesion of HUVECs to extracellular matrix components was specific and depended on the activation of thrombin receptor. Hirudin abolished this effect of thrombin. Similarly, the proteolytically inactive PPACK-thrombin had no effect, but when used in combination with thrombin prevents the inhibitory effect of thrombin. In addition, the thrombin receptor agonist peptide (TRAP) mimicked the effect of thrombin on HUVECs adhesion. The transduction mechanism involved in this action of thrombin seems to be via cAMP, since forskolin or the phosphodiesterase inhibitor 3-isobutyl-1-methyl-xanthine restored the ability of HUVECs that have been exposed to thrombin to adhere.

This novel cellular action of thrombin on endothelial cells may represent an important early event in activation of the normally quiescent endothelial cells and initiation of the angiogenic cascade.

The vascular endothelial growth factor and basic fibroblast growth factor are considered the key angiogenic factors [2, 6]. We have been investigating the possibility that thrombin may have a synergistic effect with the above angiogenic factors. We compare the rate of DNA synthesis of HUVECs exposed to thrombin and subsequently treated with VEGF or bFGF. We find that thrombin causes a dose dependent potentiation of DNA synthesis by HUVECs. There is an increase in the rate of DNA synthesis by thrombin from 50-100% over the controls. Similarly, exposure of HUVECs to VEGF or bFGF causes an even greater stimulation of DNA synthesis ranging from 250-500% over the control. What is of interest is that brief treatment of HUVECs with thrombin and subsequently exposure to VEGF or bFGF leads to a stimulation of DNA synthesis which exceeds by far the expected additive effect by thrombin and VEGF or bFGF alone (see table 1).

Table 1. Synergistic effect of thrombin with VEGF or bFGF on DNA synthesis by HUVECs

Treatment	% change over control ± SE
Thrombin (1.5 IU/ml)	77±6
VEGF (5 ng/ml)	125±9
bFGF (5 ng/ml)	239±29
Thrombin/VEGF	329±18
Thrombin/bFGF	422±32

The exposure of HUVECs to thrombin can be as brief as 15 minutes but a further incubation of HUVECs with or without thrombin for at least 8 hours is required for these effects of thrombin on DNA synthesis to become evident. This led us to hypothesize that thrombin may upregulating the expression of VEGF and bFGF receptors. Indeed preliminary experiments with quantitative RT-PCR show that the VEGF receptors KDR and Flt-1 are upregulated by exposure to thrombin. These thrombin mediated effects are specific (hirudin abolishes these action of thrombin) and require the functioning of the catalytic site of thrombin (PPACK-thrombin is without effect). The activated thrombin receptor is involved since TRAP has the same effect as thrombin itself (see table 2)

Table 2. Synergistic effect of TRAP with VEGF or bFGF on DNA synthesis by HUVECs

Treatment	% change over control ± SE
TRAP (10μM)	45±6
VEGF (5 ng/ml)	289±17
bFGF (5 ng/ml)	515±32
TRAP/VEGF	516±30
TRAP/bFGF	859±42

The above results suggest one more mechanism by which thrombin promotes angiogenesis. By increasing the sensitivity of endothelial cells to the mitogenic effects of the key angiogenic factors VEGF and bFGF, thrombin may act as an important positive modulator of the angiogenic cascade.

The question then arises which of the multitude of affects of thrombin on endothelial cells is most important and relevant to the in vivo situations. The relative contribution and importance of these cellular actions of thrombin in the promotion of angiogenesis is likely to depend on the particular site and the pathophysiology involved. Thrombin may orchestrate temporally and specially these events in order to activate, amplify or maintain the angiogenic process. The localization of thrombin on endothelial cells of capillaries in wound healing and other situations where angiogenesis is activated [20] makes this possibility plausible.

4. Discussion and Conclusion

Promotion of angiogenesis by thrombin may explain not only the metastatic spread of cancer but also suggests a role of thrombin in other conditions such as inflammation, diabetic retinopathy, wound healing, endometrial changes, atherosclerosis etc. where angiogenesis is involved [3].

In addition to cancer in all the above situations, where angiogenesis is activated, we have bleeding and blood coagulation, therefore thrombin generation. A very common clinical observation is that new capillaries grow within the blood clots in large veins where thrombin is trapped and slowly released. Thrombin then may be an important factor that transduces the angiogenic signal to activate angiogenesis in all these conditions.

This new role of thrombin opens up many therapeutic possibilities that need to be explored and worked out experimentally. The fact that thrombin which does not catalyse fibrin formation, therefore can not causes blood coagulation, promotes angiogenesis, implies that there is a possibility of developing inhibitors of the angiogenesis-promoting effect of thrombin, with no effect on blood coagulation. Such agents have potential therapeutic applications in pathological situations where uncontrolled angiogenesis is part of the pathology of the disease e.g. cancer, diabetic retinopathy etc. Conversely, the fact that TRAP is a promoter of angiogenesis opens up the possibility of using γ-thrombin, TRAP and other non-thrombogenic analogs of thrombin in situations where promotion of angiogenesis may be desirable. This may be a novel therapeutic approach for non-healing wounds and ulcers in diabetic or older patients and also in myocardial infarctions.

Acknowledgement

This work was supported by grant from ECC Biomed 2 BMH4-CT96-0669 entitled "Molecular mechanisms of angiogenesis associated to cancer progress" and a grant from General Secretarial of Greek Ministry of Energy and Technology.

References

[1]   Dimitripoulou, C., Maragoudakis, M.E. and Konerding, M.A. Effects of thrombin and D609 on the chick chorioallantoic membrane: a quantitative microvascular corrosion study. J. Vasc.Res., 1998, (submitted).

[2]   Ferrara, N. The biology of vascular endothelial growth factor, In: Molecular, Cellular and Clinical Aspects of Angiogenesis, ed. M.E. Maragoudakis, Plenum Press, Vol. 285: 73-85, 1996.

[3]   Folkman, J. Angiogenesis in cancer, vascular, rheumatoid and other disease. Nature Med. 1995; 1, 27-31.

[4]   Garcia, J.G.N., Aschner, J., and Malik, A.B., Regulation of thrombin-induced endothelial cell prostaglandin synthesis and barrier function. In: Berliner, L.J., ed. Thrombin: Structure and Function. New York: Plenum Publishing, 1991: 397-430.

[5]   Grant, R.J.A., A.S. Turnell, R.W Grabham. Cellular consequences of thrombin-receptor activation, Biochem. J. 313: 353-368, 1996

[6]   Gualandris, E., M.P. Molinari-Tosatti, M. Ziche, D. Ribatti and M. Presta. Autocrine role of basic fibroblast growth factor in angiogenesis and angioproliferative diseases, In: Angiogenesis: Models, Modulators and Clinical Applications, ed. M.E. Maragoudakis, Plenum Press, Vol. 298: 98-112,1998

[7]   Haralabopoulos, G., Grant, D.S., Kleinman, H.K., and Maragoudakis M.E. Thrombin promotes endothelial cell alignment in Matrigel in vitro and angiogenesis in vivo. Am.J.Physiol., 1997; 273 (Cell Physiol.): C239-C245.

[8]   Kanthou, C., V.V. Kakkar and O. Benzakour. Cellular and molecular effects of thrombin in the vascular system, In: Angiogenesis: Models, Modulators and Clinical Applications, ed. M.E. Maragoudakis, Plenum Press, Vol. 298:163-282, 1998

[9]   Maragoudakis, M.E., N.E. Tsopanoglou, E. Sakkoula, E. Pipili-Synetos. On the mechanism of promotion of angiogenesis by thrombin, FASEB J. 9:A587, 1995

[10]   Nierodzik, M.L., F. Kajumo and S. Karpatikin. Effect of thrombin treatment of tumor cells on adhesion of tumor cells to platelets in vitro and tumor metastasis in vivo. Cancer Res. 52: 3267-3272, 1992

[11]   Papadimitriou E., Manolopoulos V., Hayman G.T., Maragoudakis M.E., Unsworth B., Fenton J.W. II, and Lelkes P.I. Thrombin modulates vectorial secretion of extracellular matrix proteins in cultured endothelial cells. Am. Physiol. Soc. 1997; 272 (Cell Physiol. 41) C1112-C1122.

[12] Rabiet, M.J., Plantier, J.L., Rival, Y., Genoux, Y., Lampugnani, M.G., and Dejana, E. Thrombin-induced increase in endothelial permeability is associated with changes in cell-to-cell junction organization. Arterioscler. Thromb. Vasc. Biol., 1996; 16, 488-496.

[13] Rickles, F.R. and R.L. Edwards. Activation of blood coagulation in cancer: Trousseau's syndrome revisited. *Blood* 64:14-31, 1983

[14] Sloan, B.F., J. Rozhin, K. Johnson, H. Taylor, J.D. Crissman, and K.V. Honn. Cathepsin B: Association with plasma membrane in metastatic tumors. *Proc. Natl. Acad. Sci.* (USA) 83:2483-2487, 1986.

[15] Sorensen, H.T., K.L. Mellem, F.H. Steffensen, J.H. Olsen, and G.L. Nielsen. The risk of a diagnosis of cancer after primary deep venous thrombosis or pulmonary embolism, *N. Engl. J. Med.* 338: 1169-1173, 1998.

[16] Tapparelli, C., Metternich, R., Ehrhardt, C. and Cook, N.S. Synthetic low molecular weight thrombin inhibitors: Molecular design and pharmacological profile. TIPS, 1993. 14: 366-376.

[17] Trousseau A. Phlegmasia alba dolens in Trousseau A. Lectures in clinical medicine, delivered in Hotel-Dieu, Paris, London, New Sydenham, Society 281-285, 1872.

[18] Tsopanoglou N.E. and M.E. Maragoudakis. On the mechanism of thrombin-indicated angiogenesis: Inhibition of attachment of endothelial cells on basement membrane components, *Angiogenesis J.* 1(2): 192-200, 1998

[19] Tsopanoglou, N.E., E. Pipili-Synetos, and M.E. Maragoudakis. Thrombin promotes angiogenesis by a mechanism independent of fibrin formation, *Am. J. Physiol.* 264 (Cell Physiol. 33): C1302-1307, 1993.

[20] Zacharsky L-R., V.A. Memoli, W.D. Morain, J.M. Schlaeppi, and S.M. Rousseau. Cellular localization of enzymatically active thrombin in intact human tissues by hirudin binding, *Thrombosis & Haemostasis*, 73, 793-797, 1995.

[21] Zucker, S., C. Conner, B. Massimo, H. Ende, M. Drew, M. Seiki, and W.F. Bahou. Thrombin induces the activation of progelatinase A in vascular endothelial cells, *J. Biol. Chem.* 270: 23730-23738, 1995.

Abstracts of Oral Presentations

Vascular Endothelium: Mechanisms of Cell Signaling
J.D. Catravas et al. (Eds.)
IOS Press, 1999

Inhibition of Epithelial Tumor Cell Replication by the α3 chain of Type IV Collagen Is Initiated Through Its Interaction with Integrin Associated Protein (CD47) and Integrin β3

T.A. Shahan**, S. Pasco*, A. Fawzi*, J.C. Mombisse*, G. Bellon*,
and <u>N.A. Kefalides</u>**
** *University of Pennsylvania, Philadelphia, PA and *University of Reims, Reims,*
France

Previous studies from our laboratories demonstrated that the noncollagenous (NCl) domain of the α3 chain of basement membrane collagen from anterior lens capsule (ALC-COL IV) inhibits activation of polymorphonuclear leukocytes through its −SNS- trimer (Monboisse et al. J. Biol. Chem, **269**, 25475, 1994). Recently we have shown that the same region of the NC1 domain promotes adhesion and inhibits replication of melanoma cells (Han et al. J. Biol Chem, **272**, 20395, 1997). In the present study ALC-COL IV or -SNS- containing synthetic peptides (10 µg/ml) added to culture medium not only inhibited the replication of melanoma cells, but also inhibited breast-, pancreas-, stomach-tumor cells up to 67%, and prostate tumor cells by 15% compared to controls. ALC-COL IV and a peptide, α3(IV)185-203, also caused an immediate rise in intracellular cAMP levels in all cell types tested. From melanoma cells we have isolated 4 receptor proteins which bound to the α3(IV)179-208 peptide of 33, 52, 74 and 95 kDa, of which the 52 kDa and 95 kDa proteins were shown to be CD47 and integrin β3 by western analysis. Cells treated with CD47 and integrin β3 reactive antibodies prevented −SNS- containing peptides from inhibiting cell replication as well as the rise in cAMP. Pretreating the cells with unlabeled ligand (-YYSNS-) inhibited the purification of both CD47 and integrin β3, from an affinity column suggesting that the interaction is highly specific for the bioactive trimer (-SNS-). Pretreatment of cells with pertussis toxin also prevented the inhibitory effect of ALC-COL IV or its peptides on tumor cell replication and the cAMP increase. The cAMP competitive inhibitor, Rp-cAMPS, was shown to suppress the inhibitory effect of ALC-COL IV and cAMP analogs. In the presence of the protein kinase-A inhibitor H-89, ALC-COL IV failed to inhibit tumor cell replication. These data suggest that ALC-COL IV, through the NC1 domain of the α3-chain inhibited tumor cell replication through a signal transduction pathway involving G-proteins, cAMP-dependent protein kinases and the CD47-integrin β3 complex.

Vascular Endothelium: Mechanisms of Cell Signaling
J.D. Catravas et al. (Eds.)
IOS Press, 1999

[123]I-Vascular Endothelial Growth Factor165 (^{123}I-VEGF165) Binding Sites in Tumor Cells: Implication for Tumor Scintigraphy

S.R. Li[1], C. Bischof[1], S. Kapiotis[2], M. Peck-Radosavljevic[3], P. Angelberger[5], H.A. Weich[6], P.Valent[4] and I. Virgolini[1]

Departments of [1]Nuclear Medicine, [2]Medical Laboratory Diagnostics, [3]Gastroenterology & Hepatology and [4]Haematology, University of Vienna; [5]Institute of Chemistry, Research Center Seibersdorf, Austria; and [6]Society for Biotechnological Research, Department of Gen Expression, Braunschweig, Germany

Angiogenesis is suggested to be a prerequisite of tumor growth and metastases formation. The vascular endothelial growth factor (VEGF) is one of the most potent angiogenic factors, which acts directly o endothelial cells via tyrosine kinase receptors. To provide the basis for VEGF receptor scintigraphy of well vascularized primary tumors and their metastases, the binding of ^{123}I-labeled -VEGF165 (^{123}I-VEGF165) to human umbilical vein endothelial cells (HUVEC) and various human tumor cell lines (mast cell line HMC-1, epidermoid mammary carcinoma cell line A431, basophil cell line KU-812, monocyte cell line U937, human hepatic endothelioma cell line HEP-1, human hepatoma cell lines HEP-G2 and HEP-3B, B-lymphocyte cell line RAJI) as well as to primary human tumors (melanomas, ductal breast cancers,, renal cell cancers, meningiomas, carcinoids, hepatocellular carcinomas, thyroid cancers, pheocromocytomas, lymphangiomas, colorectal adenocarcinomas and cultured primary lung fibroblasts, n=38) was investigated. Human recombinant VEGF (E.coli-derived) was obtained by recombinant technology and was labeled with ^{123}I using the Chloramin-T method. Sodium dodecyle sulphate gradient polyacrylamid gel electrophoresis showed a single ^{123}I-Peak corresponding to the VEGF protein band. The biological activity of [123]I -VEGF165 was identical to that of unlabeled VEGF165 as determined by its ability to enhance the uptake of ^{3}H-thymidine by HUVEC and primary lung fibroblasts. Two classes of high affinity ^{123}I-VEGF165 binding sites were found on the cell surface of HUVEC (B_{max1}, 1580±320 binding sites/cell, K_{d1}, 8±2 pM; B_{max2}, 9500±840 binding site/cell, K_{d2}, 86±19 pM) and primary human lung fibroblasts (B_{max1}, 1340±210 binding site/cell, K_{d1}, 17±8 pM; B_{max2}, 8600±750 binding site/cell, K_{d2}, 74±15 pM). One class of high affinity binding sites for ^{123}I-VEGF165 was also found for HMC1, A431, HEP-1, HEP-G2, HEP-3B and U937 cells (B_{max}:3-27 sites x 10^9/mg protein, K_d:15-36pM). The binding of ^{123}I-VEGF165 was inhibited by unlabeled VEGF165 and VEGF121 but not by several other unrelated peptides (Vasoactive intestinal peptide, somatostatin-14, heparin, tumor necrosis factor-α, insulin growth factor and epidermal growth factor). This study demonstrates specific binding sites for ^{123}I-VEGF165 on HUVEC and on a variety of human tumor cells. We conclude that ^{123}I-VEGF165 may be useful for the *in vivo* localization of vascularized tumors.

Vascular Endothelium: Mechanisms of Cell Signaling
J.D. Catravas et al. (Eds.)
IOS Press, 1999

Modified LDL Decreases the Binding of Prostaglandin E$_2$, I$_2$ and E$_1$ onto Monocytes in Patients with Peripheral Vascular Disease

S.R. Li[1], Q. Yang[1], E. Koller[2], A. Kurtaran[3], C. Bischof[1], F. Rauscha[3], J. Pidlich[4] and I. Virgolini[1]

Departments of [1]Nuclear Medicine, [2]Physiology, [3]Cardiology and [4]Gastroenterology, University of Vienna, A-1090 Vienna, Austria

Recent data suggest that various eicosanoids including prostaglandins (PGs) play an important regulatory role in the development of atherosclerotic lesions. Peripheral blood monocytes have been implemented in early atherogenesis because they express receptors specific for modified low density lipoprotein (LDL). In this study we investigated and compared the binding of ^{3}H-PGE$_2$, ^{3}H-PGE$_1$ and ^{3}H-PGI$_1$ and ^{3}H-PGI$_2$ onto intact peripheral monocytes isolated from 20 patients (32-71 years) with manifested ischaemic peripheral vascular disease Stage II according to Fontaine with the results obained in 16 healthy volunteers (21-68 years). In controls, Scatchard analyses of the binding data indicated a single class of high affinity binding sites for ^{3}H-PGE$_2$ (maximal binding capacity (B$_{max}$): 11400±3200 sites/cell; dissociation constant (K$_d$):1.3±0.5 nM) and two classes of binding sites for ^{3}H-PGE$_1$ (B$_{max1}$: 11200±4900 sites/cell, K$_{d1}$: 1.5±0.5 nM; B$_{max2}$: 47800±6100 sites/cell, K$_{d2}$: 12.8±5.9 nM) as well as for ^{3}H-PGI$_2$ (B$_{max1}$: 10100±3700 sites/cell, K$_{d1}$: 1.7±0.7 nM; B$_{max2}$: 81200±5200 sites/cell, K$_{d2}$: 14.2±6.5 nM). In the patients, an absence of the higher affinity binding class and significantly (p<0.01) lower numbers of lower affinity binding sites were found for either ligand (PGE$_2$: B$_{max}$: 6600±3600 sites/cell, K$_d$: 20.5±7.0 nM). After incubation of monocytes with modified LDL (oxidized LDL), the binding of PGs was significantly (p<0.01 to p<0.001) decteased, whereas native VLDL, LDL and HDL did not interfere with PG-binding, PG-induced adenosine 3'-5'-cyclic monophosphate (cAMP) formation by monocytes was significantly (p>0.01) lower in patients (the concentrations causing 50% elevation of basal cAMP formation (ED$_{50}$) were 3.8±2.4 nM for PGE$_2$, the ED$_{50}$ for PGE$_1$ was 1.6±1.2 nM, for PGE$_1$ was 6.3±3.5 nM and 5.6±4.1 nM for PGI$_2$) as compared with controls (ED$_{50}$ for PGE$_2$ was 1.6±1.2 nM, for PGE$_1$ 4.8±2.5 nM and for PGI$_2$ 3.1+1.4 nM). After preincubation with modified LDL, the PG-induced cAMP-production by monocytes was remarkable decreased in both patients and controls (p<0.05). Our results suggest a direct effect of modified LDL on PGE$_2$, PGE$_1$ and PGI$_2$-binding onto monocytes by reducing the available number of cell surface expressed receptors. Modified LDL also reduces the sensitivity of monocytes to PGs which results in decreased cAMP production. The complex interactions between PGs and lipoproteins may play an important role during atherogenesis.

Vascular Endothelium: Mechanisms of Cell Signaling
J.D. Catravas et al. (Eds.)
IOS Press, 1999

Effects of X-ray Irradiation Doses and NO Synthase Modulations on Embryonic Angiogenesis

S. Papaioannou[1], C. Hadjimichael[1], E. Papademitriou[1], D. Kardamakis[2]
and J. Demopoulos[2]
[1]Department of Molecular Pharmacology, School of Pharmacy and [2]Department of
Radiology, School of Medicine, University of Patras, Greece

It was recently demonstrated that the antiangiogenic proteins angiostatin and endostatin are potent in dramatically reducing primary experimental tumors and their metastases [1,2], although interruption of such treatment resulted in rapid regrowth of the tumors. This direct evidence that tumor growth and metastasis are angiogenesis-dependent, also suggests that tumor elimination may need a combination of an antiangiogenic and cytotoxic treatment, reminding Hercules' attack on The Hydra. We have earlier suggested such an approach, combining antiagiogenic treatment with irradiation and chemotherapy, along with the elucidation of irradiation molecular mechanisms toward an efficacious treatment of tumors [3-5]. These mechanisms have not been adequately elucidated in spite of the clinical importance of irradiation. Recent evidence indicates that oxygen-derived free radicals [6] and nitric oxide (NO) are involved [7, 3]. Earlier data from our laboratories suggest that X-ray irradiation has an antiangiogenic effect on the rapidly growing chorioallantoic membrane of the chicken embryo (CAM) in vivo and the NO synthase inhibitor N^G - nirto - L - arginine methylester (L-NAME) reverses this effect, which is NO-dependent [3, 4]. The present work is an extension of the earlier work to study the effect of X-ray dosage on CAM and the effects of NO synthase inhibitors L-NAME and N^G - nitro - arginine (L-NA), as well as the NO donor sodium nitroprusside (SNP) and the NO synthase substrate L-arginine (L-Arg). In recent additional work we have also re-examined the effects of the plastic discs or rings, as well as cortisone, on the vascular density index of the 9 - or 14 - day CAM in vivo.

The angiogenesis method of CAM was used with some modifications (40 of the initially described one by Folkman [8]. This method was used because of the rapid angiogensis of the CAM on the 9th day of the embryo development that resembles actively growing tumors, whereas the angiogenesis rate of the 14-day CAM is minimal. For the kinetic studies, immediately after irradiation with X-rays (0-15 Gy, 20 KV, 0,1 mm A1), sterile plastic discs of 1 cm diameter were used to cover the irradiated CAM area, as well as an adjacent area (non-irradiated), which served as the control. For the subsequent irradiation dose-response and other studies the discs were placed on the CAM approximately 20 min post-irradiation. Discs contained regularly 100 µg cortisone acetate to prevent local inflammation [4, 8], as well as L-NAME, L-NA, SNP, or L-Arg. The egg incubation was interrupted with formalin up to 96 hours post-irradiation of the 9-day CAM for the kinetic studies or 24 hours post-irradiation routinely. CAM angiogenesis was quantitated as vascular density index (V.D.I.) [9] or by computer assisted image analysis allowing the determination of small 930-100 µm) and large (300-900 µm) diameter vessels.

The kinetic studies revealed that the maximum antiangiogenic effect of irradiation (10 Gy) on the 9-day CAM occurred 24 hours post-irradiation, whereas the irradiation of the 14-day CAM did not inhibit angiogenesis or vascular density. On the basis of these findings the following non-kinetic studies were carried out 24 hours post-irradiation. The kinetic studies also showed that the small vessels of the 9-day CAM are more radiosensitive that the medium size ones, whereas the large vessels are not appreciably affected. There was no significant effect on the 14-day CAM. Irradiation dose-response studies on the 9-day CAM showed that irradiation at 2, 5, 10 and 15 Gy significantly antiangiogenic effect of irradiation at all four doses, whereas D-NAME showed a limited incomplete inhibition of that irradiation effect. Similar studies on the 14-day CAM showed that all four doses of irradiation had no significant effect on the V.D.I. L-NAME showed a limited angiogenic effect at 2 and 5 Gy, L-NA showed a limited antiangiogenic effect at the same irradiation doses and D-NAME had no effect on the V.D.I. of the 14-day CAM at 0-15 Gy irradiation. SNP (5μg/disc) and L-Arg (12.2 μg/disc) resulted in partial disinhibition of the 9-day CAM antiangiogenic effect at all four of the X-ray doses, with the exception of the antiangiogenic effect of SNP on the non irradiated CAM. Both compounds failed to further increase the X-ray-induced antiangiogenicity of the 9-day CAM. The effect of SNP or L-Arg on the V.D.I. of the irradiated 14-day CAM was essentially insignificant for SNP and of limited antiangiogenic effect for L-Arg at 2 and 15 Gy.

The complete inhibition of the antiangiogenic effect at all doses of irradiation by both L-NAME and a second NO synthase inhibitor L-NA reconfirms our earlier data that the above effect is NO-dependent in the rapidly proliferating CAM. If this mechanism holds true for pathologically proliferating tissues (e.g. tumors), NO generating drugs (e.g. nitrovasodilators) and the recent potent antiangiogenic agents [1, 2] may be appropriately combined with irradiation to enhance tumor cytotoxicity by means of the released NO and the vasodilation-induced oxygenation of the tumors [10]. Superoxide dismutase (SOD), an endogenous superoxide scavenger, partially inhibits the irradiation-induced antiangiogenicity, confirming that superoxide free radicals are released during irradiation of the rapidly proliferation CAM. Nevertheless L-NAME & L-NA completely protect this tissue from irradiation-induced antiangiogenicity, suggesting that its NO dependency is dominant.

Recent experiments on the effects of discs with or without cortisone, or the effects of rings instead of discs on the 9- or 14-day non-irradiated cAM revealed interesting results, regarding the effects of these changes on CAM angiogenesis: For the 9-day CAM in the absence of disc or cortisone, the V.D.I. 24 hours later was 154.8 while in the presence of disc without cortisone it was 103.0 (p<0.001). in the presence of disc without cortisone the V.D.I. was 110.0, whereas in the presence of the disc and cortisone it was 88.5 (p<0.01). In the absence of any disc or ring or cortisone the V.D.I. was 136.8 whereas in the presence of a plastic ring it was 134.0 (p<0.05). The effect of cortisone was also not significant when compared with the V.D.I. of the 9-day CAM in the presence of a ring without any cortisone. It appears that the presence of disc with or without cortisone resulted in significant reduction of V.D.I. compared to their controls, whereas this is not the case for the use of rings with our without cortisone. Essentially similar effects were observed in the 14-day CAM. This is interpreted to mean that, in spite of the (adjacent) have been studied with discs and cortisone. Additional work is in progress to further elucidate the effects of the ring method with or without cortisone.

References

[1]   M.S. O' Reilly, L. Homgren, Y. Shing, C. Chen, R.A. Rosenthal, M. Moses, N.S. Lane, Y. Cao, E.H. Sage and J. Folkman. Angiostatin: A Novel Angiogenesis Inhibitor That Mediates The Suppression Of Metastases By A Lewis Lung Carcinoma. *Cell* **79** (1994) 315-328.

[2]   M.S. O' Reilly, T. Boehm, Y. Shing, N. Fukai, G. Vasios, W.S. Lane, E. Flynn, J.R. Birkhead, B.R. Olsen and J. Falkman. Endostatin: An Endogenous Inhibitor of Angiogenesis and Tumor Growth. *Cell* **88** (1997) 277-285.

[3]   S. Papaioannou, O. Hatjiconti, C. Katsarou, P. Ravazoula, J. Demopoulos and M. Maragoudakis. Inhibition of Nitric Oxide Synthase Reverses the Antiangiogenic Effect of X-ray Irradiation on Chick Embryo Chorioallantoic Membrane. In: J. Catravas, A. Callow and U. Ryan (eds), Vascular Endothelium: Responses to Injury. ISBN: 0-306-45282-0. Plenum Press, New York & London, 1994, pp. 306-308.

[4]   O. Hatjicondi, P. Ravazoula, D. Kardamakis, J. Dimopoulos and S. Papioannou. In Vivo Experimental Evidence that the Nitric Oxide Pathway Is Involved in The X-ray-Induced Antiangiogenicity. *Brit. J. Cancer* **74** (1996) 1916-1923.

[5]   S. Papaioannou, O. Hatjicondi, P. Ravazoula, C. Hadjimichael, D. Kardamakis and J. Demopoulos. The Effects of X-ray Irradiation on Angiogenesis. In: J.D. Catravas, A.D. Callow and U.S. Ryan (eds), Vascular Endothelium: Pharmacologic and Genetic Manipulations. ISBN: 0-306-45819-5. Plenum Press, New York & London, 1998.

[6]   K.M. Price, K.A. Horner and N.J. McNally. Interaction of Hydrogen Peroxide and Ionizing-Radiation-Induced Damage. In: J. Denecamp and D.G. Hirst (eds), Radiation Science of Molecules Mice and Men. *Br. J. Radiol.* 1992 suppl. **24** pp. 28-31.

[7]   N.V. Voevodskaya and A.F. Vamin. Gamma Irradiation Potentiates L-Arginine Dependent Nitric Oxide Fromation in Mice. *Biochem. Bophys. Res. Commun.* **186** (1992) 1423-1428.

[8]   J. Folkman. Tumor Angiogenesis. *Adv. Cancer Res.* **43** (1985) 175-203.

[9]   S.A. Harris-Hooker, S.A. Gajdusek, S.M. Wicht and T.N. Swartz. Neovascularization Responses Induced by Cultured Aortic Endothelial Cells. *J. Cell Physiol.* **114** (1983) 302-310.

[10]   Denecamp. Inadequate Vasculature in Solid Tumors: Consequences of Cancer Research Strategies. *Brit. J. Pathol.* Suppl **24** (1992) 111-119.

Vascular Endothelium: Mechanisms of Cell Signaling
J.D. Catravas et al. (Eds.)
IOS Press, 1999

Role of G proteins and the p38 Mitogen Activated Protein (MAP) kinase in Lipopolysaccharide (LPS)-induced signaling in human endothelial cells (EC)

Moshe Arditi, Aninda Das, Yiping Jin
*Childrens Hospital Los Angeles, Division of Infectious Diseases, Southern California
School of Medicine, Los Angeles, CA 90027*

LPS can induce the activation of vascular EC, including expression of various adhesion molecules and secretion of numerous pro-inflammatory cytokines and chemokines, which in turn play a significant role in the pathogenesis of endotoxic shock. However, the LPS receptor on EC is not known and signal transduction pathways for LPS-induced EC activation and cytokine release are not completely understood. We have previously shown that LPS induces the tyrosine phosphorylation of MAP kinases, including ERK1, ERK2, p38 MAP kinase, and c-jun N terminal kinase (JNK) in EC. In this study we measured IL-6 release as a paradigm for LPS-induced activation of human brain microvessel EC (HBMEC) and human dermal microvessel EC (HDMEC) following preincubation of EC with various specific biochemical inhibitors in quadruplicate experiments. LPS induced a dose-dependent and serum- (soluble-CD14-) dependent IL-6 release in both EC types. The p21 Ras pathway inhibitor (alpha HFPA, 0.4 μM) and the MAP kinase kinase (MEK) inhibitor [i.e. ERK1/ERK2 pathway inhibitor, (PD98059) at 100 μM] failed to inhibit LPS-induced IL-6 release from ECs, while the MEK inhibitor did inhibit LPS-induced increase in ERK2 activation in EC. However, the tyrosine kinase inhibitor (Herbimycin A, 1 - 5 μg/ml), the p38 MAP kinase inhibitor (SB203580,1-10 μM), and the G protein binding peptide Mastoparan (1-20 μM) resulted in a dose-dependent inhibition of LPS-induced IL-6 release from both EC types, with maximal inhibition of 92%, 90%, and 100% respectively. Mastoparan, a 14-residue peptide, stimulates GDP/GTP exchange on G proteins through a mechanism similar to that of G protein-coupled receptors, and binds to G proteins at the receptor-binding site. Presumably, this peptide structurally mimics a receptor's G protein binding domain. Pretreatment of ECs with the Pertussis toxin (100 ng/ml) resulted in 45% inhibition in LPS-induced IL-6 release from ECs. These results suggest that the p38 MAP kinase pathway is the predominant signaling pathway in LPS-induced IL-6 release from HBMEC and HDMEC and that this pathway may involve a heterotrimeric G protein-coupled receptor. G protein agonists or antagonists may have a potential therapeutic role in modulating endothelial cell responses in endotoxic shock.

(This work has been supported by grants from NIH-AI 40275, MA, and AHA CS1019, MA).

Vascular Endothelium: Mechanisms of Cell Signaling
J.D. Catravas et al. (Eds.)
IOS Press, 1999

The Effects of Hypoxia on Endothelial Cells: Biochemical and Molecular Aspects

C. Michiels, E. Minet, T. Arnould, N. Berna, I. Ernest, J. Remacle
Laboratoire de Biochimie et Biologie Cellulaire, FNDP, 61 rue de Bruxelles, 5000 NAMUR, Belgium

Ischemia is a common situation involved in several pathologies. Besides the reperfusion injury, which is now well, established, ischemia and/or hypoxia by itself also induces cell changes. However, the biochemical and molecular mechanisms of the cellular response to hypoxia are still relatively unknown.

In order to study this response, we developed an *in vitro* model where human umbilical vein endothelial cells were submitted to a severe hypoxia. We observed that before affecting viability, hypoxia is able to strongly activate the endothelial cells. Hypoxia induces an increase in the cytosolic calcium concentration, which is then responsible for the activation of phopholipase A_2. Phospholipase A_2 activity releases arachidonic acid which is transformed in endothelial cells into prostaglandins and lyso-PAF which leads to PAF (platelet-activating factor). The synthesis of both PAF and prostaglandins is actually induced by hypoxia.

We also investigated the mechanism responsible for the increase in calcium concentration: the Na^+-glucose cotransport activity is increased when glycolysis is activated by hypoxia, this leads to an influx of Na^+. Na^+ is then exchanged with Ca^{++} through the Na^+/Ca^{++}-exchanger, leading to the increase in calcium concentration. No decrease in the intracellular pH is observed.

Th physiological consequences of the endothelial cell activation are numerous. We showed that endothelial cells release chemotactic factors for neutrophils under hypoxic conditions. PGF_2 was identified as responsible at least in part for this activity. We also observed that hypoxia-activated endothelial cells have an increased adhesiveness for neutrophils and are able to activate them to release reactive oxygen species and inflammatory mediators. These results suggest that ischemia by itself is able to lead to a local inflammation and that endothelial cells play an important role in this process.

Secondly, the regulation of gene transcription by hypoxia is under investigation. We have demonstrated that the bHLH-PAS transcription factor HIF-1 is activated by hypoxia in endothelial cells (HMEC-1). This has been shown using a gene reported approach as well by gel shift assay. In these cells, hypoxia induces a decrease in ATP content between 60 and 90 min but after 120 min of hypoxia, the ATP content recovers to reach control values. In parallel, an increase in glucose uptake is observed. We propose that hypoxia, through the activation of HIF-1, induces the expression of glycolytic enzymes which are part of the adaptative response of the cells to hypoxia allowing the cells to survive in such conditions. Current investigations are aimed to better characterize this response.

Acknowledgments

CM is a Senior Associate of FNRS (Fonds National de la Recherche Scientifique, Belgium) and EM is a fellow of FRIA (Fonds pour la Recherche dans l'Industrie et l'Agriculture, Belgium)

Vascular Endothelium: Mechanisms of Cell Signaling
J.D. Catravas et al. (Eds.)
IOS Press, 1999

211

The Nitric Oxide Receptor, Soluble Guanylyl Cyclase: Functional Expression, Revised Isozyme Family, Pharma-Cological Modulation And Endothelial Localization

Ulrike Zabel,[1] Volker O. Melichar,[1] Peter Kugler,[2] Victor W.M. van Hinsbergh,[3] Harald H. H. W. Schmidt[1]

[1]Dept. of Pharmacology and Toxicology and [2]Dept. Anatomy, Julius-Maximilians-University, Würzburg, Germany; [3]Gaubius Laboratory TNO-PG, Leiden, The Netherlands

Endothelium-derived nitric oxide (NO) is a key antithrombotic and vasodilatory mediator and vasoprotectant. While NO synthases have been extensively studied in the past years, very little is known about the molecular receptor of NO, soluble guanylyl cyclase (sGC). sGC is a heterodimeric (α/β) heme protein which in response to NO converts GTP to the second messenger cGMP, and functions also as the receptor for nitrovasodilator drugs. Three distinct cDNAs of each subunit (α_1- α_3; β_1- β_3) have been reported from various species. From human sources, none of these have been expressed as functionally active enzyme. Here we describe the expression of human α/β heterodimeric sGC in Sf9 cells yielding active recombinant enzyme (rhsGC), that was stimulated by the nitrovasodilator sodium nitroprusside (SNP) or the NO-independent activator 3-(5'-hydroxymethyl-2'-furyl)-1-benzylindazole (YC-1). Carbon monoxide (CO) was inactive on sGC in broken cells and a weak stimulator in intact cells. At the protein level, both α and β subunits were detected in human tissues, suggesting coexpression also *in vivo*. Moreover, re-sequencing of the human cDNA clones (originally termed α_3 and β_3; Giuili et al. (1992) *FEBS Lett.* 304, 83-88) revealed several sequencing errors in human α_3, correction of which eliminated major regions of divergence to rat and bovine α_1. As human β_3 also displays more than 98 % similarity to rat and bovine β_1 at the amino acid level, α_3 and β_3 represent in fact the human homologs of rat and bovine α_1 and β_1, and the isozyme family is reduced to two isoforms for each subunit (α_1, α_2; β_1, β_2). Having access to the human key enzyme of NO signalling will now allow to study novel sGC-modulating compounds with therapeutic potential. One such compound is YC-1, a novel type of sGC-activator that does not release NO. The vasomotor activity of YC-1 was studied in isolated rabbit aortic rings and compared to that of NO donors. Similar to NO, YC-1 caused concentration-dependent, endothelium-independent relaxations, which were greatly reduced by the sGC inhibitor ODQ. Surprisingly, NO and YC-1 actions displayed different kinetics when pre-incubated with aortic rings. YC-1 had a long-lasting inhibiting effect of YC-1 on the phenylephrine (PE)-induced contractile response, which was not fully reversible even after extensive washout of YC-1, and was accompanied by a long-lasting elevation of intracellular cGMP. In contrast, NO had no effect on the vasoconstrictor potency of PE, and increases in intravascular cGMP levels were readily reversed after washout of the NO donor compound. Here we demonstrate for the first time that YC-1 is an unspecific inhibitor of phosphodiesterases, as it inhibits cGMP breakdown in aortic extracts and the activity of phosphodiesterase isoforms 1-5 *in vitro*. We conclude that YC-1 causes a persistent elevation of intravascular cGMP *in vivo* also by inhibition of cGMP breakdown.

Thus, YC-1 is a highly effective vasodilator compound, with prolonged duration of action unprecedented for any previously known sGC activator. YC-1 is a promising therapeutic lead compound for the development of novel drugs, which might replace the currently used, short-lived and tolerance-prone nitrovasodilators. With respect to the vascular distribution of sGC it is open whether the NO receptor is only present in classical NO target cells, vascular smooth muscle and platelets, or also in the vascular endothelial cells which generate NO. Initial studies investigating endothelial cells from different vascular beds (aorta to microvessels) were negative, ie neither sGC immunoreactive protein nor sGC activity could be detected. However, subsequent immunocytochemistry and analysis of primary and earlier passage cells revealed that sGC is expressed to high levels in vascular endothelium but rapidly downregulated upon culture of endothelial cells. The mechanisms for this are presently under investigation.

Vascular Endothelium: Mechanisms of Cell Signaling
J.D. Catravas et al. (Eds.)
IOS Press, 1999

Regulation of Gas Phase Nitric Oxide (NO) by Ventilation and Pulmonary Blood Flow in Human Lungs

Nándor Marczin and Magdi Yacoub

^{1}Department of Cardiothoracic Surgery, National Heart and Lung Institute, Imperial
College of Science Technology and Medicine, The Royal Brompton and Harefield
Hospital, Harefield, United Kingdom

NO have been demonstrated in exhaled breath of animals and humans and have been increasingly used as markers of a variety of lung pathologies. Despite recent progress in understanding of the physiological regulation of NO, fundamental aspects remain unresolved such as the local and systemic origin of NO, its distribution alongside the airways and regulation of alveolar concentrations. To clarify these issues we investigated the influence of ventilation and pulmonary blood flow on NO concentrations in the lower airways of patients undergoing open heart surgery in exclusion of NO from ambient air and upper airways. This study reveals that concentrations of NO in the lower airways increase as ventilation decrease, suggesting importance of ventilation in eliminating NO from human lungs. In the absence of air flow, NO accumulated rapidly in the main airways reaching plateau levels of app.10 times of end tidal levels within 30 seconds. Breath holding maneuvers followed by inspiration or expiration reveal that alveolar concentrations of NO remain low despite accumulation of NO in the main airways during breath holding, suggesting that NO is continuously removed from the alveoli. Rapid reduction in pulmonary arterial blood flow at instrumentation of cardiopulmonary bypass results in increased NO concentrations in the airways suggesting that pulmonary blood flow is responsible for tonic removal of NO from the lower airways and that NO is not delivered from systemic sources but produced locally within the lungs. The potential significance of these observations on one lung ventilation was tested in patients undergoing thoracic surgery. Measurement of NO concentrations in the non-dependent and dependent lungs demonstrate that one lung ventilation creates a NO gradient between non-ventilated and ventilated lungs in the magnitude of 20-50 fold in favour of the non ventilated lung. This provides the basis for a hypothesis that accumulation of the selective pulmonary vasodilator NO in unventilated lung regions might contribute to the pathophysiology of right to left transpulmonary shunt and hypoxemia in a variety of lung pathologies.

References

[1]   Pinsky DJ. The vascular biology of heart and lung preservation for transplantation. *Thromb. Haemost* 1995; **74**:58-65

[2]   Dusting GJ, Macdonald PS. Endogenous nitric oxide in cardiovascular disease and transplantation. *Ann. Med.* 1995; **27**:395-406

[3]   Kharitonov SA, Barnes PJ. Exhaled nitric oxide: A marker of airway inflammation? *Curr. Opin. Anaest.* 1996, 9:542-548

[4]   Date H, Triantafillou AN, Trulock EP, Pohl MS, Cooper JD, Patterson GA. Inhaled nitric oxide reduces human lung allograft dysfunction. *J. Thorac. Cardiovasc. Surg.*1996; **111**:913-919.

[5]   Marczin N, Riedel B, Royston D, Yacoub M. Intravenous nitrite vasodilators and exhaled nitric oxide. *Lancet* 1997, **349**:1742

Vascular Endothelium: Mechanisms of Cell Signaling
J.D. Catravas et al. (Eds.)
IOS Press, 1999

Losartan as an antiatherogenic agent

T. M. Scott

Faculty of Medicine, Memorial University of Newfoundland,
St. John's, Newfoundland, Canada.

In recent years many drugs prescribed as antihypertensives have been found to have antiatherogenic properties. These include ACE inhibitors, calcium channel blockers and angiotensin II receptor antagonists. Although there are many factors implicated in the structural changes of atherogenesis, including lipid peroxidation, production of growth factors and inflammation, angiotensin II acting through the AT_1 receptor is considered to be a primary determinant of vascular structure [8]. Angiotensin II is able to produce vascular smooth muscle [4], smooth muscle cell hyperplasia [7, 6] or a rearrangement of vascular smooth muscle cells [1] depending on the model [5]. Angiotensin II also contributes to the control of growth through the release of growth promoting factors such as platelet-derived growth factor and basic fibroblast growth factor, and antiproliferative factors such as transforming growth factor [2] or through AT_2 -mediated apoptosis. Losartan, the first orally available AT_1 antagonist to be used clinically, might therefore be expected to be antiatherogenic, acting though the mechanism of an AT_1 antagonist, through its ability to inhibit LDL lipid-peroxidation, through its ability to lower blood pressure or possible through other as yet unknown mechanisms related to the actions of angiotensin II.

Atherosclerosis can take the form of a fatty streak in the intima of elastic vessels, eventually forming a plaque, or it may be a response to injury to the vessel wall resulting in a thickened intima and plaque formation. The major changes in both cases occur in the endothelium, the intima and the media. We have carried out a pilot study of the antiatherogenic action of Losartan using both models of atherosclerosis. The ability of Losartan to inhibit the development of atherosclerosis in the uninjured aorta and to reduce the response to injury in the injured common carotid artery in the hyperlipidemic rabbit model was examined.

Ten male New Zealand White rabbits were fed a high cholesterol diet (1% cholesterol) for three weeks. The right common carotid artery was injured by freezing a 2mm section with forceps cooled in liquid nitrogen. Five rabbits then continued on the high cholesterol diet for a further six weeks, while five rabbits received Losartan (10mg/kg/day) in addition to the high cholesterol diet for a further six weeks. Serum cholesterol was measured at initiation, at three weeks and at nine weeks. At sacrifice blood pressure was measured, followed by perfusion of the vascular system with Zamboni's fixative. The aorta and common carotid arteries were removed. The aorta was cut open and the segment between the origin of the left subclavian artery and the first pair of intercostal arteries was stained with sudan IV to reveal lipid deposits. The extent of lipid plaque was determined and expressed as a percentage of the area of the aortic segment. The right and left common carotid arteries were removed into Karnovsky's fixative. The injured segment and a comparable segment from the uninjured left carotid were processed for 1um sections and electron microscopy. The thickness of the intima at the injured site was compared for Losartan treated and untreated animals, and with the uninjured side.

The plaque area in the cholesterol-fed rabbits was 71+7%, while in the cholesterol-fed Losartan-treated rabbits the plaque area was reduced to 47+14%. The intimal thickness in the injured common carotid artery of cholesterol-fed rabbits was 175+7um, while in the cholesterol-fed, Losartan-treated rabbits the intimal thickness was 85+3um. The intima of the injured artery in both series of rabbits showed thickening of the endothelium, the presence of foam cells and phenotypically embryonic smooth muscle cells, and an increase in extracellular matrix.

This pilot study has confirmed that Losartan therapy can inhibit plaque formation in hypercholesterolemia in the aorta, and reduces intimal thickening following injury. These findings are contrary to those reported by [3] in hyperlipidemic rabbits, but consistent with the findings of [9]. The mechanism of action of Losartan as an antiatherogenic agent has not been fully elucidated, although most evidence suggests that the AT_1 receptor is involved. It is likely that Losartan and AII are able to influence only certain aspects of the control of smooth muscle growth and migration. It would therefore be expected that the timing of Losartan therapy in relation to the time course of plaque development or repair following injury would be critical to the end result. This study has shown that Losartan three weeks after initiation of hyperlipidemia is effective in reducing plaque, and that Losartan treatment beginning at the time of vascular injury is able to limit intimal thickening. The temporal relationship of Losartan action to the natural history of plaque formation and intimal thickening requires further study.

References

[1]   Baumbach G, Heistad DD. (1989). Remodeling of cerebral arterioles in chronic hypertension. Hypertension 13:968-972.

[2]   Dahlfors G, Chen Y, Wateson M, Arnqvist HJ. (1998). PDGF-BB-induced DNA synthesis is delayed by angiotensin II in vascular smooth muscle cells. Am. J. Physiol. 274:H1742-1748.

[3]   Fennessy PA, Campbell JH, Mendelsohn FAO, Campbell GR. (1996)Angiotensin-converting enzyme inhibitors and atherosclerosis: relevance of animal models to human disease. Clin. Exp. Pharm. Phys.23:Suppl.1, S30-32.

[4]   Geisterfer AT, Peach MJ, Owens GK. (1988). Angiotensin II induces hypertrophy, not hyperplasia, of cultured rat aortic smooth muscle cells. Circ. Res. 62:749-756.

[5]   Owens GK. (1993). Determinants of angiotensin II induced by hypertrophy versus hyperplasia in vascular smooth muscle. Drug Dev. Res. 29:83-87.

[6]   Paguet JL, Baudouin-Legros M, Brunelle G, Meyer P. (1990). Angiotensin II induced proliferation of aortic myocytes in spontaneously hypertensive rats. J. Hypertens. 8:565-572.

[7]   Resnik TJ, Scott-Burden T, Baur U, Buhler FR. (1987). Increased proliferation rate and phosphoinosite turnover in cultured smooth muscle cells from spontaneously hypertensive rats. J. Hypertens. 5:S145-148.

[8]   Unkelbach M, Auch-Schwelk W, Unkelbach E, Jautzke G, Fleck E. (1998) Regulation of aortic wall structure by the renin-angiotensin system in Wistar rats. J. Cardiovasc. Pharmacol. 31:31-38.

[9]   Van Kleef EM, ingerle J, Daemen MJAP. (1996) Angiotensin II-induced progression of neointimal thickening in the balloon-injured rat carotid artery is AT_1 receptor mediated. Arterioscler. Thromb. Vasc. Biol. 16:857-863.

Vascular Endothelium: Mechanisms of Cell Signaling
J.D. Catravas et al. (Eds.)
IOS Press, 1999

Inhibitory Effects of Lipoteichoic Acid, a Gram Positive Bacterial Cell Wall Product, on Lps-Induced Adhesion Molecule Expression and Chemokine Generation from Lung Microvascular Endothelial Cells

Anne Burke-Gaffney[1], **Paul G. Hellewell**[2] **& Kate Blease**[1]

[1]*Applied Pharmacology, Imperial College School of Medicine at the National Heart and Lung Institute, Dovehouse St., London.* [2]*Section of Medicine-Vascular Biology, Clinical Science Centre, Northern General Hospital, Sheffield*

Severe bacterial infection, often due to the presence of several different bacteria, may disrupt normal host defense mechanisms and spread from lung tissue into the blood. One defense mechanism that may be disrupted is recruitment of neutrophils, across the endothelial lining of blood vessel, to sites of infection. This process is governed by the interaction of cell adhesion molecules (CAM) on neutrophils and endothelial cells and also the actions of chemokines on neutrophils. Insufficient neutrophil recruitment to the site of infection may allow bacteria to multiply unchecked and pass into the blood. Cell wall products, such as lipopolysaccharide (LPS) from gram negative, or lipotechoic acid (LTA) from gram positive bacteria, normally increase endothelial CAM expression and chemokine release [1, 2] thus facilitating neutrophil recruitment and controlling infection. It is not known, however, what effects LPS and LTA, in combination, have on these control mechanisms. We hypothesize that, under certain conditions, these bacterial cell wall products may interact to suppress CAM expression and chemokine release and this may be one way in which normal host defense mechanisms are evaded.

In this study we investigated the effects of LPS and LTA, alone and together, on expression of the endothelial CAM, ICAM-1 (at 24h) and E-selectin (at 6h) and also release of the neutrophil chemokine, IL-8 (24h), from human lung microvascular endothelial cells (HLMVEC; Clonetics). CAM were detected by ELISA. Functional consequences of CAM expression were assessed by measuring adhesion of human peripheral blood neutrophils to LTA and/ or LPS-stimulated HLMVEC monolayers. Neutrophils, isolated by plasma/Percoll gradient centrifugation were labelled with a fluorescent dye (Calcein-AM, 10μM) and incubated (37°C, 30 min) with HLMVEC. Results are expressed as percent adherent cells over total cells added per well (1.25×10^5). IL-8 release into culture supernatants was quantified by radioimmunoassay. Effects on CAM or IL-8 mRNA were also determined, using a semi-quantitative R-PCR technique.

The effects of increasing concentrations of LTA (0.3 to 30μg/ml) on CAM expression and IL-8 release were bell-shaped, with a maximal response at 3μg/ml. LPS alone (0.01 and 0.1μg/ml) caused a significant increase in CAM expression and IL-8 release, that was inhibited in the presence of increasing concentrations of LTA. The inhibitory effect was not due to cell death, as assessed by cell viability assays. Inhibitory effects on CAM expression where paralleled by similar effects on neutrophil adhesion. For example, adhesion increased following stimulation of endothelial cells with LPS

(0.1µg/ml; 6h; 35±2%) was reduced to basal levels (18±1%) in the presence of LTA (30µg/ml). LTA also inhibited LPS-induced CAM or IL-8 mRNA, but this inhibition was reversed in the presence of the protein synthesis inhibitor, cycloheximide. LTA-induced repressor proteins may therefore mediate the inhibitory effects of LTA on LPS-induced CAM expression and IL-8 release.

These results suggest that the presence of cell wall products from gram negative and gram positive bacteria, together at sites of infection, may inhibit rather than increase endothelial CAM expression and chemokine release. These effects may lead to reduced neutrophil migration and thus less control of the bacterial infection. We have identified, therefore, a mechanism that may, in part, account for the ability of bacteria to evade host defense mechanisms and spread from the lungs to the blood and other organs. This process may ultimately result in a condition known as septic shock, the most common cause of death in hospital intensive care units. Understanding the mechanisms that allow bacteria to spread to the blood is important in developing treatments to prevent septic shock and it's lethal consequences.

KB holds a British Heart Foundation studentship. ABG is supported by the National Asthma Campaign, U.K.

References

[1]   Blease, K., Seybold, J., Adcock, I.M, Hellewell, P.G. & Burke-Gaffney, A. (1998a). *Am. J. Respir. Cell Mol. Biol.* **18**, 620-630.
[2]   Blease, K., Burke-Gaffney, A. and Hellewell, P. G. (1998b). *FASEB J.* **12**, A1005.

218

Vascular Endothelium: Mechanisms of Cell Signaling
J.D. Catravas et al. (Eds.)
IOS Press, 1999

VE Cadherin: A Cell Adhesion Receptor Essential for the Biological Functions of Blood Vessels

Danielle GULINO and **Thierry VERNET**

Macromolecule Engineering Laboratory, Jean-Pierre Ebel Institute of Structural Biology,
CEA/CNRS. 41 avenue des Martyrs - 38027 Grenoble Cedex 1 - France
Tel: 33 (0)4 76 88 92 04 - Fax: 33 (0)4 76 88 54 94. gulino@ibs.fr and vernet@ibs.fr

The traffic of molecules and cells between blood and tissues is regulated by a monolayer of contiguous cells lining all blood vessels: the vascular endothelium. The selective permeability of this cellular interface plays a critical role during the inflammatory response. Cohesion of the endothelial cells (EC) is ensured by adhesive proteins located at the inter-endothelial cell-cell junctions. One of these proteins, designated as VE cadherin (Vascular Endothelium cadherin), was isolated in 1992 by [1]. This 140 kDa transmembrane glycoprotein belongs to the cadherin cell adhesion receptor family whose adhesive properties result from Ca++-dependent auto-assembly of the same type of cadherin molecules through the inter-cellular space (homophilic interactions).

We have raised a series of polyclonal antibodies against recombinant VE cadherin fragments. To establish the physiological role of VE cadherin in endothelium, these antibodies, which specifically recognize the inter-endothelial junctions, were incubated with cells isolated from human umbilical vein cords. When added to confluent EC, AntiVE cadherin antibodies transiently generate interstices between cells resulting in a concomitant reversible increase of the permeability of EC monolayers. This result establishes the role played by VE cadherin in the maintenance of the endothelium integrity. Disorganisation of cell-cell contacts induces a small but significant increase of VE cadherin RNA leading to a rapid resynthesis of the molecule. Resynthesis of VE cadherin, which precedes the restoration of endothelium integrity, might take place following transmigration of leucocytes through the endothelial wall.

Modulation of homotypic interactions between VE cadherins likely plays a central role in endothelial cell-cell junction dynamics. Consequently, in parallel with our studies on the physiological role of VE cadherin, we have recently analysed the mechanism by which molecules of VE cadherin autoassemble. The basic structure of cadherins is constituted by an N-terminal extracellular domain composed of five homologous modules of about 100 amino acids (EC1-EC5) followed by a single transmembrane region and a conserved C-terminal cytoplasmic tail. Structural data for N and E cadherins show that the EC1 module dimerises, although the mode of assembly of the other four modules has not been clearly established. We have produced in E. coli and purified, the EC1 module and a fragment of the ectodomain encompassing the four N-terminal modules of VE cadherin (Cad 1-4), all deprived of disulfide bounds. The folding and oligomerization status of these recombinant fragments was evaluated by circular dichroism, gel filtration chromatography and analytical centrifugation. Despite of its correct folding, EC1 was shown to remain monomeric in solution up to a concentration of 350 mM, even in the presence of calcium. In contrast, Cad 1-4 monomers assembled into a Ca++-dependent 10.2 S complex whose molecular mass is compatible with an hexameric structure. At a

1.1 M concentration, half of the Cad1-4 molecules are monomeric and half are engaged into the complex. The complex, observed by electron microscopy, displays a hexagonal structure with a central cavity. These strutures assemble into honey comb-like structures. The relative orientation of each monomer within the hexamers and the biological significance of this molecular arrangement remain to be established. Taken together, these results underlines the synergy existing between the different extracellular modules of VE cadherin in promoting calcium-dependent homotypic interactions. Determination of the tridimensional structure of various modular arrays of VE cadherin is in progress and will provide additional information on the mechanism of cadherin assembly.

References

[1]   M.G. Lampugnani, M. Resnati, M. Raiteri, R. Pigott, A. Pisacane, G. Houen, L.P. Ruco, E. Dejana. (1992) J. Cell Biol., 118: 1511 - 1522

[2]   D. Gulino, E. Concord, E. Delachanal, Y. Genoux, M. Alemany, T. Vernet (1996). 6th European Bia Symposium, p. 55-61

220

Vascular Endothelium: Mechanisms of Cell Signaling
J.D. Catravas et al. (Eds.)
IOS Press, 1999

ICAM-1 and VCAM-1 Expression Induced by TNF-a Are Inhibited by A Glutathione Peroxidase Mimic

Patrizia D'Alessio(*), **Marc Moutet**(±), **Evelyne Coudrier**(§),
Sophie Darquenne(±) and **Jean Chaudière**(II)

(*) INSERM U75 CHU Necker Laboratoire de Biochimie Pharmacologique et Métabolique 75730 Paris Cedex 15 France (±) OXIS International SA 94385 Bonneuil s/Marne France (§) Institut Curie Laboratoire de Morphogénèse et Signalisation Cellulaire UMR 144 CNRS 75231 Paris France (II) UFR de Biologie Paris VII 75251 Paris France

Address correspondence to: Patrizia d'Alessio, M.D. Ph.D., Laboratoire de Biochimie Métabolique et Pharmacologique, Inserm U 75, CHU Necker, 156, rue de Vaugirard, 75730 Paris Cedex 15 France. Phone: 33-1-40615345, FAX: 33-1-40615585, E-mail: dalessio@necker.fr

Abstract

Intercellular adhesion molecule-1 (ICAM-1) and vascular cell adhesion molecule-1 (VCAM-1) are respectively involved in the endothelial recruitment of neutrophils and in that of lymphocytes or tumor cells, in response to specific signals. We have used the glutathione peroxidase (GPx) mimic BXT-51072 to assess the possibility that endogenous hydroperoxides play a role in the Tumor Necrosis Factor-a (TNFa)-induced expression of ICAM-1 and VCAM-1 by monolayers of human endothelial cells. The GPx mimic BXT-51072 strongly inhibits the TNFa-induced and cycloheximide-sensitive expression of ICAM-1 and VCAM-1. It also inhibits the TNFa-induced reorganization of the actin network and the associated formation of stress fibers. Actin reorganization induced by cytochalasin D treatment did not inhibit ICAM-1 expression. Our results are compatible with specific and synergistic effects of endogenous hydroperoxides on the biosynthesis and processing of cell adhesion molecules and cytoskeleton components.

1. Background

ICAM-1 is an adhesion molecule expressed constitutively by endothelial cells. Upon stimulation by cytokines and bacterial lipopolysaccharide (LPS), its expression contributes to the initiation of the inflammatory reaction. ICAM-1 mediates the adhesion and diapedesis of all classes of leukocytes to and through endothelium. Linkage with the cytoskeleton localizes ICAM-1 within regions of the endothelial cell membrane to facilitate leukocyte adherence/transmigration during the inflammatory reaction. In COS cells transfected with human ICAM-1 cDNA, the cytoplasmic domain of ICAM-1 binds to the cytoskeleton through its linkage with a-actinin - a cytoskeleton protein which would act as an anchor of actin filaments in the cell membrane [1]. Structural modifications of the cytoskeleton may play an important role in the topological distribution of ICAM-1 at the cell surface [2].

Like ICAM-1, VCAM-1 is an adhesion molecule of the immunoglobulin supergene family. VCAM-1 supports the adhesion of lymphocytes, monocytes, basophils and eosinophils, but not that of neutrophils to endothelial cells. VCAM-1 is important for the development of T-cell rich infiltrates, contributing to specific memory T-cell extravasation at sites of inflammation: it appears in acute immune cell-mediated inflammatory reactions. In vivo, VCAM-1 is known to be expressed in delayed hypersensitivity and allograft rejection [3]. Also, there is increasing evidence of ongoing immune stimulation during human atherogenesis where both VCAM-1 and ICAM-1 have been shown to provide costimulatory signals for T cell activation [4]. Beside its role in cell-cell and cell-matrix adhesion, VCAM-1 is also involved, thanks to its versatile receptor a4b1 integrin, in tumor metastasis extravasation. VLA-4 molecules expressed by tumor cells initiate their adhesion to endothelial cells through interaction with VCAM-1 molecules expressed by the latter [5].

When the recruitment of leukocytes at vascular sites is required for host defence or for tissue remodelling in response to injury, the inflammatory cytokine Tumor Necrosis Factor-a (TNF-a) released by activated macrophages, stimulates the expression of ICAM-1 and VCAM-1 by endothelial cells. The incubation of an endothelial monolayer with TNF-a induces a high level of expression of such adhesive molecules by endothelial cells, as well as the extensive reorganization of actin filaments with the appearance of stress fibers.

Once activated, leukocytes also release reactive oxygen species, such as superoxide and hydrogen peroxide. TNF-a itself stimulates the endothelial production of peroxides [6] and that of hydrogen peroxide in particular. Hydrogen peroxide acts as a redox regulator of cell signaling [7] and it has also been shown to interfere with actin polymerization [8]. In endothelial cells exposed to hydrogen peroxide, a reversible S-protein thiolation [9] is accompanied by cell shrinkage and loss of cell to cell contact due to structural reorganization of the cytoskeleton.

Glutathione peroxidases (GPx) are selenoenzymes which catalyze the reduction of hydrogen peroxide and organic hydroperoxides in the cytosolic and mitochondrial compartments of the cell. In a previous study, we found that a marked protection of human endothelial cells could be obtained with the new GPx mimic BXT-51072 [10, 11] from the toxicity of either hydroperoxides, TNF-a-activated neutrophils or TNF-a alone.

In this work, we have studied the relationships between the endothelial expression of ICAM-1 and VCAM-1, and modifications of the actin network, upon stimulation with TNF-a. Furthermore, we have used the GPx mimic BXT-51072 to assess the possibility that endogenous hydroperoxides play a role in such relationships. The present study shows that this GPx mimic is indeed able to inhibit the structural modifications of the endothelial cytoskeleton induced by TNF-a. Moreover, this compound inhibits the TNF-a-induced expression of the adhesion molecules ICAM-1 and VCAM-1 by endothelial cells. Interestingly, such effects were not observed with ebselen, a selenoorganic compound which was first shown to exhibit GPx activity.

2. Discussion

Circulating leukocytes reach tissues by crossing the endothelium. Following infection or trauma, inflammatory cytokines, such as TNF-a or Il-1, induce the endothelial expression of adhesion molecules for circulating leukocytes.

Leucocytes recruited by endothelial cells may release peroxides. Moreover, it has been shown [6] that TNF-a increases the production of endogenous peroxides of mitochondrial origin, i.e., hydrogen peroxide. Thus endothelial antioxidant enzymes might be critically involved in the regulation of the endothelial response to both endogenous and exogenous peroxides. In particular, glutathione peroxidases (Se-GPx) play a prominent role in endothelial cells and the latter are known to efficiently recycle the reduced form of glutathione [12, 9]. In a previous study [11], we showed that ultrastructural modifications of endothelial cells induced by exogenous hydrogen peroxide were extensive. They consisted mainly in a disruption of the cell monolayer with a marked decrease in cell density. A pre-treatment with the GPx mimic preserved the integrity of the cell monolayer and inhibited the morphological alterations induced by subsequent stimulation with hydrogen peroxide.

In this study, we focused on two main effects of TNF-a on endothelial cells, i.e. the induced expression of adhesive molecules and alterations of the cytoskeleton [13]. We reported previously that the GPx mimic BXT-51072 also inhibited the TNF-a induced release of Il-8 as well as the expressions of E- and P-selectin [10]. Here we have shown that this GPx mimic counteracts the effects of TNF-a stimulation on the cytoskeleton structure as well as on the expression of the adhesive molecules ICAM-1 and VCAM-1 in endothelial cells. Such results suggest that an increase in intracellular hydrogen peroxide and/or other hydroperoxides would mediate such effects of TNF-a.

The drastic reorganization of actin filaments which is observed upon incubation of endothelial cells with TNF-a and the enhanced expression of ICAM-1 are concomitant. However, as suggested by the results obtained in the presence of cytochalasin D, actin reorganization does not seem to be a prerequisite of the expression of ICAM-1 at the cell surface (Figure 1). This suggests that the two processes are not coupled to each other.

The GPx mimic BXT-51072 used in this study prevented TNF-a induced actin reorganization as well as ICAM-1 and VCAM-1 expressions to a large extent. The effects of BXT-51072 on endothelial actin fibers, observed following TNF-a stimulation, suggested that this compound might interfere with the adhesion transducing unit constituted by actin/a-actinin/ICAM-1 [1]. A similar type of structural organization was reported for ELAM-1 [14]. However, the experiments using actin-disrupting agents show that ICAM-1 expression is independent from the state of the actin filament network. Consequently, the inhibitory effect on ICAM-1 expression, observed following treatment with the GPx mimic, is independent from that observed on actin filament reorganization. Nevertheless, upon TNF-a stimulation, association of ICAM-1 with the complex made of actin and a-actinin may account for the surface anchoring of a part of ICAM-1. This would be illustrated by the enhanced ICAM-1 expression following co-incubation with TNF-a and cytochalasin D.

TNF-a stimulates the intracellular production of H_2O_2, which is known to activate NF-kB-dependent gene transcription. Glutathione peroxidase was recently shown to down-regulate this process [15]. This could explain the major effect of the GPx mimic BXT-51072 on the biosynthesis of adhesion molecules. The much more potent effects of BXT-51072 compared with those of ebselen, are consistent with its higher GPx activity, as well as with its much stronger protective effects when endothelial cells are exposed to exogenous hydroperoxides [16]. Moreover, we have shown that the sulfur analog of BXT-51072, which exhibits a very weak GPx activity, had no effect on endothelial pro-inflammatory responses following TNF-a stimulation [17]. This is consistent with an important role of the GPx activity of BXT- 51072, but the intracellular compartmentation of this GPx mimic is unknown.

However, one cannot exclude the possibility that other effects could play a major role, such as direct interference of this seleno-organic compound with enzymes of the lipoxygenase pathway or with thiol/disulfide exchanges. Although the involvement of such mechanisms in the regulation of cell adhesion molecule expression is not demonstrated, it is well established that cytoskeletal rearrangements can be regulated by 5- or 12-lipoxygenase [18, 19] as well as by S-thiolation [20, 21, 22].

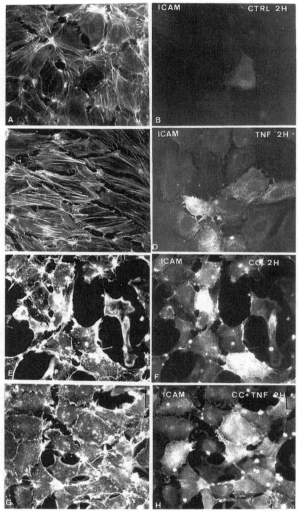

Figure 1.Structure of the endothelial actin network and ICAM-1 expression, as assessed by double immuno-fluorescent labeling of F-actin and ICAM-1. On the left side: actin filaments labeled with rhodamine / phalloidine. On the right side: ICAM-1 detected with a mouse monoclonal anti-ICAM-1 antibody and with a fluorescein-conjugated rabbit anti-mouse IgG. Observations performed by means of optical microscopy (original magnification x 630).

A: actin filaments in endothelial cells (control cells) following 2 hours of incubation with complete medium (20% FCS). **B**: ICAM-1 expression in endothelial cells following 2 hours of incubation with complete medium (20% FCS). **C**: actin filaments in endothelial cells following 2 hours of TNF-a stimulation **D**: ICAM-1 expression in endothelial cells following 2 hours of incubation with TNF-a. **E**: actin filaments in endothelial cells following 30 minutes of cytochalasin D treatment, washing, and then 2 hours of further cytochalasin D treatment. **F**: ICAM-1 expression in endothelial cells following 30 minutes of cytochalasin D treatment, washing, and then 2 hours of further cytochalasin D treatment. **G**: actin filaments in endothelial cells following 30 minutes incubation with cytochalasin D, washing with PBS and 2 hours of further incubation with TNF-a and cytochalasin D. **H**: ICAM-1 expression in endothelial cells following 30 minutes incubation with cytochalasin D, washing with PBS and 2 hours of further incubation with TNF-a and cytochalasin D.

Based on the effects of the GPx mimic BXT-51072 used in this study, it is tempting to speculate that actin reorganization and the expression of cell adhesion molecules are both under primary control of the peroxide tone. Actin reorganization is independent from protein synthesis, as shown with cycloheximide (Figure 2), and ICAM-1 surface expression does not depend on actin filament reorganization, as shown with cytochalasin D. Therefore, we propose that, upon TNFa-stimulation, the inhibition of two distinct pathways, both depending on hydroperoxides, may account for the effects of the GPx mimix BXT-51072 observed on adhesion molecules and cytoskeleton components in endothelial cells.

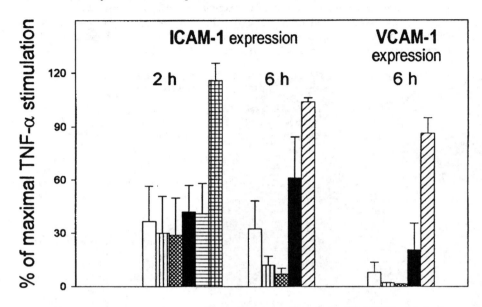

Figure 2. Effect of cycloheximide, cytochalasin D and the GPx mimics BXT 51072 and ebselen on the endothelial expression of ICAM-1 and VCAM-1 induced by TNF-a. HUVEC were exposed or non-exposed (control cells) to 1 ng/ml TNF-a for 2 or 6 hours and then fixed. The cell surface expression of ICAM-1 and VCAM-1 was determined by primary binding with a mouse monoclonal antibody to human ICAM-1 and human VCAM-1, respectively, which was followed by secondary binding with an alkaline phosphatase-conjugated rabbit anti-mouse IgG. Results are expressed as percentages of the maximal cell adhesion molecule expression measured in the presence of TNF-a alone. *Open bars*: Control cells. For experiments with cycloheximide, HUVEC were incubated with 10 mg/ml cycloheximide for 2 and 6 hours in the absence (*vertical hatched bars*) or in the presence (*crossed hatched bars*): of TNF-a. For experiments with cytochalasin D, HUVEC were pre-treated with 0.5 mM cytochalasin D for 30 minutes and then incubated for 2 hours in the presence of 0.5 mM cytochalasin D alone (*horizontal hatched bar*) or 0.5 mM cytochalasin D plus TNF-a (*grid hatched bar*). GPx mimics were tested at 10 mM by pre-treating HUVEC for 1 h and further co-treating them during TNF-a stimulation. *Closed bars*: BXT-51072 + TNF-a. The expression of cell adhesion molecules observed in the presence of BXT-51072 alone (% as above described) are 30.4±18.6 and 34.1±18.0 for ICAM-1 at 2 and 6 hours, respectively, and 7.3±6.0 for VCAM-1). *Slash hatched bars*: Ebselen + TNF-a. The expression of cell adhesion molecules observed in the presence of ebselen alone (% as above described) are 47.5±15.2 and 12.7±6.7 for ICAM-1 and VCAM-1 at 6 hours, respectively.

References

[1]   Carpen, O.; Pallai, P.; Stauton, D.E.; Springer, T.A. Association of Intercellular Adhesion Molecule-1 (ICAM-1) with actin-containing cytoskeleton a-actinin. *J. Cell Biol.* **5**:1223-1234; 1992.

[2]   Helander, T.S.; Carpen, O.; Turunen, O.; Kovanen, P.E.; Vaheri, A.; Timonen, T. ICAM-2 redistributed by ezrin as a target for killer cells. *Nature* **382**:265-268;   1996.

[3]   Briscoe, D.M.; Schoen, F.J.; Rice, G.E.; Bevilacqua, M.P.; Ganz P. Induced expression of endothelial-leukocyte adhesion molecules in human cardiac   allografts.*Transplantation.*   **51**:537-539; 1991.

[4]   Libby, P.; Hongmei L. Vascular cell adhesion molecule-1 and smooth muscle cell activation during atherogenesis. *J. Clin. Invest.* **92**:538-539; 1993.

[5]   Kawaguchi, S.; Kikuchi, K.; Ishii, S.; Takada, Y.; Kobayashi, S.; Uede, T. VLA-4 molecules on tumor cells initiate an adhesive interaction with VCAM-1 molecules on endothelial cell surface. *Japanese J. Cancer Res.* **83**:1304-1316; 1992.

[6]   Schulze-Osthoff, K.; Bakker, A.C.; Vanhaesebroek, B.; Beyaert, R.; Jacob,   W.A.; and Fiers W. Cytotoxic activity of tumor necrosis factor is mediated by early   damage   of   mitochondrial function. *J. Biol. Chem.* **267**:5317-5323; 1992.

[7]   Schreck, R. and P.A. Bauerle. Assessing oxygen radicals as mediators in activation of inducible eukaryotic transcription factor NF-kB. *Meth. Enzymol.* **234**:151-163; 1994.

[8]   Dalle Donne, I.; Milzani, A.; Colombo, R. H_2O_2-treated actin: assembly and polymer interactions with cross-linking proteins. *Biophys.J.* **69**:2710-2719; 1995.

[9]   Schuppe-Koistinen, I.; Gerdes, R.; Moldeus, P. and Cotgreave, I.A. Studies on   the reversibility of protein-S-thiolation in human endothelial cells. *Arch. Biochem. Biophys.* **315**:226-234; 1994.

[10]   Moutet, M.; Malette, P.; Devaux, V.; Darquenne, S.; d'Alessio, P. and Chaudière, J. Endothelial protection by BXT-51072 and other glutathione peroxidase mimics. *Oxygen '95.* I-**73**:50 abstr. (1995).

[11]   d'Alessio, P.; Moutet, M.; Marsac, M.; Chaudière, J. Pharmacological modulation of endothelial cytoskeleton induced by hydrogen peroxide and TNF-a. *C.R. Soc. Biol.* **190**:289-297; 1996.

[12]   Jongkind, G.; Verkerk, A.and Baggen, R.G. Glutathione metabolism of human vascular endothelial cells under peroxidative stress. *Free Radic. Biol. Med.* **7**:507-512; 1989.

[13]   Goldblum, S.E.; Ding, X.; Campbell-Washington,J. TNF-a induces endothelial cell F-actin depolymerization, new actin synthesis, and barrier dysfunction. *Am. J. Physiol.* **264**:C894-905; 1993.

[14]   Yoshida, M.; Westlin, W.F.; Wang, N.; Ingber, D.E.; Rosenzweig, A.; Resnick, N.; Gimbrone, M.A. Leukocyte adhesion to vascular endothelium induces E-selectin linkage to the actin cytoskeleton. *J. Cell Biol.* **133**:445-455; 1996.

[15]   Kretz-Remy, C.; Mehlen, P.; Mirault, M.E.; Arrigo, A.P. Inhibition of IkBa phosphorylation and degradation and subsequent NFkB activation by glutathione peroxidase overexpression. *J. Cell Biol.* **133**:1083-1093; 1996.

[16]   Chaudière, J.; Yadan, J.C.; Erdelmeier, I.; Tailhan-Lomont, C.; Moutet, M. Design of new selenium-containing mimics of glutathione peroxidase. In: R. Paoletti editor *Oxidative Processes and Antioxidants*. New York: Raven Press Ltd; 1994:165-184.

[17]   Moutet M, d'Alessio P, Malette P, Devaux V, Chaudière J. Glutathione peroxidase mimics prevent TNF-a and neutrophil-induced endothelial alterations, Free Radic. Biol. Med., in press.

[18]   Peppelenbosch, M.P.; Tertoolen, L.G.J.; Hage, W.J.; de Laat, S.W. Epidermal   Growth   Factor-induced actin remodeling is regulated by 5-lipoxygenase and cycloxygenase   products.   *Cell* **74**:565-575; 1993.

[19]   Tang, D.G.; Timar, J.; Grossi, I.M.; Renaud, C.; Kimler, V.A.; Diglio, C.A.; Taylor, J.D.; Honn, K.V. The lipoxygenase metabolite, 12(S)-HETE, induces a protein kinase C-dependent cytoskeletal rearrangement and retraction of microvascular cells. *Exp. Cell Res.* **207**:361-37; 1993.

[20]   Edelhauser, H.F.; van Horn, D.L.; Miller, P.; Pederson, H.J. Effect of thiol-oxidation of glutathione with diamide on corneal endothelial function, junctional   complexes, and microfilaments. *J. Cell Biol.* **68**:567-578; 1976.

[21]   Spangenberg, P.; Till, U.; Gschmeissner, S.; Crawford, N. Changes in the distribution and organization of platelet actin induced by diamide and its functional consequences. *Brit. J. Haematol.* **67**:443-450; 1987.

[22]   Prescott, A.R.; Stewart, S.; Duncan, G.; Gowing, R.;.Warn, R.M. Diamide induces reversible changes in morphology, cytoskeleton and cell-cell coupling in lens epithelial cells. *Exp. Eye Res.* **52**:83-92; 1991.

Vascular Endothelium: Mechanisms of Cell Signaling
J.D. Catravas et al. (Eds.)
IOS Press, 1999

Regulation of Genes Involved in Lipid Homeostasis and the Pathogenesis of Atherosclerosis: The Role of Promoters, Enhancers, Hormone Nuclear Receptors and Auxiliary Factors in Apolipoprotein Gene Regulation

Vassilis Zannis, Eleni Zanni and Dimitris Kardassis
Section of Molecular Genetics, Boston University Medical Center, Boston and
Division of Basic Sciences, Department of Medicine, University of Crete, Heraklion

Human apolipoproteins participate in cholesterol homeostasis. ApoA-I participates in the reverse transport of cholesterol whereas apoC-II and apoC-III modulate the catabolism of triglyceride-rich lipoproteins. The apoA-I, apoC-III and apoA-IV genes are located within a 15 kb gene cluster on chromosome 11 and utilize common regulatory elements for their transcription [1]. A similar gene cluster exists on chromosome 19 and contains the human apoE, ApoC-IV and apoC-II genes within a 45 kb region [2].

A common feature of the proximal promoters of the apoA-I/C-III/A-IV cluster is that they contain Hormone Response Elements (HREs) which are the binding sites for homo and heterodimers of hormone nuclear receptors [1, 3-7]. In addition, the activity of the three promoters is controlled by a common enhancer located between -800 and -600 bp upstream of the apoC-III gene within the apoC-III distal promoter region. The enhancer contains multiple Sp1 binding sites as well as HREs [4-7].

In vitro mutagenesis combined with transient transfection assays and antisense methodologies established the specificities of the different HREs and showed that HNF-4 plays an important role for the promoter/enhancer activity in cell cultures. Members of the jun/ATF-2 family of transcription factors and SMAD proteins which participate in TGF-β mediated signal transduction pathways were also shown to modulate the activity of the apoA-I promoter /apoC-III enhancer cluster. Transgenic experiments established that the HRE site of the enhancer is essential for the intestinal expression of the apoA-I gene but is not required for the hepatic expression.

Similar analysis established that the 0.55 kb intergenic region between the apoC-II and apoC-IV genes is a strong cell type specific promoter and its activity is enhanced by the Hepatic Control Region-1 (HCR-1) only in hepatic cells. The apoC-II promoter contains five regulatory elements designated CIIA to CIIE. Important role in apoC-II gene regulation and transcriptional enhancement play two hormone response elements which map within elements CIIB (-102/-81) and CIIC (-159/-116) and have different specificities for orphan and ligand-dependent nuclear receptors. CIIC is recognized by ARP-1, EAR-2 and RXRα/T3Rβ heterodimers but not by HNF-4, whereas CIIB is recognized exclusively by HNF-4 [8,9].

Transienr co-transfection experiments showed that in the presence of T3, RXR/T3R heterodimers transactivated the apoC-II promoter in HepG2 and COS-1 cells. No transactivation was observed in the presence of 9-cis retinoic acid. Transactivation requires the regulatory element CIIC suggesting that this element contains a thyroid hormone response element (TRE) [9]. HNF-4 did not affect the apoC-II promoter activity in HepG2 cells. However, mutations in the HNF-4 binding site on element CIIB and inhibition of HNF-4 synthesis in HepG2 cells by antisense HNF-4 constructs decreased the apoC-II promoter activity to 25 to 40% of the control indicating that HNF-4 is a positive regulator of the apoC-II gene (9). ARP-1, another orphan nuclear receptor repressed the apoC-II promoter activity. Repression required the presence of the regulatory element CIIC. In contrast, combination of ARP-1 and HNF-4 transactivated different apoC-II promoter segments. Mutagenesis or deletion of elements CIIB or CIIC established that the observed transactivation requires DNA binding of one of the two factors and may result from HNF-4: ARP-1 interactions which elicit the transactivation function of HNF-4 [9].

The combined data indicate that $RXR\alpha/T3R\beta$ heterodimers in the presence of T3 and HNF-4 can upregulate the apoC-II promoter activity by binding to the regulatory element CIIC and CIIB respectively. In addition, ARP-1 can either have inhibitory effect by binding directly to DNA or a stimulatory effect via putative protein-protein interactions with HNF-4.

The overall data suggest that the apoC-II promoter/HCR-1 cluster can direct expression in cells of hepatic origin and it can be transactivated by orphan and ligand-dependent nuclear receptors. Optimal enhancer activity requires synergisitc interactions between factors bound to the distal HCR-1 and nuclear receptors bound to the two proximal hormone response elements.

Apolipoproteins have been implicated in the protection or the pathogenesis of atherosclerosis. Their local concentration may also affect endothelial functions. Understanding the regulatory mechanisms that control their expression may provide, in the near future, new modes of protection and/or treatment of atherosclerosis.

References

[1]   Kardassis D, Laccotrippe, M., Talianidis, I. and Zannis, V. (1996) Hypertension 27: 980-1008 (1996)
[2]   Allan, C., Walker, D. and Taylor, JM. (1995) J. Biol. Chem. 270:26278-26281.
[3]   Ladias, J.A.A., Hadzopoulou-Cladaras, M., Kardassis, D., Cardot, P., Cheng, J., Zannis V., and Cladaras, C. (1992) J. Biol. Chem. 267:15849-15860.
[4]   Talianidis, I., A. Tambakaki, J., Toursounova and V. I. Zannis. (1995). Biochemistry 34:10298-10309.
[5]   Tzameli, I. and Zannis, V. (1996) J. Biol. Chem. 271:8402-8415.
[6]   Kardassis, D., Tzameli, I., Talianidis, I. and Zannis V. (1997) Arteriosclerosis, Thrombosis & Vascular Biology. 17:222-232.
[7]   Lavrentiadou, S., Hadzopoulou-Cladaras, M., Kardassis, D. and Zannis, V. (1998) Biochemistry submitted.
[8]   Vorgia P., Zannis V. and Kardassis D. (1998) . J. Biol. Chem. 273:4188-4196.
[9]   Kardassis, D., Sacharidou, E. and Zannis, V. (1998) J. Biol. Chem. In Press.

Vascular Endothelium: Mechanisms of Cell Signaling
J.D. Catravas et al. (Eds.)
IOS Press, 1999

Transcript Profiles of Human Endothelial Cells and Smooth Muscle Cells

Olga Bandman and <u>Benjamin G. Cocks</u>
Department of Exploratory Biology, Incyte Pharmaceuticals Inc.
Palo Alto, CA, USA

A major focus of our group is the application of genomics tools, such as DNA microarray technology and high-throughput sequencing, to understanding the processes and individual gene functions in cells mediating or regulating inflammation. Monitoring the expression of thousands of genes in parallel in endothelial cells, macrophages, and vascular smooth muscle cells under various stimuli provides new information on the nature of these cells and their dynamic regulatory roles. Critical information can be distilled from the large amount of data obtained using specially designed software. Appropriate software and mining tools developed at Incyte allow efficient evaluation of these experiments in the context of an integrated database, which includes relevant clinical samples and treated primary vascular cells from different organs. In addition to confirming many published observations, we have been able to discover novel genes and new gene networks participating in vascular function and inflammatory processes.

Vascular Endothelium: Mechanisms of Cell Signaling
J.D. Catravas et al. (Eds.)
IOS Press, 1999

Direct Actions of Angiopoietin-1 on Human Endothelium: Evidence for Network Stabilization and Interaction with Other Angiogenic Growth Factors

Andreas Papapetropoulos, **David Fulton, Guillermo García-Gardeña**
and William C. Sessa
Boyer Center for Molecular Medicine, Yale University School of Medicine
New Haven, CT, USA

Angiopoietin-1 (Ang-1) is the first member of a newly described family of angiogenic proteins. The importance of Ang-1 for blood vessel formation *in vivo* was documented in experiments where the Ang-1 gene was disrupted leading to a lethal phenotype in the homozygous mutant. However, no direct actions of Ang-1 on endothelial cell (EC) phenotype have been demonstrated to date. To evaluate the ability of Ang-1 to influence vascular network structure, we used an in vitro matrix-driven angiogenesis assay. When confluent cultures of human umbilical vein EC (HUVEC) where overlaid with type I collagen they rapidly reorganized into networks consisting of tubes and cords within 3 to 6 hrs. The networks matured by approximately 12 hrs and then started to regrets leaving few traces of organized structures by 24hrs. Addition of Ang-1 to the culture medium allowed the networks to survive for up to 48hrs. The effects of Ang-1 on network stabilization resulted from activation of the Tie2 receptor, since a soluble form of the Tie2 receptor completely abrogated the effects of Ang-1.

The rapid regression of the HUVEC network in the collagen overlay assays led us to hypothesize that the stabilizing action of Ang-1 on the vascular networks may result from inhibition of cell death. Indeed, when HUVEC were cultured in the absence of endothelial cell growth supplement (ECGS), there was a $46.6 \pm 6.7\%$ decrease in the number of cells surviving after 48hrs. The addition of Ang-1 to the culture medium prevented EC death in a concentration-dependent manner. Consistent with previously published results, Ang-1 failed to stimulate EC proliferation, in contrast to both vascular endothelial growth factor (VEGF) and EGCS. In addition, Ang-1 was a weak migratory stimulus in Byden chamber assays, with high amounts (1μg/ml) required in order to stimulate migration.

To investigate the ability of Ang-1 to drive tube formation, we used the three dimensional collagen gel culture system. Under these conditions, HUVEC did not engage in network formation in the presence of Ang-1, while parallel cultures exposed to VEGF organized into complex networks of tubes within 48hrs. The different behavior of ang-1 in the two *in vitro* angiogenesis assays (3D vs. overlay) suggests that Ang-1 is not sufficient to initiate endothelial cell re-organization. Perhaps Ang-1 has a more delayed role in the neovascularization process, participating in the stabilization and maturation of vascular structures.

In order to examine if an interaction exists between Ang-1 and other known angiogenic factors, overlay cultures of HUVEC were exposed to VEGF or ECGS in the presence of Ang-1. While the morphological appearance of the network was determined by the primary mitogen (ECGS or VEGF), networks exposed simultaneously to ECGS or VEGF and Ang-1 survived for longer periods of time than cultures exposed to any of the growth factors alone.

To determine if vascular cells express angiopoietins in culture, we used reverse transcription polymerase chain reaction to amplify Ang-1 and Ang-2 from cultured human EC, smooth muscle, fibroblasts and macrophages. All cells tested, with the exception of macrophages, expressed Ang-1. On the other hand, Ang-2 was only expressed by endothelial cells (HUVEC and dermal microvascular cells).

The current model for the actions of Ang-1 in vascular development and angiogenesis suggests that ang-1 cause the release of a substance that initiates recruitment of mesenchymal cells to the developing vasculature resulting in more stable neovessel structures. The results of the present study offer an additional action by which Ang-1 can influence angiogenesis, namely by directly stabilizing EC networks and by modulating growth factor mediated reorganization of Ecs, both effects that occur in the absence of accessory cells. Understanding the molecular mechanisms of EC plasticity in vitro and in vivo.

Vascular Endothelium: Mechanisms of Cell Signaling
J.D. Catravas et al. (Eds.)
IOS Press, 1999

Complex Role of Matrilysin and Type IV Collagenases in Angiogenesis

QingXiang Amy Sang

Biochemistry Division, Department of Chemistry, Florida State University,
Tallahassee, Florida 32306-4390, U.S.A.

Matrix metalloproteinases (MMPs) are a family of highly homologous zinc endopeptidases that cleave peptide bonds of the extracellular matrix (ECM) proteins, such as collagens, laminins, proteoglycans, and fibronectin. Their proteolytic activities are regulated by tissue inhibitors of metalloproteinases (TIMPs). This family of proteinases are involved in normal morphogenesis, development, reproduction, wound healing, and neovascularization and collateral circulation. However, the imbalance of MMPs and their tissue inhibitors may contribute to pathological processes such as cardiovascular diseases, cancer metastasis and angiogenesis, and arthritis. Angiogenesis consists of a sequence of events that include dissolution of the basement membrane underlying the endothelial cell layer, migration and proliferation of endothelial cells, formation of the vascular capillary, and formation of a new basement membrane. 72 kDa gelatinase A/type IV collagenase (MMP-2) and 92 kDa gelatinase B/type IV collagenase (MMP-9) dissolve basement membrane type IV collagen and may initiate and promote angiogenesis. The two type IV collagenases are produced as inactive proenzymes (zymogens) by many types of cells including endothelia. We have demonstrated that matrilysin (MMP-7) is able to proteolytically activate pro-MMP-2 and Pro-MMP-9, thus, it may also contribute to the initiation of angiogenesis. A different paradigm is also suggested based on the reports by us and others: MMP-7, MMP-9, stromelysin (MMP-3), and metalloelastase (MMP-12) may inhibit angiogenesis by converting plasminogen to angiostatin, which is one of the most potent angiogenesis inhibitors. MMPs and TIMPs play a complex role in regulating angiogenesis. An understanding of the biochemical and cellular pathways and mechanisms of angiogenesis will provide significant information to allow the regulation of neovascularization, e.g. the stimulation of angiogenesis for coronary collateral circulation formation and the inhibition for cancer and arthritis.

(This work was in part supported by a Grant-in-Aid AHA 9601457 from the American Heart Association, Florida Affiliate to Dr. Sang)

Vascular Endothelium: Mechanisms of Cell Signaling
J.D. Catravas et al. (Eds.)
IOS Press, 1999

PULMONARY ENDOTHELIUM-BOUND ANGIOTENSIN CONVERTING ENZYME ACTICITY IN SYSTEMIC SCLERODERMA

E. Psevdi, S.E. Orfanos, D. Langleben, P.G. Vlachoyiannopoulos, I. Pakas, N. Stratigis, G. Anastasiadis, J.D. Catravas, M. Kyriakidis, H.M. Moutsopoulos, and Ch. Roussos

Critical Care Department, Evangelismos Hospital, Athens, Greece;
Departments of Pathophysiology and Cardiology, Laikon Hospital, Athens, Greece;
Department of Medicine, Division of Cardiology, Jewish General Hospital, Montreal,
Canada; Vascular Biology Center, Medical College of Georgia, Augusta, Georgia USA

Systemic scleroderma (SSc) is a chronic autoimmune disease characterized by early endothelial damage and collagen deposition in the skin and internal organs. In the lung, the diffuse (dSSc) and the limited (lSSc) subsets of SSc are characterized by pulmonary fibrosis (PF) and pulmonary hypertension (PH), respectively. The purpose of this study was to investigate: whether PCEB ACE dysfunction, an index of endothelial injury occurs in SSc, and whether it occurs prior to PH and/or PF development. Pulmonary capillary endotheliun-bound (PCEB) angiotensin converting enzyme (ACE) activity was estimated in eleven dSSc and six lSSc patients, as well as in nine adult volunteers (controls) with no lung disease, undergoing right heart catheterization for clinical purposes. By means of indicator-dilution techniques we measured the single pass transpulmonary hydrolysis of the synthetic ACE substrate ^{3}H-benzoyl-Phe-Ala-Pro (BPAP), expressed as % metabolism (%M) and $v = -\ln(1-M)$, and calculated the modified kinetic parameter A_{max}/K_m, an index of functional capillary surface area (FCSA). Mean pulmonary artery pressure (mPAP) and pulmonary vascular resistance (PVR) were estimated in six dSSc, six lSSc patients and the nine volunteers. Pulmonary fibrosis was additionally estimated by high resolution computerized tomography (CT) of the lung in sixteen SSc patients.

BPAP %M and v were decreased in SSc as compared to controls (52.4 % $\pm$ 5.1 vs 83.9 $\pm$ 1.8, p<0.001 and 0.86 $\pm$ 0.13 vs 1.87 $\pm$ 0.1, p<0.001, respectively) with no differences between dSSc and lSSc (48.4 % $\pm$ 5.8 vs 59.7 $\pm$ 9.8 and 0.74 $\pm$ 0.14 vs 1.07 $\pm$ 0.27, respectively), denoting the endothelial dysfunction in SSc. A_{max}/K_m normalized to body surface area (BSA) was also reduced in SSc (1902 $\pm$ 460 ml/min/m^2 vs. 3707 $\pm$ 417), reflecting the loss of FCSA. Similar reductions in all PCEB ACE activity parameters were observed in patients where pulmonary hemodynamics were obtained, with no differences between SSc and controls in mPAP or PVR (21.9 $\pm$ 2.1 mmHg vs 18.9 $\pm$ 1.4, and 185 $\pm$ 50 dyn sec/cm^5 vs 107 $\pm$ 14, respectively). There was no correlation between either v or A_{max}/K_m/BSA and %PF on lung CT, while in the absence of PF (0% on CT, n=6) v ranged from 1.97 to 0.33, suggestive of severe PCEB ACE activity reduction in some patients. Thus, our study provides evidence for PCEB ACE dysfunction in SSc in the absence of PH or PF.

Supported by a grant from the Greek Ministry of Health (KESY) and a grant from the Athens University.

Vascular Endothelium: Mechanisms of Cell Signaling
J.D. Catravas et al. (Eds.)
IOS Press, 1999

Angiogenic Hyaluronan Oligosaccharides interact with Endothelial Cell CD44 to Upregulate Expression of Adhesion Molecules, VEGF Receptors and IL-8

West DC, Wilson J, Lagoumintzis G. and Joyce M.
Department of Immunology, University of Liverpool
P.O.Box. 147, Liverpool L69 3BX, UK
Tel 0151 706 4358; Fax 0151 706 5814; e-mail westie@liv.ac.uk.

Hyaluronan (HA, also called hyaluronic acid or hyaluronate) is a high-molecular-weight linear polysaccharide, a glycosaminoglycan, composed of repeating 1,4- linked disaccharide units of 1,3- linked glucuronic acid and N-acetylglucosamine. Although small amounts are present in the extracellular matrix of most animal tissues, the highest concentrations are found in the avascular adult connective tissues. This distribution, combined with its high water- binding capacity and simple structure, led to the general belief that it was an inert viscoelastic lubricant, or space filling molecule [38, 14]. However, an increasing body of evidence has accumulated suggesting that HA has a significant regulatory effect on the behaviour of many cell- types, through interaction with several surface receptors [7, 17].

Localised accumulation occurs in association with tissue damage, organ rejection and in many inflammatory diseases, notably psoriasis and scleroderma, and it is a major component of many tumours [20,16]. A HA- rich matrix also develops transiently during embryogenesis, and adult tissue regeneration, coinciding with rapid cell proliferation and migration. Significantly, subsequent tissue differentiation, vasculogenesis and angiogenesis, occur concomitantly with a decrease in tissue HA levels [42]. The temporal and spatial distribution of HA during embryogenesis suggests that both the synthesis and degradation of HA play an important regulatory role in these processes, and certain pathological conditions such as tumour growth and metastasis [9, 46, 47].

Angiogenesis and HA size *in vivo*

The high concentration of HA found in avascular tissues, such as cartilage and vitreous humour, and at relatively avascular sites, such as the desmoplastic region of invasive tumours, suggests that extracellular matrix HA can inhibit angiogenesis (West and Kumar, 1989; Barsky et al., 1987). The recent finding that the vascularisation of cartilage requires prior degradation of matrix HA [9], gives added support to this hypothesis. Furthermore, *in vivo* studies indicate that high concentrations of macromolecular hyaluronan inhibit blood vessel formation in granulation tissue [2, 6] and induce regression of the capillary plexus in the developing chick limb bud [8] (Table 1).

In contrast, low-molecular-weight HA-oligosaccharides (OHA; 4-20 disaccharides in length) stimulate angiogenesis in the chick chorioallantoic membrane assay [48], in both wound healing and graft models [1, 21, West et al., in preparation], and after subcutaneous implantation or topical application. [13] Have independently confirmed the angiogenic activity of this range of OHA, using the rabbit corneal assay (Table 1).

Table. 1. Comparison of angiogenic and anti-angiogenic properties of hyaluronan oligosaccharides and macromolecular hyaluronan, respectively.

High- molecular weight hyaluronan (> 500 kDa)	Angiogenic hyaluronan oligo-saccharides (OHA; 4-20 disaccharides)
Inhibits angiogenesis in vivo:	Angiogenic in several in vivo models:
• inhibits granulation tissue formation and vascularization [2]; • inhibits vascularization of implanted fibrin gels [6]; • causes regression of the capillary plexus in chick limb buds [8]; • Endogenous HA inhibits angiogenic activity of human wound fluids in CAM assay [1], and • Inhibits cartilage vascularisation [9]	• CAM [48]; • Rabbit corneal [13]; • Rat skin: topical application [37]; • Rat skin graft [21]; • Rat polyvinyl sponge implant [West et al]; • Rabbit subcutaneous implants [West & Kumar, unpublished], and • pig full thickness wounds [1]
In vitro it inhibits:	In vitro :
• endothelial cell proliferation [51]; • endothelial migration [36, 10, 44], and • preventrs cell- cell adhesion [50] all at physiological concentrations i.e. 100- 200mg/ml.	• stimulates: endothelial proliferation [50, 1]; migration [37]; migration into collagen/ fibrin gels [43, 29, Burbridge & West unpublished data], and tube formation [13, 34]. • Induces synthesis of proliferation- associated proteins, type VIII collagen, uPA and PAI-1 [50, 35, 29].

Recent studies on the relationship between angiogenesis and tissue HA metabolism in a rat sponge-implant wound healing model (West et al., in preparation), a freeze-injured rat skin-graft model [21], and sheep foetal wounds [46] suggest that tissue angiogenesis coincides with the degradation of matrix hyaluronan, indicated by both a rapid fall in tissue HA size and content, and an increase in hyaluronidase levels. Furthermore, [27] have shown that the addition of exogenous streptomyces hyaluronidase to foetal wounds, decreases wound HA content and increased both fibroplasia and capillary formation.

Paradoxically, increased levels of hyaluronan are often found in human and animal tumours [16] showing increased angiogenesis, especially metastatic tumours. Our studies on a bone metastasising form of Wilm's tumour, Bone Metastasising Renal Tumour of Childhood (BMRTC) showed that it secretes high levels of low molecular weight HA. In contrast, Wilm's tumours, which are rarely metastatic, produce high levels of high molecular weight HA [18]. Recently, we have analysed the HA content/size and hyaluronidase activity of syngeneic murine and rat tumours, and human xenograft tumours, but although HA levels were generally increased, there was a significant shift to a lower molecular mass, compared with normal tissues. The size of HA also exhibited a loose inverse relationship to the relative levels of tumour HA and hyaluronidase activity [40, 39]. A similar situation was also encountered when cultured tumour cell lines were examined i.e. the most angiogenic, usually metastatic lines, also had low- molecular- weight HA, both in the medium and on the their cell- surface, as well as high hyaluronidase activity. The size of the HA produced by the most angiogenic cell- lines suggested that not only would the endogenous angiogenic cytokines be active, but the HA degradation products could actively stimulate angiogenesis, metastasis and result in a poor tumour prognosis [29, 39, 47]. Support is given to this hypothesis by a recent report by [23] showing an association between elevated hyaluronidase levels and prostate cancer progression. [22] Have found a potential "neutral" surface-associated hyaluronidase, similar to the glycosylphosphatidylinositol (GPI)- anchored sperm PH-20 hyaluronidase, expressed by angiogenic tumour cell-lines. Our own initial results confirm the presence of PH-20 hyaluronidase on the most angiogenic tumour cell-lines. Furthermore, the recent finding that normal serum hyaluronidase, which apparently differs from the tumour enzyme [33], also contains the GPI-anchor, suggests that cell-surface hyaluronidase(s) are present on many cell-types [12, 13]. Thus *in vivo* studies suggest that, in many tumours, inflammatory diseases and probably during wound healing, local hyaluronidase activity will degrade macromolecular HA to produce angiogenic HA oligosaccharides, in addition to removing the inhibitory effect of macromolecular HA.

In vitro studies

Examination of the effect of macromolecular HA on cultured endothelial cells have shown that it significantly inhibits endothelial proliferation and migration [49, 50, 51, 52] and disrupts newly formed monolayers, at physiologically relevant concentrations ($\geq$ 50µg/ ml) i.e. concentrations found in avascular tissues and transiently during tissue remodelling. The inhibitory effect decreases with reducing HA size. Significantly, the HA- mediated inhibition can not be reversed by the addition of exogenous growth factors, such as basic Fibroblast Growth Factor (bFGF) [50, 52]. [43] Have recently confirmed these findings in a 3-dimensional collagen gel endothelial cell culture system. Furthermore, high concentrations (1mg/ml) of HA have been reported to inhibit the migration of human adipose capillary endothelial cells into fibrin gels, *in vitro*, and blood vessel formation in fibrin gels implanted subcutaneously in guinea pigs [6, 10]. In own studies, using rat aorta cultured in a serum-free collagen gel matrix [30], preliminary data suggests that macromolecular HA selectively inhibits endothelial capillary formation (Burbridge and West, unpublished results).

In parallel studies, OHA 2-8 kDa (4-20 disaccharides) specifically stimulate both proliferation, and to a lesser extent migration, of rat, bovine and human endothelial cells [50, 51, 36]. However, in the rat aortic model, OHA stimulated capillary formation, which is thought to be mainly due to endothelial migration (Burbridge and West, unpublished results). [13] Have reported that aniogenic OHA markedly stimulated endothelial tube formation, on "matrigel", and two recent studies have shown that OHA (4-20 disaccharides in length) stimulate angiogenesis in 3-dimensional collagen and fibrin matrices [29, 43]. [43] Also confirmed that the 3-disaccharide oligosaccharide is not angiogenic, confirming the lower limit to the angiogenic size range to be the octasaccharide.

Mode of action of HA-oligosaccharides

Receptor binding

Several workers, including ourselves, have reported that endothelial cells possess high affinity HA-binding proteins, or receptors, on their cell surface, that both bind and internalise HA [51, 45, 41, 26]. In our initial studies, we used macromolecular HA (10^6 Da) and detected 2,000 receptors/cell, with a Kd of 10^{-10} M. The low receptor number suggested that the macromolecular HA may be giving a reduced degree of binding due to steric exclusion. Subsequently, we have repeated this study, using a defined 42 kDa HA fraction, and have found approximately 10^5 receptors/ cell and a Kd of 2 x 10^{-10} M [45, 41]. I^{125}- labeling of human and bovine endothelial cell- surface proteins, followed by HA-affinity chromatography and SDS- PAGE analysis, has identified six major cell-surface HA- binding proteins, between 78 and 125 kDa, with a minor band at 46 kDa [52, 45]. Western blotting with anti- CD44 and anti- ICAM-1 antibodies indicates that the 78 and 90 kDa bands are non-variant CD44 (the lack of splice variants was confirmed by PCR) and the bands at 90-125 kDa appear to be ICAM-1 isoforms [West, unpublished results]. Other cell-surface HA- receptors, such as RHAMM and hyaluronectin, have been characterised, but antibodies to these do not appear to stain human or bovine endothelial cells.

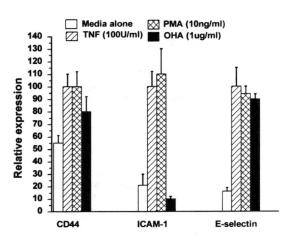

Figure 1. Comparison of the effect of OHA on human endothelial cell CD44, ICAM-1 and E-selectin expression. Cultured human umbilical vein endothelial cells were incubated with TNFα, PMA or OHA for 12 hours. Relative surface expression was determined by FACS analysis.

CD44 appears to play an important role in the angiogenic process as anti-CD44 antibodies have been reported to inhibit the migration and tube formation of bovine and porcine endothelial cells *in vitro* [3, 43]. Although it binds HA oligosaccharides of this size range, it also binds the HA- hexasaccharide which is not angiogenic and, because of this, appears unlikely to be the primary "angiogenic" receptor for the active oligosaccharides. However, [32, 31] have reported that HA-oligosaccharides, between the hexasaccharide and 440 kDa, activate cultured macrophages by binding to CD44. However the role of CD44 was not conclusively proven. The other putative receptor, ICAM-1, was originally identified as a HA- receptor on rat liver sinusoidal endothelial cells by [24], but a recent publication

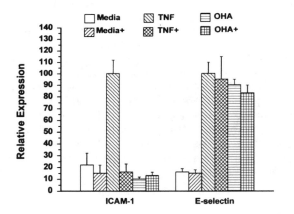

Figure 2. Comparison of the effect of ISIS 1939 antisense oligonucleotide on OHA and TNFα induction of ICAM-1 and E-selectin. Cultured human umbilical vein endothelial cells were incubated with 100 nM of ISIS 1939 (Bennett et al., 1994), in the presence of Lipofectin, for 4 hr. This was replaced by 100nM ISIS 1939 in medium and OHA or TNFα added. After 12 hrs stimulation, the expression of ICAM-1 and E-selectin were determined as in Fig.1. The sense oligonucleotide corresponding to ISIS 1939 was without significant effect.

from the same group suggests that ICAM-1 is binding to the hydrophobic spacer arm and is not a HA-receptor [25].

Effect of cytokines on endothelial receptor and protein expression

Preliminary studies have shown that OHA induces proliferation related proteins, stimulates the phosphorylation of a 32 kDa protein and increases Type I and VIII collagen synthesis by 4-6 fold [50, 35]. [29] Have reported that OHA, but not macromolecular HA, induce urokinase- type plasminogen activator (uPA) and plasminogen activator inhibitor (PAI) within a few hours. These data indicate that both OHA and HA interact directly with endothelial cells, respectively inducing and inhibiting the metabolic pathway initiating angiogenesis.

Recently, we examined the effect of the angiogenic cytokines VEGF and bFGF on endothelial cell expression of ICAM-1 and E-Selectin, with OHA, TNF-α and phorbolmyristyl acetate (PMA), using flow cytometry. As expected, TNF-α and PMA maximally upregulated ICAM-1 and E-selectin expression (400%), after 12 hours (Fig.1). VEGF increased both ICAM-1 and E-Selectin expression by 150%, whilst bFGF upregulated ICAM-1 expression 200% but had only a marginal effect on E-selectin. Similar findings were recently reported by [28]. OHA greatly increased E-Selectin expression (350%) and down-regulated ICAM-1. The latter result was surprising and was initially thought to be due to phagocytosis of the ICAM-1, possibly with bound HA-oligosaccharide.

To determine the role of ICAM-1 in OHA induction of angiogenesis, we have inhibited of endothelial cell ICAM-1 expression using the ISIS 1939 antisense oligonucleotide [4]. (Fig.2) Although the ISIS 1939 oligonucleotide completely inhibited any TNFα induced increase in ICAM-1 expression; it failed to inhibit the upregulation of E-selectin by OHA. These data indicate that endothelial CD44, and not ICAM-1, must play a major role in OHA stimulation of angiogenesis.

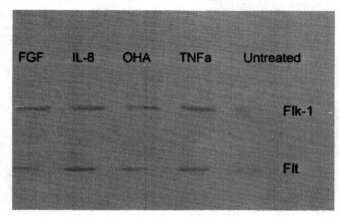

Figure 3. Effect of cytokines on endothelial VEGF- receptor expression. Human umbilical vein endothelial cells were stimulated with either bFGF (1ng/ ml), TNFα (100 U/ ml, 1L-8 (10ng/ ml) or OHA (1µg/ ml) for 12 hours. After solubilisation, SDS-electrophoresis and transfer to nitrocellulose membrane, the membranes were probed with primary polyclonal rabbit antibodies to Flk-1 and Flt and developed with peroxidase-conjugated goat- anti- rabbit Ig and 3,3- diaminobenzidine.

[29] Have recently reported that angiogenic OHA acts synergistically with VEGF, arguably the main angiogenic cytokine in tumours, but not basic Fibroblast growth factor (bFGF). Our own preliminary results, using rat aorta cultured in a serum-free collagen gel matrix, indicate that whilst both VEGF and OHA stimulate microvessel growth in this model, their combined effect is at best additive and not synergistic. (Burbridge and West, unpublished results). In contrast, we have recently found that OHA does upregulate Flk-1

and Flt VEGF- receptor expression by cultured human endothelial cells after 12 hours (Fig.3.), a possible route for synergy.

OHA induced NFκB activation

The induction of E- selectin by OHA, together with the rapid (within one hour) increase in IL-8 mRNA levels (West and Noble, preliminary data), suggested that endothelial NFκB activation may play a role in OHA stimulation of angiogenesis. The upregulation of IL-8 was previously reported for HA- stimulated murine macrophages [31] and appears to indicate a rapid CD44- mediated activation of the NFκB transcription factor and reduction of IκBα expression.

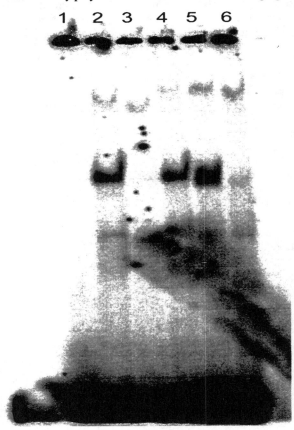

Cultured human umbilical vein endothelial cells were treated with OHA (10 μg/ ml) or macromolecular HA (100 μg/ ml) for various times. Protein extracts were preincubated with a ^{32}P- labelled consensus- NFκB binding-region (Santa Cruz) and subjected to electrophoretic mobility shift analysis (EMSA). OHA rapidly activated NFκB (Fig.4) yielding a dimeric band in EMSA. The bands were abolished when competed with 25- fold of unlabelled binding region, but not a mutant binding region (Santa Cruz). Macromolecular HA does not activate NFκB, but initial data suggests a significant down regulation over four hours, whereas in OHA stimulated cells the level of activated NFκB continues to increase (Wilson & West, unpublished data). In contrast, [5] recently reported that OHA induces the immediate early response genes c-fos, c-jun, jun-B, Krox-20 and Krox-24 in bovine aortic endothelial cells, whilst high-molecular-weight HA did not. However,

Figure 4. Mobility- shift analysis of NFκB activation by HA and OHA. Cells were treated with OHA (10μg/ ml) or HA (2 x 10⁶Da; 100μg/ ml) for 1 hr. Cell protein extracts were treated with a ^{32}P-labelled consensus- NFκB binding- region (Santa Cruz) and subjected to electrophoretic mobility shift analysis (EMSA). To define the specificity of binding samples were treated with a twenty-five fold excess of unlabelled consensus oligonucleotide or a mutant variant. Lane [1] consensus- NFκB binding- region alone, [2] untreated cells, [3] untreated cells + unlabelled oligonucleotide, [4] HA treated cells, [5] OHA treated cells, and [6] OHA treated cells + unlabelled oligonucleotide.

[19] reported that in response to 12(R)-hydroxyeicosatrienoic acid, an angiogenic arachidonic acid metabolite, they found rapid activation of both NFκB and, to a lesser extent, the AP-1 transcription factor.

Conclusions

Studies on high-molecular-weight HA suggest that it is inhibitory to new blood vessel formation and that its degradation is a necessary prerequisite to tissue vascularisation. Recently, at least two GPI-linked cell-surface hyaluronidases have been indentified and, at least in tumours, their expression coincides with matrix HA degradation. OHA stimulates angiogenesis *in vitro* and in many *in vivo* models. This stimulation of angiogenesis is probably by direct action on the vascular endothelium and appears to involve binding to CD44, with subsequent rapid activation of the NFκB and AP-1 transcription factors.

Acknowledgements

The authors thank the North West Cancer Research Fund (DCW, MJ).

References

[1]   Arnold, F., Jia, C.Y., He, C.F., Cherry, G.W., Carbow, B., Meyer-Ingold, W., Bader, D. and West, D.C., 1995, Hyaluronan, heterogeneity and healing: The effects of ultra-pure hyaluronan of defined molecular size on the repair of full thickness pig skin wounds. *Wound Rep Reg.* **3**: 10-21.

[2]   Balazs, E.A., and Darzynkiewcz, Z., 1973, The effect of hyaluronic acid on fibroblasts, mononuclear phagocytes and lymphocytes, in: *Biology of the fibroblast* (E. Kulonen, and J. Pikkarainen, eds), pp. 237-52, Acad Press, New York

[3]   Banerjee, S.D. and Toole, B.P., 1992, Hyaluronan-binding protein in endothelial morphogenesis. *J Cell Biol.* **119**: 643-52.

[4]   Bennett, C.F., Condon, T.P., Grimm, S., Chan, H., and Chiang M-Y., 1994, Inhibition of endothelial cell adhesion molecule expression with antisense oligonucleotides. *J. Immunol.* **152**: 3530-40.

[5]   Deed, R., Rooney P., Kumar, P., Norton, J.D., Smith, J., Freemont, A.J. and Kumar, S., 1997, Early-response gene signalling is induced by angiogenic oligosaccharides of hyaluronan in endothelial cells. Inhibition by non-angiogenic, high-molecular-weight hyaluronan. *Int J. Cancer.* **71**: 251-6.

[6]   Dvorak, H.F., Harvey, S., Estralla, P., Brown, L.F., McDonagh, J., and Dvorak, A.M., 1987, Fibrin containing gels induce angiogenesis, *Lab Invest.* **57**: 673-86.

[7]   Entwistle, J., Hall, C.L. and Turley, E.A., 1996, HA Receptors: Regulators of signalling to the cytoskeleton. *J. Cellular Biochem.* **61**: 569-77.

[8]   Feinberg, R.N. and Beebe, D.C., 1983, Hyaluronate in vasculogenesis, *Science.* **220**: 1177-1179.

[9]   Fenwick,S.A., Gregg,P.J., Kumar,S., Smith,J. and Rooney,P., 1997, Intrinsic control of vascularisation in developing cartilage rudiments. *Int.J.Exp Pathol.* **78**: 187-96.

[10]   Fournier, N. and Doillon, C.J., 1992, In vitro angiogenesis in fibrin matrices containing fibronectin or hyaluronic acid. *Cell Biol Int Reports.* **16**: 1251-63.

[11]   Frost, G.I., Csoka, T. and Stern, R., 1997, Purification, cloning and expression of human plasma hyaluronidase. *Biochem. Biophys. Res Commun.* **236**: 10-15.

[12]   Frost, G.I., Csoka, T. and Stern, R., 1996, The hyaluronidases: A chemical, biological and clinical overview. *Trends In Glycoscience And Glycotechnology.* **8**: 419-34.

[13]   Hirata, S., Akamarsu, T., Matsubara, T., Mizuno, K. and Ishikawa, H., 1993, *Arthritis & Rheum.* **36**:S247.

[14]   Jackson, R.L., Busch, S.J. and Cardin, A.D., 1991, Glycosaminoglycans: Molecular properties, protein interactions, and role in physiological processes. *Physiol. Rev.* **71**: 481- 538.

[15]   Kinsella, A.R., Lepts, G.C., Hill, C.L. and Jones, M., 1994, Reduced E-cadherin expression correlates with increased invasiveness in colorectal carcinoma cell lines. *Clin Exp Metastasis.* **12**: 335-342

[16]   Knudson, W., Biswas, C., Li, X.-Q., Nemec, R.E. and Toole, B.P., 1989, The role and regulation of tumour-associated hyaluronan. in: *The Biology of Hyaluronan*, Ciba Foundation Symposium **143** (D. Evered, and J. Whelan, eds), pp. 150-169, John Wiley and Sons, Chichester

[17]   Knudson, C.B. and Knudson, W., 1993, Hyaluronan- binding proteins in development, tissue homeostasis, and disease. *FASEB J.* **7**: 1233- 41.

[18]   Kumar, S., West, D.C., Ponting, J. and Gattamaneni, H.R., 1989, Sera of children with renal tumour contain low molecular mass hyaluronic acid. *Int. J. Cancer.* **44**: 445-8.

[19]   Laniado-Schwartzman, M., Lavrovsky, Y., Stoltz, R.A., Conners, M.S., Falck, J.R., Chauhan, K. and Abraham, N.G., 1994, Activation of nuclear factor B and oncogene expression by 12 (R)-hydroxyeicosatrienoic acid, an angiogenic factor in microvessel endothelial cells. *J. Biol Chem.* **269**: 24321-7.

[20]   Laurent, T.C. and Fraser, J. R. E., 1992, Hyaluronan. *FASEB J.* **6**, 2397-404.

[21]   Lees, V.C., Fan, T-P.D. and West, D.C., 1995, Angiogenesis in a delayed revascularization model is accelerated by angiogenic oligosaccharides of hyaluronan, *Lab Invest.* **73**:259-266.

[22]   Liu, D., Pearlman, E., Diaconu, E., Guo, K., Mori, H., Haqqi, T., Markowitz, S., Willson, J., and Sy, M-S., 1996, Expression of hyaluronidase by tumor cells induces angiogenesis in vivo. *Proc. Natl. Acad. Sci. U.S.A.* **93**: 7832-7837.

[23]   Lokeshwar, V.B., Lokeshwar, B.L., Pham, H.T. and Block, N.L., 1996, Association of elevated levels of hyaluronidase, a matrix- degrading enzyme, with prostate cancer progression. *Cancer Res.* **56**: 651-657.

[24]   McCourt, P.A.G., Ek, B., Fosberg, N. and Gustafson, S., 1994, Intracellular adhesion molecule-1 is a cell surface receptor for hyaluronan. *J. Biol Chem.* **269**: 30081-4.

[25]   McCourt, P.A.G. and Gustafson, S., 1997, On the adsorption of hyaluronan and ICAM-1 to modified hydrophobic resins. *Int. J. Biochem. Cell Biol.* **29**: 1179-89.

[26]   Madsen, K., Schenholm, M., Jahnke, G. and Tengblad, A., 1989, Hyaluronate binding to intact corneas and cultured endothelial cells. *Invest Opth Vis Sci.* **30**: 2132-7.

[27]   Mast, B.A., Haynes, J.H., Krummel, T.M., Diegelman, R.F. and Cohen, I.K., 1992, In vivo degradation of fetal wound hyaluronic acid results in increased fibroplasia, collagen deposition, and neovascularization. *Plastic. Reconstructive Surgery.* **89**: 503-9.

[28]   Melder, R.J., Koenig, G.C., Witwer, B.P., Safabakhsh, N., Munn, L.L. and Jain, R.K., 1996, During angiogenesis, vascular endothelial growth factor and basic fibroblast growth factor regulate natural killer cell adhesion to tumour endothelium. *Nature Medicine.* **2**: 992-997.

[29]   Montesano, R., Kumar, S., Orci, L. and Pepper, M.S., 1996, Synergistic effect of hyaluronan oligosaccharides and vascular endothelial growth factor on angiogenesis in vitro. *Lab Invest.* **75**: 249-62

[30]   Nicosia, R.F., and Ottinetti, A., 1990, Growth of microvessels in serum-free matrix culture of rat aorta. *Lab Invest.* **63**: 115-22.

[31]   Noble, P.W., McKee, C.M., Cowman, M. and Shin, H.S., 1996, Hyaluronan fragments activate an NFkB/IkBα autoregulatory loop in murine macrophages. *J Exp Med.* **186**: 2373-2378.

[32]   Noble, P.W., Lake, F.R., Henson, P.M. and Riches, D.W.H., 1993, Hyaluronate activation of CD44 induces insulin-like growth factor-1 expression by tumor necrosis factor-α-dependent mechanism in murine macrophages. *J Clin Invest.* **91**: 2368-2377.

[33]   Podyma, K.A., Yamagata, S., Sakata, K. and Yamagata, Y., 1997, Differences of hyaluronidase produced by human tumor cell lines with hyaluronidase present in human serum as revealed by zymography. *Biochem. Biophys. Res Commun.* **241**: 446-452.

[34]   Rahmanian, P., Pertoft, H., Kanda, S., Christofferson, R., Claesson-Welsh, L. and Heldin, P., 1997 hyaluronan oligosaccharides induce tube formation of brain endothelial cell line *in vitro*. *Exp. Cell Res.* **237**: 223-30.

[35]   Rooney, P., Wang, M., Kumar, P. and Kumar, S., 1993, Angiogenic oligosaccharides of hyaluronan enhance the production of collagen by endothelial cells. *J. Cell Sci.* **105**: 213-8

[36]   Sattar, A., Kumar, S. and West D.C., 1992, Does hyaluronan have a role in endothelial cell proliferation of the synovium. *Semin. Arth. Rheum.* **21**: 43-49.

[37]   Sattar, A., Rooney, P., Kumar, S., Pye, D., West, D.C., Scott, I. and Ledger, P., 1994, Application of angiogenic oligosaccharides of hyaluronan increase blood vessel numbers in rat skin. *J. Invest Dermatol.* **103**: 576-579

[38]   Scott, J. E., 1995, Extracellular matrix, supramolecular organization and shape. *J. Anat.* **187**: 259-269.

[39]   Shaw, D.M. (1996) Ph.D. Thesis, University of Liverpool

[40]   Shaw, D.M., West, D.C. and Hamilton, E., 1994,Hyaluronidase and hyaluronan in tumours and normal tissues, quantity and size distribution. *Int J Exp Pathol.* **75**: A67

[41]   Smedrod, B., Pertoft, H., Eriksson, S., Fraser, J.R.E. and Laurent, T., 1984, Studies in vitro on the uptake and degradation of sodium hyaluronate by rat liver endothelial cells. *Biochem J.* **223**: 617-26.

[42]   Toole, B.P., 1982, Glycosaminoglycans in morphogenesis, in *Cell Biology of the Extracellular Matrix* (Hay, E.D., ed), Plenum Press, New York, pp. 259- 294.

[43]   Trouchon, V., Mabilat, C., Bertrand, P., Legrand, Y., Smadia-Joffe, F., Soria, C., Delpeche, B. and Lu, H., 1996, Evidence of involvement of CD44 in endothelial cell proliferation, migration and angiogenesis in vitro. *Int. J. Cancer.* **66**: 664-668

[44]   Watanabe, M., Nakayasu, K. and Okisaka, S., 1993, The effect of hyaluronic acid on proliferation and differentiation of capillary endothelial cells. *Nippon Ganka Gakkai Zasshi.* **97**: 1034-9.

[45]   West, D.C., 1993, Hyaluronan receptors on human endothelial cells: the effect of cytokines. in: *Vascular Endothelium: Physiological Basis of Clinical Problems II* (J.D. Catravas, ed), pp.209-210, Plenumm Press, New York.

[46]   West, D.C., Shaw, D.M. and Joyce, M., 1997, Tumour angiogenesis and metastasis: The regulatory role of hyaluronan and its degradation products. In: *Angiogenesis: Models, modulators and clinical applications* (M.E. Maragoudakis, ed), pp337-347, Plenum Press, New York.

[47]   West, D.C. and Shaw, D.M., 1998, Tumour hyaluronan in relation to angiogenesis and metastasis. In: *The chemistry, biology and medical applications of hyaluronan and its derivatives* (T.C. Laurent, ed), Werner- Gren International Series. **72**: 227-233, Portland Press Ltd, London.

[48]   West, D.C., Hampson, I.N., Arnold, F. and Kumar, S., 1985, Angiogenesis induced by degradation products of hyaluronic acid, *Science.* **228**: 1324-8.

[49]   West, D.C. and Kumar, S., 1988, Endothelial proliferation and diabetic retinopathy. *Lancet.* **1**: 715-6.

[50]   West, D.C., and Kumar, S., 1989a, Hyaluronan and angiogenesis, in: *The Biology of Hyaluronan,* Ciba Foundation Symposium **143** (D. Evered,. and J. Whelan, eds), pp. 187-207, John Wiley and Sons, Chichester

[51]   West, D.C. and Kumar, S., 1989b, The effect of hyaluronate and its oligosaccharides on endothelial proliferation and monolayer integrity. *Exp Cell Res.* **183**: 179-96.

[52]   West, D.C. and Kumar, S., 1991, Tumour-associated hyaluronan: a potential regulator of tumour angiogenesis. *Int J Radiol.* **61/62**: 55-60.

[53]   West, D.C, Shaw, D.M., Lorenz, P., Adzick, N.S/ and Longaker M., 1996, Fibrotic healing of adult and late gestation fetal wounds correlates with increased hyaluronidase activity and removal of hyaluronan. *Int. J. Biochem Cell Biol.* **29**: 201-10.

Abstracts of Poster Presentations

Vascular Endothelium: Mechanisms of Cell Signaling
J.D. Catravas et al. (Eds.)
IOS Press, 1999

245

Lipopolysaccharide (LPS)-induced signaling in human endothelial cells (EC).
Roles of G proteins and the p38 MAP kinase pathway

Aninda Das, Yiping Jin and <u>Moshe Arditi</u>

Childrens Hospital Los Angeles, Division of Infectious Diseases, Southern California School of Medicine, Los Angeles, CA 90027

LPS can induce the activation of vascular EC, including expression of various adhesion molecules and secretion of numerous pro-inflammatory cytokines and chemokines, which in turn play a significant role in the pathogenesis of endotoxic shock. However, the LPS receptor on EC is not known and signal transduction pathways for LPS-induced EC activation and cytokine release are not completely understood. We have previously shown that LPS induces the tyrosine phosphorylation of MAP kinases, including ERK1, ERK2, p38 MAP kinase, and c-jun N terminal kinase(JNK) in EC. In this study we measured IL-6 release as a paradigm for LPS-induced activation of human brain microvessel EC (HBMEC) and human dermal microvessel EC (HDMEC) following preincubation of EC with various specific biochemical inhibitors in quadruplicate experiments. LPS induced a dose-dependent and serum- (soluble-CD14-) dependent IL-6 release in both EC types. The p21 Ras pathway inhibitor (alpha HFPA, 0.4 µM) and the MAP kinase kinase (MEK) inhibitor [i.e. ERK1/ERK2 pathway inhibitor, (PD98059) at 100 µM] failed to inhibit LPS-induced IL-6 release from ECs, while the MEK inhibitor did inhibit LPS-induced increase in ERK2 activation in EC. However, the tyrosine kinase inhibitor (Herbimycin A, 1 - 5 µg/ml), the p38 MAP kinase inhibitor (SB203580,1-10 µM), and the G protein binding peptide Mastoparan (1-20 µM) resulted in a dose-dependent inhibition of LPS-induced IL-6 release from both EC types, with maximal inhibition of 92%, 90%, and 100% respectively. Mastoparan, a 14-residue peptide, stimulates GDP/GTP exchange on G proteins through a mechanism similar to that of G protein-coupled receptors, and binds to G proteins at the receptor-binding site. Presumably, this peptide structurally mimics a receptor's G protein binding domain. Pretreatment of ECs with the Pertussis toxin (100 ng/ml) resulted in 45% inhibition in LPS-induced IL-6 release from ECs. These results suggest that the p38 MAP kinase pathway is the predominant signaling pathway in LPS-induced IL-6 release from HBMEC and HDMEC and that this pathway may involve a heterotrimeric G protein-coupled receptor. G protein agonists or antagonists may have a potential therapeutic role in modulating endothelial cell responses in endotoxic shock.

(This work has been supported by grants from NIH-AI 40275, MA, and AHA CS1019, MA).

Vascular Endothelium: Mechanisms of Cell Signaling
J.D. Catravas et al. (Eds.)
IOS Press, 1999

Shear Stress activates a Chloride-Selective Membrane Current in Vascular Endothelial Cells

A.I. Barakat[1], E. Clark[1], P.A. Pappone[1], and P.F. Davies[2]
[1]University of California, Davis, CA and [2]University of Pennsylvania, Philadelphia

Changes in membrane potential are one of the earliest known physiological responses to fluid mechanical shear stress in endothelium. We report a shear stress-activated chloride-selective membrane current in bovine aortic endothelial cells (BAECs). Using membrane potential-sensitive fluorescent dye recordings of single cells, steady laminar shear stress induced membrane depolarization following the initial hyperpolarization previously reported by Olesen et al. (*Nature,* 331: 168-170, 1988). A similar sequence was noted using whole-cell patch-clamp recordings. In current-clamp experiments on confluent BAEC monolayers using normal Ringer's solution, 15 of 23 cells responded with depolarization. However, in low Cl⁻ Ringer's, which maximized the depolarizing response, 6 of 7 cells responded. The depolarization did not desensitize appreciably after 4 minutes of continued flow and it often persisted for several minutes after termination of flow. Voltage-clamp recordings of single cells revealed a flow-activated current with a reversal potential of -18 mV -- close to the equilibrium potential of Cl⁻ (E_{Cl}) in these experiments (-36 mV). The reversal potential of the current shifted with E_{Cl} upon replacing external Cl⁻ with aspartate (reversal potential of +28 mV, E_{Cl} = +31 mV). In contrast, when E_{Na} was made more negative by replacing external Na⁺ by the impermeant cation N-methyl-D-glucamine (MNDG), the reversal potential of the current did not shift similarly. These data suggest a flow-induced current that is largely mediated by chloride.

Supported by Whitaker Foundation RG-97-0114 (A.I.B.) and NHLBI HL-07237 (P.F.D.).E.C. supported by NSF Research Training Grant 9602226.

Vascular Endothelium: Mechanisms of Cell Signaling
J.D. Catravas et al. (Eds.)
IOS Press, 1999

The Anticoagulant Factor Protein S Acts as A Survival Factor for Cultured Human Vascular Smooth Muscle Cells (HVSMC)

Omar Benzakour and Chryso Kanthou
Molecular and Cell Biology Laboratory, Thrombosis Research Institute, Manresa Road
London SW3 6LR, UK

The anticoagulant factor protein S is a homologue of the growth arrest specific protein, Gas6, which was demonstrated to exhibit growth promoting and cell survival properties. We have previously shown that PS is mitogenic for HVSMC and that these cells secrete PS. Here we investigated the effect of PS on HVSMC survival. HVSMC were gown in the presence of serum and were switched to serum-free medium before the addition of agents that induced cell death such as H_2O_2 and sodium nitroprusside (SNP) in the presence of either PS, platelet-derived growth factor-BB (PDGF-BB) or diluent. Total cell death was assessed by the trypan blue exclusion assay and apoptosis was determined using annexin V staining followed by FACS analysis. Additionally, cell supernatants were assessed for lactate dehydrogenase activity. Cultured HVSMC in serum-free medium present a low level (3 to 5%) of spontaneous cell death at both 4 and 24 h. Cell death rises to 15-50% in the presence of H_2O_2 or SNP. Pretreatment of cells with PS resulted in a significant decrease in cell death (10-30%). Under similar conditions, PDGF-BB, which is a more potent HVSMC mitogen than PS, inhibited cell death to a lesser extent than PS. These observations suggest that HVSMC survival is independent from mitogenic stimulation and may involve the activation of specific survival signalling pathways. Hence, the activation of the components of the MAP kinase pathway, ERK1/2, JNK/SAPK and p38 under the conditions of the apoptosis assay were studied by Western blotting using antibodies which recognise the phosphorylated/activated protein forms. The above apoptosisinducing agents led to a rapid activation of the JNK whereas PS induced ERK1/2 activation. Therefore, in addition to its role in the coagulation cascade, PS may be an important VSMC survival factor.

Vascular Endothelium: Mechanisms of Cell Signaling
J.D. Catravas et al. (Eds.)
IOS Press, 1999

TYROSINE NITRATION IN BLOOD VESSELS OCCURS WITH INCREASING NITRIC OXIDE CONCENTRATION: IMPLICATIONS FOR NITROVASODILATOR THERAPY

C. Amirmansour, P. Vallance and R.G. Bogle
Centre for Clinical Pharmacology & Toxicology, Wolfson Institute for Biomedical Research, University College London, London W1P 5NL, U.K.

Blood vessels generate free radical species including nitric oxide (NO) and superoxide anion (O_2^-). In contrast to the extensively characterised biology of NO, the biosynthetic pathways and roles of O_2^- remain unclear. NO and O_2^- react at almost diffusion limited rate to form peroxynitrite ($ONOO^-$). This acts as a powerful oxidant leading to the generation of other reactive species and can result in cell damage. In addition $ONOO^-$ reacts with proteins resulting in nitration of tyrosine residues and formation of 3-nitrotyrosine (NT). NT has been detected in human atherosclerotic plaques and in acute lung injury (see [1] for a review). The aim of this study was to estimate O_2^- production from isolated rabbit aortic rings *in vitro* and identify its possible enzymatic sources and to test the hypothesis that an increase in NO, generated from an NO donor would be sufficient to combine with endogenous O_2^- to form $ONOO^-$.

Aortic rings were isolated from male New Zealand white rabbits. O_2^- production was measured using lucigenin chemiluminescence. All tissues were treated with diethyldiothiocarbamate (10mM) to inhibit endogenous superoxide dismutase SOD; [2]. NT was detected by Western blotting using a specific polyclonal anti-rabbit IgG (TCS Biologicals, U.K.)

Basal O_2^- production from aortic rings was 0.9 ± 0.01 pmol/min/mg protein. The effect of potential substrates on O_2^- production was assessed. NADH and NADPH significantly increased O_2^- production to 9.8 ± 1.0 and 1.5 ± 0.1 pmol/min/mg protein respectively whereas xanthine, arachidonic acid or succinate and antimycin A had no effect (n=3). NADH- stimulated O_2^- production was inhibited by 85% in the presence of SOD (15×10^3 units/ml). Incubation of aortic rings with the NO donor S-nitrosoglutathione (GSNO) resulted in a concentration-dependent quenching of O_2^- chemiluminescence. The quenching of the signal was proportional to NO release and thus the most likely product formed was $ONNO^-$. $ONOO^-$ formation was assessed indirectly by determining NT in rabbit aorta. Basally and in the presence of NADH a single band of NT immunoreactivity was detected. Incubation of aorta with GSNO alone or with NADH resulted in the appearance of other NT bands. Incubation of albumin with GSNO did not result in NT formation whereas SIN-1, a co-donor of NO and O_2^-, resulted in significant NT formation which was blocked by oxyhaemoglobin or SOD.

Addition of exogenous NO results in NT formation in aortic rings. NT formation is likely to result from the reaction of NO and O_2^- resulting in $ONOO^-$. Formation of $ONOO^-$ and nitration of tyrosine residues potentially could lead to vascular damage and might represent unexpected adverse effects of long-term nitrate therapy.

This work was supported by the British Heart Foundation.

References

[1] Beckman, J.S. and Koppenol, W.H. (1996). Nitric oxide, superoxide and peroxynitrite: the good, the bad and the ugly. *Am. J. Physiol.*, **271**, C1424-C1437.

[2] Pagano, P.J., Tornheim, K. and Cohen, R.A. (1993). Superoxide anion production by rabbit thoracic aorta: effect of endothelium-derived nitric oxide. *Am. J. Physiol.*, **265**, H707-H712

Vascular Endothelium: Mechanisms of Cell Signaling
J.D. Catravas et al. (Eds.)
IOS Press, 1999

INFLUENCE OF NITRIC OXIDE (NO) ON HUMAN AORTIC SMOOTH MUSCLE CELL (HASMC) PROLIFERATION, CELL CYCLE AND APOPTOSIS

Ruth Bundy, Nandor Marczin, Adrian Chester, Magdi Yacoub
Department of Cardiothoracic Surgery, NHLI
Imperial College of Science, Technology and Medicine
London, UK

NO is known to inhibit growth of animal cells, however its influence on HASMC remains unknown. We investigated the effect of NO donors on proliferation, serum-induced mitogenesis, and cell cycle progression and on apoptosis. Proliferation was evident as cell number doubled over 4 days and was reduced (51.4, 51.1 and 43.8%) by 250 M S-nitroso-glutathione (GSNO), S-nitroso-penicillamine (SNAP) and sodium nitroprusside (SNP), respectively. To investigate mitogenesis, ongoing DNA synthesis and DNA content were monitored by ^{3}H-thymidine uptake and flow cytometry. Cells synchronised at G_1/S phase by hydroxyurea (HU) progressed through S phase 1-4 hrs after washout of HU. GSNO inhibited both DNA synthetic rate and increase in DNA content in a concentration dependent manner (82.8 ± 4.9; 15.1 ± 2.9 and 2.5 ± 0.2 % of control for 100, 250 and 1000 M), whereas, only high concentrations (1 mM) of SNAP caused inhibition. The effects of S-nitrosothiols were prevented by 10 M hemoglobin suggesting the principal role of NO. This inhibition of DNA synthesis by NO was partially reversed by the addition of 2-deoxyadenosine and 2-deoxyguanosine, suggesting the involvement of ribonucleotide reductase (RR). N-acetyl-L-cysteine (NAC) reversed the inhibition of DNA synthesis and S phase progression in a concentration dependent manner, however, its analogue N-acetyl-L-serine (NAS) which lacks the sulphydryl moiety had no effect. NAC had no effect on inhibition of DNA synthesis by HU, an inhibitor of the tyrosyl radical on RR or the inhibition by desferrioxamine, an inhibitor of the iron centre. These data suggest that NO inhibition of RR may be distinct from that of HU and desferrioxamine and may act on the redox sensitive sulphydryl on the R1 subunit. To investigate if NO donors also influenced G_0/G_1 progression, cells were synchronised at G_0 by serum starvation. In control cells ^{3}H-thymidine uptake increased 18-24 hours after restimulation with serum. Both GSNO and SNAP (250 M) virtually eliminated DNA synthesis. Time course experiments also suggest that NO donors influence a relatively early event during G_1 progression. Assessment of apoptosis by TUNEL revealed that apoptosis was caused only by high mM concentrations of NO.

Vascular Endothelium: Mechanisms of Cell Signaling
J.D. Catravas et al. (Eds.)
IOS Press, 1999

Endothelium-Derived Metabolites of Cytochrome P450 Produce Relaxation of Coronary Small Arteries by Opening Ca"-Dependent IC Channels (Kc.)

Shawn G. Clark, **Natalie Clarke and Leslie C. Fuchs**
Vascular Biology Center and Department of Pharmacology and Toxicology
Medical College of Georgia, Augusta, Georgia 30912, USA

Previously, we reported that acetylcholine (ACh)-induced relaxation that was resistant to inhibition of nitric oxide synthase (NOS) was mediated by opening of K^+ channels in hamster coronary small arteries (150-250 µm). The present study was designed to determine if this vasodilatory response to ACh was due to release of endothelium-derived metabolites of cytochrome P450 acting via opening of Ca^{2+}-dependent K^+ channels (K_{Ca}). Intraluminal diameter was continuously recorded in isolated coronary arteries (150-250 µm) obtained from male Golden Syrian hamsters. All vessels were maintained at a constant intraluminal pressure of 40 nmfflg and pretreated with indomethacin (IO ptM). To assess the role of large (BK_{Ca}) and small (SK_{Ca}) channels in regulating relaxation, coronary arteries were pretreated with a combination of charybdotoxin (CTX, 0.1µM) and apamin (AP, 0.5µM). Relaxation to Ach (10^{-9} to $3x10^{-5}$ M) was completely abolished by CTX/AP. In endothelium-denuded coronary arteries, relaxation to ACh was also completely abolished indicating that the Independent relaxation is mediated by release of endothelium-derived relaxing factors. The role of the cP450 pathway in mediating relaxation to ACh was determined with inhibitors of cP450 that act through different mechanisms. Miconazole (20µM), which forms a nitrogenous ligand to the heme iron of P450, proadifen (30 µM), which is converted to a reactive intermediate that sequesters cytochrome in a catalytically inactive complexed state, and 1-aminobenzotriazole (I mM), which causes autocatalytic destruction of cP450, significantly inhibited relaxation to ACh that was resistant to inhibition of NOS. These results indicate that endothelium-derived cP450 metabolites contribute to ACh-induced opening of K_{Ca}, channels and vascular relaxation of hamster coronary small arteries.

Vascular Endothelium: Mechanisms of Cell Signaling
J.D. Catravas et al. (Eds.)
IOS Press, 1999

Roles for VEGF in Neutrophil-Endothelial Cell Interactions

Valerie C. Cullen, Glare M. O'Connor* and Alan K. Keenan
Dept of Pharmacology and "Dept of Medicine and Therapeutics, University College Dublin, Belfield, Dublin 4, Ireland

Although the processes involved in neutrophil-endotheial cell (EC) adhesive interactions are well understood, the mechanisms by which neutrophils traverse the vascular endothelium and migrate into the underlying interstitium remain unclear. Both in vivo and in vitro investigations have shown that such neutrophil migration is coupled to an increase in endothelial permeability to plasma proteins such as alburninl. EC permeability is also increased by the mutifunctional cytokine vascular endothelial growth factor (VEGF) as part of its overall angiogenic activity in the endothelium, and this has been postulated to occur in an NO-dependent way[2]. Furthermore, VEGF has recently been localised to the specific granules of human neutrophils and has been shown to be released from them in response to the chemotactic agents fMLP and PMA[3]. In the present study, we hypothesised that neutrophilderived VEGF may play a mechanistic role in neutrophil-EC interactions.

The chemotactic peptide fMLP was used to activate isolated neutrophils in vitro. Such activation caused a dose-dependent release of nitric oxide as measured by an iso-electric probe (10.5 and 2.5 pmol/min/l06 cells with lo-8M and 10^{w6}M respectively). Moreover, this agent mediated a significant increase in VEGF secretion from isolated neutrophils as determined by ELISA (1.78 f 0.13 fold over the basal value of 194.13 & 57.10 pg/ml). Three other chemotactic stimuli, namely PMA, IL-S and LTB4, also elevated VEGF release from neutrophils (3.3 + 0.87, 1.50 f 0.03 and 1.32 + 0.10 fold respectively).

Human pulmonary artery endothelial cells (HPAEC) were employed as a physiologically relevant target system for the direct characterisation of VEGF effects. HPAEC monolayers were established on collagen-coated polycarbonate supports. A 15 min treatment of these monolayers with 1, 10 or 100 ng/ml VEGF caused a 1.21 + 0.0.08, 1.43 f 0.07 or 1.55 + 0.06 fold increase in EC permeability to trypan blue-labelled bovine serum albumin respectively. In conclusion, chemotactic stimuli may evoke from neutrophils the release of substances which modulate the permeability of the endothelial monolayer.

This work was supported by the Irish Health Research Board and by a UCD President's Research Award.

References

[1]   Cepiminas C, Noseworthy R, Kvietys P. Transendothelial neutrophil migration, Role of neutrophil-derived proteases and relationship to transendothelial protein movement. Circ Res 1997; 81: 618626.

[2]   Mac Wu H, Huang Q, Yuan Y, Granger H. VEGF induces NO-dependent hyperpermeability in coronary venules. Am J Physiol 1996; 271: H2735-H2739.

[3]   Gaudry M, Bregerie 0, Andrieu V, El Benna J, Pocidalo M-A, Hakim J. Intracellular pool of vascular endothelial growth factor in human neutrophils. Blood 1997; 90: 4153-4161.

Vascular Endothelium: Mechanisms of Cell Signaling
J.D. Catravas et al. (Eds.)
IOS Press, 1999

Demonstration of Increased Leukocyte-Endothelial Interaction in the Systemic Microcirculation Following Localized Ischemia-Reperfusion, *in vivo* Microscopy Animal Model

H. Sobral do Rosdrio, C. Saldanha, J. Martins e Silva
Institute of Biochemistry, Faculty of Medicine of Lisbon, Lisbon, Portugal

Introduction: The role of leukocytes in the mechanisms of local tissue injury after ischemia-reperfusion (I/R) has for long been characterized. However, their role in the pathophysiology of the systemic inflammatory injury following localized LIR has not yet been fully analyzed. The objective of this work was to evaluate the dynamics of leukocyte behavior in the systemic microcirculation in an experimental model of I/R using *in vivo* light microscopy.

Materials: Male Wistar rats 8-12 weeks old (n= 1 6) were used, and divided in 2 groups: 1) bilateral hindlimb ischemia (120 minutes) followed by reperfusion (90 minutes) - Group A; 2) sham-operated controls - Group B. In both groups the dynamics of leukocyte-vessel wall interaction was assessed by *in vivo* light microscopy of the mesenteric microcirculation during 120 minutes (in Group A, for the last 30 minutes of ischemia and the 90 minutes of reperfusion); the parameters measured were the number of rolling and adherent leukocytes to the post-capillary venules. Data analysis was performed using non-parametric tests, with significative differences if $p < 0.05$.

Results: No differences were found between the two groups at the end of the ischemia period. After reperfusion, however, we identified that: 1) Group A showed a slight increase in the rolling leukocytes against a decrease in controls (at minute 90 of reperfusion: 55.04 ± 39.08 *vs* $16.18 \pm 3,36$; $p < 0.01$); 2) Group A showed a significative increase in adherent versus controls (at minute 90 of reperfusion: 37.61 ± 9.55 *vs* 14.63 ± 4.32; $p < 0.01$), but reaches a peak (for the adherent leukocytes) at 70 minutes post-reperfusion (20.89 ± 3.18 *vs* 8.46 ± 3.37; $p < 0.001$).

Conclusions: We demonstrate an increased leukocyte-vessel wall interaction in the systemic microcirculation following a localized I/R lesion. Although the focus on the study of the pathophysiology of the systemic inflammatory injury following localized I/R has been on the release of soluble mediators from the reperfused territory (such as proinflammatory cytokines, araquidonic acid derivatives, reactive oxygen species), the increased leukocyte-endothelial interaction observed in this experiment should be in favor for a role of leukocytes (mainly neutrophils) in the systemic organ injury that follows. The mechanisms involved in their role in the development of this systemic tissue injury following I/R must be farther characterized.

Vascular Endothelium: Mechanisms of Cell Signaling
J.D. Catravas et al. (Eds.)
IOS Press, 1999

255

Effect of Butyrate on Endothelial Cell Apoptosis: Comparison with Lymphoid and Colonic Epithelial Tumour Cell Lines

B.C. Edmonds, P.D. Zalewski and N.W.R Wickham
Departments of Medicine and Haematology-Oncology
The Queen Elizabeth Hospital, AUSTRALIA

Under normal resting conditions, endothelial cells in vivo exhibit a quiescent phenotype (0.1% replications per day) despite the endothelium being constantly exposed to numerous activating signals and potentially toxic stimuli. Thus, endothelial cell apoptosis does not occur frequently in vivo. Butyrate is a naturally occurring molecule that can induce apoptosis at physiological concentrations in many tumor cell lines in vitro while having no apparent toxicity to normal tissue in vivo.

The aim of this study was to determine whether human umbilical vein endothelial cells (HUVECS) are susceptible to apoptosis when treated with butyrate in vitro and to compare this result with the response to butyrate previously documented in lymphoid and colonic epithelial tumor cell lines. Confluent, first passage HUVECs were treated with a range of butyrate concentrations for 18 hours then cell lysates were prepared and assayed for caspase-3-like activity, a quantitative biochemical marker of apoptosis.

HUVECs treated with 4mM butyrate, an optimal concentration for induction of apoptosis in tumor cell lines, were relatively resistant to apoptosis, levels of caspase-3-like activity being only 1.2 fold higher than negative controls. In contrast, a 14-fold increase in activity occurred with 4mM butyrate treatment in Jurkat T lymphoma cells and a six-fold increase in activity was observed in LIM1215 colon carcinoma cells. Even at higher concentrations of butyrate (up to 64mM) there was no increase in the amount of apoptosis induced by butyrate in HUVECS. However, HUVECs were capable of undergoing apoptosis when deprived of serum and growth factors as evidenced by a three-fold increase in caspase-3-like activity after serum deprivation.

These studies provide in vitro evidence that butyrate can induce apoptosis much more efficiently in tumor cells than in normal, untransformed cells (HUVECs). The quiescent phenotype of endothelial cells may confer resistance to apoptosis induced by butyrate, implying that differences in the response to butyrate may occur between resting endothelium and proliferating endothelium. This has important implications for tumor angiogenesis because proliferating endothelial cells may mimic tumor cells in their susceptibility to apoptosis induced by butyrate. A difference in susceptibility to butyrate could potentially be exploited therapeutically by targeting butyrate to induce apoptosis selectively in neoangiogenic blood vessels.

Vascular Endothelium: Mechanisms of Cell Signaling
J.D. Catravas et al. (Eds.)
IOS Press, 1999

Proangiogenic Effect of E1A Oncoprotein

Claudia Giampietri[1], Massimo Levrero[2,3], Angelina Felici[1], Maurizio C. Capogrossi[1,4], and Carlo Gaetano[1]

[1]*Laboratorio di Patologia Vascolare, Istituto Dermopatico dell'Immacolata, Istituto di Ricovero e Cura a Carattere Scientifico, 00167 Rome, Italy.* [2]*Laboratorio di Espressione Genica, Fondazione Andrea Cesalpino, Universita' degli Studi di Roma "La Sapienza", 00161 Rome, Italy.* [3]*Istituto di Medicina Interna, Universita' di Cagliari, 09124 Cagliari, Italy.* [4]*Laboratory of Cardiovascular Science, National Institute on Aging, National Institutes of Health, Baltimore, Maryland, USA*

The viral oncoprotein E1A interacts with members of the retinoblastoma and p300/CBP gene families, altering cell phenotype and reactivating proliferation of terminally differentiated cells. Angiogenesis is a growth factor-dependent process sustained by the reactivation of proliferation of quiescent endothelial cells and, at least in part, it mimics the effect of E1A in differentiated cells. Therefore the aim of the present study was to examine the effect of E1A on endothelial cell's function and to investigate the mechanisms of angiogenesis at molecular level. Bovine aortic endothelial cells (ECs) were transfected either with wild type E1A (wtE1A) or with different E1A mutants. We found that transient overexpression of wtE1A proteins greatly accelerated ECs' ability to form capillary-like structures on reconstituted basement membrane proteins (Matrigel). In contrast, the E1A mutant dl646N, lacking the CR1 domain of E1A, did not modulate the development of capillary-like structures. ECs' invasion, examined in a modified Boyden chamber assay, revealed that wtE1A-transfected ECs exhibited an enhanced ability to invade, compared to both dl646N and mock transfectants. Zymograms and RT-PCRs showed that matrix metalloproteinase-9 (MMP-9) protein and m-RNA were induced in wtE1A, but not in dl646N- transfected cells. ELISA tests for bFGF revealed an increase of this growth factor in the conditioned media from wtE1A-transfected ECs but not in those collected from E1A dl646N-transfected cells. The results demonstrate a role for E1A oncoprotein as inducer of *in vitro* angiogenesis in adult ECs. This observation, associated with the enhanced MMP-9 activity and bFGF production, is apparently dependent on the integrity of the CR1 domain and suggests a potential role for p300 and Rb family proteins as regulators of nuclear events leading to the angiogenic switch.

Vascular Endothelium: Mechanisms of Cell Signaling
J.D. Catravas et al. (Eds.)
IOS Press, 1999

Endothelin-l-Induced Contraction of Mesenteric Small Arteries is Dependent on Ryanodine- Sensitive Ca 21 Stores

Ararat D. Giulumian, Leslie C. Fuchs and László G. Mészáros
Vascular Biology Center and Departments of Pharmacology and Physiology and Endocrinology, Medical College of Georgia, Augusta GA 30912, USA

The role of ryanodine-sensitive Ca^{2+} stores in endothelin-1 (ET-1)-induced vascular contraction is unknown. This study determined the effect of the ryanodine receptor Ca^{2+} release channel (RYRC) inhibitor, dantrolene, on contraction of rat isolated small mesenteric arteries (250-300 m intralumianl diameter). Application of dantrolene (10^{-7} – 10^{-6} M) induced relaxation of the vessels that were preconstricted by endothelin-I (ET-1), but not vessels preconstricted by the -adrenoceptor agonist, phenylephrine (PE), or by KCL-induced depolarization. The effect of dantrolene was insensitive to K^+ channel inhibition with tetraethylammonium (10 M) or inhibition of nitric oxide synthase activity with N-nitro-L-arginine (1mM), indicating that it was not mediated by release of endothelium-derived relaxing factors. When administered prior to ET-1, dantrolene (3 M) had no effect on basal vascular tone, but significantly inhibited contraction to ET-1. Finally, activation of the RYRC with ryanodine had no significant effect on ET-1 -induced contraction. In conclusion, this study provides evidence that Ca^{2+} release from the sarcoplasmic reticulum via the RyRC occurs in association with ET-1, but not PE or KCL, signaling in small mesenteric arteries.

Vascular Endothelium: Mechanisms of Cell Signaling
J.D. Catravas et al. (Eds.)
IOS Press, 1999

INCREASED MORTALITY IN CRITICALLY ILL PATIENTS WITH DECREASED PULMONARY CAPILLARY ENDOTHELIUM BOUND ANGIOTENSIN CONVERTING ENZYME ACTIVITY

C. Glynos, S.E Orfanos, A. Psevdi, P. Kaltsas, P. Sarafidou, J.D. Catravas, A. Armaganidis, and Ch. Roussos
Critical Care Department, Evangelismos Hospital, University of Athens Medical School Athens, Greece;
Vascular Biology Center, Medical College of Georgia, Augusta, Georgia USA

Pulmonary capillary endotheliun-bound (PCEB) angiotensin converting enzyme (ACE) activity was estimated in 29 mechanically ventilated critically-ill patients suffering from various pathological conditions associated with acute respiratory distress syndrome (ARDS) development, with lung injury score (LIS) ranging from 0 (no injury) to 3.7(ARDS). By means of indicator-dilution techniques we measured the single pass transpulmonary hydrolysis $v = -\ln\{1-M\}$ (where M = metabolism) of the synthetic ACE substrate ^{3}H-benzoyl-Phe-Ala-Pro (BPAP), and calculated the modified kinetic parameter A_{max}/K_m, an index of functional capillary surface area (FCSA). Both v and A_{max}/K_m decreased with increasing LIS ($r = -0.785$, $p<0.001$ and $r = -0.641$, $p<0.001$, respectively), denoting a correlation between PCEB ACE activity depression and the clinical severity of acute lung injury (ALI). In our population, two distinct groups of A_{max}/K_m values, above and below the observed mean (3378 mL/min) may be formed: a *high* group of nine patients (5045 to 10149 mL/min) and a *low* group of twenty patients (385 to 3144 mL/min). Eight patients (8/9) in the *high* group survived, while only two (2/20) survived in the *low* group ($p<0.001$, Fisher's exact test). We conclude that high PCEB ACE activity expressed by the FCSA index A_{max}/K_m, a parameter depending on both enzyme mass available for reaction and enzyme functional integrity, might distinguish survivors from nonsurvivors in critically-ill patients suffering from ALI/ARDS.

Supported by a grant from the European Union and the Greek General Secretariat of Research and Technology (PENED 1997).

Vascular Endothelium: Mechanisms of Cell Signaling
J.D. Catravas et al. (Eds.)
IOS Press, 1999

Involvement of Map-Kinases in the Control of cPLA$_2$ and Arachidonic Acid Release in Endothelial Cells

H. Halldórsson, K. Magnúsdóttir, J.W. E. van den Hout, I. Guðmundsdóttir and G. Thorgeirsson

Department of Pharmacology, University of Iceland, Reykjavík, Iceland

Human umbilical vein endothelial cells respond to a variety of stimuli by a short burst of arachidonic acid (AA) release and prostacyclin production. This response involves phospholipase C activation and a consequent Ca^{++} increase and phosphorylation of proteins including cytosolic phospholipase A$_2$ (cPLA$_2$), the enzyme responsible for the AA release. We have used inhibitors to study the pathways leading to phosphorylation of cPLA$_2$ and MAP-kinases, as well as release of AA and production of prostacyclin after stimulation with different agonists. We find that all agonists causing prostacyclin produciton activate MAP-kinases p42/p44 (ERK) and cause phosphorylation of cPLA$_2$. However, the importance of this, as well as the signal pathway to ERK activation seems to be agonist dependent. Thus, the MEK 1 inhibitor PD98059 at 20 µM caused 80%, 40% and 10% inhibition of AA release after treatment with aluminium fluoride (AlF), histamine and thrombin respectively. Downmodulation or inhibition of protein kinase C also greatly inhibited the AA response to AlF, but only slightly inhibited the response to histamine and had no effect on the thrombin repsonse. These results were reflected in the effects of these treatments on ERK actvity. In contrast the thrombin response is more sensitive than the histamine response to the tyrosine kinase inhibitor genistein and to pertussis toxin. The p38 inhibitor SB203580 at 20 µM caused 35-50% inhibition of the response to all agonists.

Genistein, PD98059 and SB203580 all inhibited prostacyclin production regardless of the agonist used as well as by externally applied arachidonic acid, suggesting inhibition of cyclooxygenase or prostacyclin synthase in addition to their effects on proteinkinases. Finally the unspecific protein kinase staurosporine at 0,2 µM completely inhibited ERK activation and cPLA$_2$ phosphorylation in response to both histamine and thrombin, without any inhibiton of AA release.

We conclude that although stimulation of HUVECs to produce prostacyclin causes phosphorylation of cPLA$_2$ by ERK and possibly p38 and other protein kinases this has only a minor effect on the ammount of prostacyclin produced, presumably because a rise in Ca^{++} is the most important signal. Despite the minor effects of the manipulations they suggest differences in signalling between thrombin and histamine the former relying more on G$_{\beta\gamma}$ and tyrosine phosphorylation the latter more dependent on G$_{\alpha q}$ PKC, somewhat analogous to the differences in pathways described by Hawes et al (J. Biol. Chem; 270; 17148-17153 (1995)) between Gi and Gq mediated signalling in COS sells.

260

Vascular Endothelium: Mechanisms of Cell Signaling
J.D. Catravas et al. (Eds.)
IOS Press, 1999

Effects of Growth Factors on Healing Process

K. Ultibsyram[1], C.Ertan[2], P.Korkusuz3, N.Cakar[3], N.Hasirci[1]
[1]*Middle East Technical University Department of Chemistry, 06531 Ankara Turkey*
[2]*Middle East Technical University, Medical Center, 06531 Ankara, Turkey*
[3]*Hacettepe Univ.* Faculty *of Medicine,* Histology *and Embryology, 06531 Ankara Turkey*

Introduction

For deep and non-healing wounds, an immediate coca of the wound surface with a spongy material that protects the loss of body fluid, prevents the bacterial attack and at the same time creates a support for the proliferating cells, is important. These materials are generally made of polymers.

In the present study, a bilayer wound covering material with an elastic polyurethane upper layer and spongy gelatin lower layer was constructed. Into some preparations, Epidermal Growth Factor (EGF) was added. Addition of EGF was achieved either directly in free form or indirectly by entrapping EGF in gelatin microspheres. All covering materials prepared were tested on full-thickness skin defects (0.5 cm^2) created on rabbits. The animals were kept in separate cages, At certain time intervals, the areas of the wounds were measured and recorded as were as the specimens of the wound area were biopsied and sent for histological examinations.

In-vivo experiments showed that, in case of the application of coverings with EGF, the wounds healed completely in three weeks without any scar formation. The other wounds had longer healing time with scar formations. Histological examinations supported faster tissue regeneration for EGF containing coverings.

References

[1] Yamas IV and Burke JF, Design of an artificial skin. I Basic design principles, J.Biomater.Res, 14:65-81,1980.
[2] Bruin P, Jonkman M.F, Meijer HJ and Pennings AJ, A new porpus polyetherurethane wound covering, J.Biomed Mater Res, 24:217-226,1990.
[3] Burke JF, Yannas IV and Quinby WC, Successful use of physiologically acceptable artificial skin in the treatment of extensive burn injury, Ann Surg, 1 94:413-428,1981.

Vascular Endothelium: Mechanisms of Cell Signaling
J.D. Catravas et al. (Eds.)
IOS Press, 1999

Preconditioning In Hypercholesterolemic Rabbits *in vivo*

E.K. Illodromitis, E.Bofills, L.Kaklamams, G.K. Karavolias, A. Papalois,
D.Th. Kremastinos
2nd Dept of Cardiology, Onassis Cardiac Surgery Center, Athens, GREECE

Preconditioning (PC) in hypercholesterolermic rabbits has not been thoroughly investigated; we studied the role of PC on infarct size in hypercholesterolermic rabbits 'in vivo. Sixteen male rabbits were fed for 8 weeks with 0.2 % cholesterol (chol) rich diet. All the animals were divided into 2 groups (Gp); Gp A was subjected to 30 M'M sij-,tained ischemia (isc) followed by 180 min reperfusion (rep) and Gp B to one cycle of PC (5 min isc-10 min rep) followed by 30 min isc and 180 min rep. A second series of 15 rabbits fed a normal diet were similarly divided into 2 Gp, C and D which were subjected to 30 min isc without or with prior PC respectively. Blood samples were drawn at baseline and before the procedure for chol levels and segments from the aorta and the carotid artery were taken at the end for histologic examination. Infarcted (1) and risk areas (R) were delineated with the aid of Zn-Cd fluorescent particles and TTC staining and their ratio expressed in %. Results: Mean chol was 58.3±8.7 mg % at baseline and 1402±125 mg% at 8 weeks (p<0.0001) in Gp A and B and 57.5±5.8 mg% before the procedure **in** Gp C and D. % I/R: Gp A 39.3±6.3, Gp B 16.7±3.9 (p<0.01), Gp C 41.4±7.5 and Gp D 10.8±3.3 (p<O. 0 1). Thus, PC equally protects hypercholesterolemic and normal rabbits against infarction *in vivo*.

Vascular Endothelium: Mechanisms of Cell Signaling
J.D. Catravas et al. (Eds.)
IOS Press, 1999

Pretreatment with Angiotensin II as a Preconditioning Analogue *in vivo*

E.K. Illodromitis, E. Bofills, E. Sbarouni, D.V. Vlahakos, G. K. Karavollas, D.Th. Kremastinos

2ⁿᵈ Dept of Cardiology, Onassis Cardiac Surgery Center, Athens, GREECE

Although anglotensin II (Ang) infusions exert direct vasoto-xic effects in vivo, in ex vivo experiments **it** protects against infarction via PLC and PKC activation. To investigate if Ang can mimic preconditioning (PC) with one cycle of 5 min ischemia (isc) and 10 min reperfusion (rep), 5 min infusion of Ang solutions in pressor (5 g /ml) or non-pressor (1 g/ml) concentrations were administered intravenously (IV) or directly into the left atrium (LA) of male anesthetized rabbits. All animals were then subjected to 30 min isc followed by 120 min rep. Groups (Gp) A and B received a 5 min Ang infusion (5 g /ml) IV or in LA respectively in order to increase mean blood pressure (BP) at least 60 mm Hg above baseline. Gp C served as control, without any intervenvention before the sustained isc and Gp D and E received a 5 min Ang infusion (1 g/ml) IV or in LA respectively without any pressure response. Infarcted ( ) to risk (R) areas are expressed in percent (%I/R). Results: Gp A 31.2±4.8, Cip B 52.2±6.9*, Gp C 39.6±6. 1, Gp D 42.1±5.9, Gp E 48.9±3.5* (* $P < 0.05$ vs Gp A). Ang failed to mimic isc PC in vivo. Moreover, direct LA administration of Ang seems to increase infarct size regardless the systemic pressor response. In fact, systemic hypertension due to the IV infusion ameliorates the direct Ang toxicity.

Vascular Endothelium: Mechanisms of Cell Signaling
J.D. Catravas et al. (Eds.)
IOS Press, 1999

Nitric Oxide-Angiotensin II Interaction in Modulation of Vascular Smooth Muscle Signalling: A Possible Role for ROS?

Siobhan Kelleher, Stephen Wilson and Alan K. Keenan

Dept of Pharmacology University College Dublin, Belfield, Dublin 4, Ireland

Endothelium-derived nitric oxide (NO) is routinely scavenged by superoxide anion produced in the vascular wall [1].   One source of such superoxide anion is the NADH/NADPH oxidase family of enzymes whose activity is stimulated by angiotensin II (AII) in vascular smooth muscle [2]. This study examined NO-AII interactions in the context of the development of tolerance to NO donors, a process variously attributed to compensatory activation of the renin-angiotensin system [3] and to increased scavenging of NO by vascular-derived superoxide anion [4].

Rat aortic smooth muscle cells were used as a model system in which to investigate tolerance (measured as a decrease in NO donor-stimulated cGMP production following a 12 hrs exposure to the same drug). The NO donors used were sodium nitroprusside (SNP), S-nitroso-N-acetyl-D,L-penicillamine (SNAP) and isosorbide dinitrate (ISDN). In some experiments AII was present during the 12 hrs incubation period ± SOD. Flow cytometric analysis was used to detect reactive oxygen species (ROS) in cells via oxidation of 2,7-dichlorofluorescin-diacetate (DCFH-DA) to fluorescent dichlorofluorescin (DCF).

A reduction in CGNW responsiveness was observed in cells pre-exposed for 12 hrs to 1.0 mM ISDN, 20 M SNP or 10 M SNAP. The SNP-mediated reduction was significantly offset in cells pre-exposed in the presence of 0.1 M AII alone, but not when 1000 U/ml superoxide dismutase (SOD) was also present during the preexposure period. In contrast however SOD alone had no effect on the development of tolerance to SNP.

In separate experiments SOD increased basal CGNW production by cells over a 15 min period, suggesting that a tonic release of superoxide by cells was occurring. In experiments designed to confirm that basal release of superoxide or a downstream radical was occurring, flow cytometric analysis of ROS production was first carried out following a 15 min exposure of cells to 1.0 mM ISDN, 10 M SNP, or 50 M SNAP. The fold increases in ROS recorded were 3.6 ± 0.37 (n=3, $p<0.05$), 2.9 ± 0.3 (n=5. $p<0.01$), or 2.5 ± 0.3 (n=5, $p<0.05$) respectively. These increases were significantly attenuated in cells pre-exposed to 1.0 mM ISDN, 20 M SNP or 10 M SNAP for 12 hrs.

We conclude that ROS do not appear to mediate the development of tolerance to NO donors in this study. The protective effect of AII against the development of tolerance has not previously been reported and may be due to increased smooth muscle cell NO production via induction of INOS. The loss of such protection in the presence of SOD may be due to AII degradation by H_2O_2 produced from dismutation of cellular superoxide.

This work was supported by the Irish Health Research Board (SK) and the Irish Heart Foundation (SW)

References

[1] Gryglewski RJ, Palmer RMJ, Moncada S. Superoxide anion is involved in the breakdown of endothelium-derived vascular relaxing factor. Nature 1986; 320:454.

[2] Griendling KK, NEnieri CA, Ollerenshaw JD, Alexander RW. Angiotensin 11 stimulates NADH and NADPH oxidase activity in cultured vascular smooth muscle cells. Circ Res 1994; 74:1141-1148.

[3] Packer M, Lee W, Kessler PD, Gottlieb SS, Medina N, Yushak M. Prevention and reversal of nitrate tolerance in patients with congestive heart failure. N Engl J Med 1987; 317:799-804.

[4] Munzel T, Sayegh H, Freeman BA, Tarpey MM, Harrison DG. Evidence for enhanced vascular superoxide anion production in nitrate tolerance. J Clin Invest 1995;95:187-194

Vascular Endothelium: Mechanisms of Cell Signaling
J.D. Catravas et al. (Eds.)
IOS Press, 1999

Inhibition of Angiogenesis by Blockers of Volume-Regulated Anion Channels

Vangelis G. Manolopoulos, Sandra Liekens*, Thomas Voets, Eric De Clercq*, Guy Droogmans, and Bernd Nilius
Laboratory of Physiology, Medical School, Campus Gasthuisberg, and *Rega Institute for Medical Research, Katholieke Universiteit Leuven, B-3000 Leuven, BELGIUM

In endothelial cells, we have identified an outwardly rectifying Cl⁻ current, $I_{Cl,swell}$, which is activated by osmotic cell swelling (for a review see Nilius *et al.*, 1997). The molecular identity of the volume-regulated anion channel (VRAC) mediating this current has not yet been identified, but there is evidence that the VRAC channel in endothelial cells may differ from that in other cell types. Very little is known also about the physiological role of VRAC in endothelial cells. One important endothelial cell function is the formation of new blood vessels from preexisting ones, termed angiogenesis. This process is essential in a variety of physiological and pathological functions, most notably solid tumor growth (Folkman, 1995). The angiogenic cascade consists of several sequential and highly-coordinated steps including basement membrane proteolysis, migration of individual endothelial cells, and endothelial cell proliferation.

We have identified several potent blockers of VRAC in endothelial cells, including the established anion channel blocker NPPB, anti-estrogens such as tamoxifen and clomiphene, and certain clinically relevant phenol derivatives such as mibefradil and quinine. We found that NPPB (50 μM), mibefradil (1-30μM), and tamoxifen (1-30 μM), inhibit the proliferation of calf pulmonary artery endothelial cells. Further, we have used these compounds to study the possible involvement of VRAC in angiogenesis. For these studies, three well-characterized models of angiogenesis were used, including both an *in vivo* model (the chorioallantoic membrane assay) and two *in vitro* models (the matrigel and rat aorta-ring assays). The technical aspects of these models in our hands have been described elsewhere (Liekens et al, 1997). We found that the volume-regulated anion channel blockers NPPB (100 μM), mibefradil (20 μM), and tamoxifen (20 μM), inhibit tube formation of rat microvascular endothelial cells plated on a thin gel of matrigel by 58.4 ± 9.6%, 54.3 ± 4.6%, and 39.7 ± 3.1%, respectively. Furthermore, NPPB, mibefradil, and clomiphene caused a dose-dependent inhibition of microvessel formation in the rat aorta-ring assay. Finally, NPPB, mibefradil, and clomiphene dose-dependently inhibited microvessel formation in the chorioallantoic membrane assay.

Taken together, these results provide strong evidence that VRAC blockers are potent inhibitors of angiogenesis, and allow us to suggest a novel functional role for the volume-regulated anion channels in endothelial cells, namely the regulation of angiogenesis. This regulation may take place at the level of endothelial cell proliferation, although it is likely that VRAC is involved also on other steps of the angiogenic cascade.

References

[1] Folkman, J. (1995) Angiogenesis in cancer, vascular, rheumatoid and other disease.*Nature Med.* **1**: 27-31

[2] Liekens, S., Neyts,J., Degreve, B., & De Clercq, E. (1997) The sulfonic acid polymers PAMPS [Poly(2-acrylamido-2-methyl-1-propanesulfonic acid)] and related analogues are highly potent inhibitors of angiogenesis.*Oncol. Res.* **9**: 173-181

[3] Nilius, B., Eggermont, J., Voets, T., Buyse, G., Manolopoulos, V. & Droogmans, G. (1997) Properties of volume-regulated anion channels in mammalian cells. *Prog. Biophys. Mol. Biol.* **68**: 69-119

Vascular Endothelium: Mechanisms of Cell Signaling
J.D. Catravas et al. (Eds.)
IOS Press, 1999

Regulation of Tissue Factor Expression in Endothelial Cells by Vascular Endothelial Growth Factor

D. Mechtcheriakova, A. Wlachos, H. Holzmüller, B.R. Binder and E. Hofer
Department of Vascular Biology and Thrombosis Research at Vienna
International Research Cooperation Center, University of Vienna, Austria

Tissue factor (TF), in addition to its function as high affinity receptor for the serum protease factor VII and as major cellular initiator of the coagulation cascade, has been proposed to play an important role during vasculogenesis and angiogenesis. We have previously analyzed the regulation of the TF gene by inflammatory mediators using reporter gene and electrophoretic mobility shift assays. These studies demonstrated that the NFKB-like site in the TF promoter is essential for transcriptional upregulation during inflammatory activation (T. Moll et al., J. Biol. Chem. 270, 3849-3857 (1995)). Now we have investigated whether vascular endothelial cell growth factor-A (VEGF-A) would upregulate TF expression and which transcription factors would be induced in this process. The obtained data, in accordance with the suggested role of TF in the angiogenic response, show that TF and TF MRNA are strongly upregulated following treatment of human umbilical vein or human skin microvascular endothelial cells with VEGF-A. In contrast, several adhesion molecules upregulated by inflammatory cytokines, e.g. E-selectin, V-CAM1 and I-CAM, are not affected at all by VEGF-A. Furthermore, treatment of the cells with a combination of VEGF-A and TNF-A leads to additive upregulation of TF on the endothelial cells, suggesting that TF induction is regulated differently during the inflammatory and angiogenic response. Additional data indicate that NFCB and AP1 factors appear to be not of primary importance in TF induction by VEGF. We have shown that this induction is mediated by a GC-rich region within the TF promoter.

(Supported by Austrian Science Foundation SFB5/10)

Vascular Endothelium: Mechanisms of Cell Signaling
J.D. Catravas et al. (Eds.)
IOS Press, 1999

Characterization of Murine Monoclonal Anti-Endothelial Cell Antibodies (Aeca) Produced by Idiotypic Manipulation with Human Aeca

N. Del Papa , E- Raschi, Y. Levy*, B. Gilburd*, J. George*, [†], R. Mallone[‡], M. Damianovich*, M. Blank*, A. Radice[§], Y. Renaudineau*[¶], P. Youinou[¶], A. Wiik[∥], F. Malavasi[‡], <u>P.L. Meroni</u>, Y. Shoenfeld*

*Dept. Internal. Med., , IRCCS-Policlinico, Univ. of Milan, Italy. *Dept. Medicine 'B', and Res.Unit of Autoimm. Dis., Tel-Hashomer and Sackler Faculty of Medicine, Tel-Aviv Univ., Sheba Medical Center.‡Lab. Cell Biol., Dept.Genetic, Biology & Biochemistry, Univ. of Turin, Italy. §Dept. Nephrol., S. Carlo Hosp., Milan, Italy. ¶Lab. Immunol., Univ. of Brest, France. ∥Statens Seruminstitut, Copenhagen, Denmark*

The IgG fraction of human AECA obtained from a patient with Wegener's granulomatosis was used as immunogen to raise AECA mAbs in mice selected among those which developed vasculitis-like lesions after immunization. Three mAbs (BGM, 3C8 and 7G2), selected by cyto-ELISA and flow cytometry analyses, featured a specific reactivity with HUVEC and the mouse endothelial cell line H5V; on the contrary, HEp2 cells, the murine melanoma B16 cell line, the extracellular matrix as well as several other antigens tested were not recognized. BGM mAb, an IgG$_3$ precipitating a 70 kD structure from HUVEC, was able to induce endothelial cells to secrete amounts of Interleukin-6 significantly higher than irrelevant controls or mAbs binding different endothelial antigens (*i.e.*, CD31, CD29, ICAM-1 and HLA Class I). Even if not displaying any antibody- or complement-dependent cytotoxicity, BGM mAb induced significant levels of ADCC (13 $\pm$ 2.5 % vs. 0.6 $\pm$ 0.03 %). To the best of our knowledge, BGM is the first murine mAb specific for human endothelial cells generated by idiotypic manipulation; secondly, its biological properties further support the notion of a pathogenic role for AECA in autoimmune-mediated diseases.

Vascular Endothelium: Mechanisms of Cell Signaling
J.D. Catravas et al. (Eds.)
IOS Press, 1999

Human β2-Glycoprotein I Binds To Endothelial Cells Through A Cluster of Lysine Residues that Are Critical for Anionic Phospholipid Binding and Offers Epitopes for Anti- β2-Glycoprotein I Antibodies*

Del Papa N, *Sheng YH, Raschi E, *Kandiah DA, [†]Tincani A, [‡]Khamashta MA, [‡]Atsumi T, [‡]Hughes GRV, [§]Ichikawa K, [§]Koike T,, [†]Balestrieri G, *Krilis SA, and Meroni PL

*Dept. Internal. Med.,IRCCS Policlinico, Univ. of Milan - Italy; *Dept. of Immunol., Allergy & Infect. Dis., The St. George Hospital, Univ. of South Wales , Kogarah Australia; , [†]Clin. Immunol. Unit, Spedali Civili-Brescia - Italy; [‡]Lupus Res. Unit, St Thomas' Hospital, London - UK; [§]Dept. of Med. II, Hokkaido Univ. School of Medicine, Sapporo-Japan*

Beta 2 glycoprotein I (β2GPI) is a phospholipid binding protein recognized by serum autoantibodies from the anti-phospholipid syndrome (APS) both in cardiolipin (CL) and β2GPI-coated plates. We found that : a) recombinant wild-type β2GPI bound to human umbilical cord vein endothelial cells (HUVEC) and was recognized by both human monoclonal IgM and affinity purified polyclonal IgG anti-β2GPI APS antibodies and b) a single amino acid change from Lys^{286} to Glu significantly reduced endothelial adhesion. Double and triple mutants (from $Lys^{284,287}$ to $Glu^{284,287}$, from $Lys^{286,287}$ to $Glu^{286,287}$ and from $Lys^{284,286,287}$ to $Glu^{284,286,287}$) completely abolished endothelial binding. A synthetic peptide (P1) spanning the sequence Glu^{274}-Cys^{288} of the β2GPI fifth domain still displayed endothelial adhesion. Another peptide (P8), identical with P1 except that Cys^{281} and Cys^{288} were substituted with serine residues, did not bind to HUVEC. Anti-β2GPI antibodies, once bound to P1 adhered to HUVEC, induced E-Selectin expression and up-regulated Interleukin 6 (IL-6) secretion. Control experiments carried out with irrelevant antibodies as well as with the P8 peptide, did not show any endothelial antibody binding nor E-Selectin and IL-6 modulation. Our results suggest that: a) β2GPI binds to endothelial cells through its fifth domain, b) the major phospholipid binding site that mediates the binding to anionic phospholipids is also involved in endothelial binding, c) HUVEC provide a suitable surface for β2GPI binding comparable to that displayed by anionic phospholipids dried on microtitre wells and d) the formation of the complex between β2GPI and the specific antibodies leads to endothelial activation *in vitro*.

Vascular Endothelium: Mechanisms of Cell Signaling
J.D. Catravas et al. (Eds.)
IOS Press, 1999

269

Regulation of Hepatic Apolipoprotein Gene Transcription by Smad Family Members

K. Pardali, **V. Zannis** and **D. Kardassis**
Division of Basic Sciences, School of Medicine, University of Crete and I.M.B.B.
Heraklion 71110, GREECE

We have reported recently that SMADs, which participate in TGF mediated signal transduction cooperate with the ubiquitous transcription factor Sp1 to activate hepatic transcription of the p21/WAF1 gene. This indicated that SMADs might act as general transactivators of promoters whose transcription depends on Sp1 and possibly other factors. Here we report that in transient transfections of HepG2 cells, SMADs transactivate the human apolipoprotein C-III promoter (-890/+24)which contains multiple Sp1 sites within the distal -790 to -500 region. Among the various SMAD proteins tested, SMADs 3 and 4 showed the greatest transactivation potential (25-fold). A synthetic promoter containing the distal apoC-III (-790/-500) promoter region fused with the minimal AdML promoter was transactivated by SMAD3/4 proteins (4-fold). The proximal apoC-III (-163/+24) promoter region that does not contain Sp1 binding sites was also transactivated by SMAD3/4 proteins (10-fold). Both the proximal and distal regions contain binding sites for the orphan nuclear receptor HNF-4 that are critical for apoC-III promoter function. Therefore, we tested putative functional and physical interactions between SMADs and HNF-4. It was found that: a) transactivation of the apoC-III promoter by SMADs was severely reduced in HepG2 cells expressing antisense HNF-4, b) SMADs transactivated Hormone Response Element (HRE)-dependent synthetic promoters synergistically with HNF-4 and c) SMAD3 physically interacted with HNF-4 in vitro protein-protein interaction assays. These findings suggest that i) SMAD proteins can modulate gene transcription by novel mechanisms which involve their physical and functional interaction with hormone nuclear receptors such as HNF-4 and ii) factors which regulate the expression of SMAD proteins in hepatic cells could play an important role in cholesterol homeostasis and lipoprotein metabolism.

Vascular Endothelium: Mechanisms of Cell Signaling
J.D. Catravas et al. (Eds.)
IOS Press, 1999

Tissue Inhibitor of Metalloproteinase-4 in Human Breast Cancer and Endothelial Cells

QingXiang Amy Sang*, Xinyun Xu*, Y. Eric Shi** and Hui Li*
*Chemistry and Biochemistry, Florida State University, Tallahassee, Florida 32306-4390;
**Pediatrics and Pathology, Long Island Jewish Medical Center, New Hyde Park, New York, 11040, U.S.A.*

Angiogenesis is a fundamental process by which new capillaries are formed from preexisting blood vessels and it plays a very important role in both normal and pathological processes such as coronary collateral circulation, cancer growth, invasion, and metastasis, and rheumatic diseases. Angiogenesis requires breakdown of the extracellular matrix (ECM) by proteinases. Angiogenic switching is accompanied by up-regulation of matrix metalloproteinase (MMP) bioactivity and down-regulation of tissue inhibitors of metalloproteinases (TIMPs). The TIMP family may regulate ECM turnover and tissue remodeling by forming tight binding inhibitory complexes with MMPs. Recently, tissue inhibitor of metalloproteinase-4 (TIMP-4) has been reported. TIMP-4 may inhibit breast cancer cell invasion and angiogenesis. The kinetic studies of the inhibition of the MMPs by recombinant TIMP-4 protein (rTIMP-4p) was performed in a continuous fluorimetric assay with a quenched fluorescent peptide substrate. The inhibition kinetics of rTIMP-4p were analyzed against human fibroblast collagenase (MMP-1), human fibroblast gelatinase A (MMP-2), human fibroblast stromelysin (MMP-3), matrilysin (MMP-7), and human neutrophil gelatinase B (MMP-9). The inhibitor concentrations that inhibited 50% of MMP activities (IC50) were determined to be 19, 3, 45, 8, and 83 nM for MMP-1, MMP-2, MMP-3, MMP-7, and MMP-9, respectively. Therefore, TIMP-4 is a potent inhibitor of all five MMPs tested and it has preference for MMP-2 and MMP-7. We have also prepared polyclonal and specific antibody directed against an unique peptide sequence of TIMP-4. This antibody has been characterized in TIMP-4 transfected human breast cancer cell line, MDA-MB-435. Our preliminary studies have also demonstrated that human endothelial cells (HUV-EC-C and ECV304) produce pro-MMP2 pro-MMP9, and MT1-MMP, as well as TIMP-4. The expression and function of TIMP-4 during angiogenesis are under investigation.

(Supported in part by grants from American Heart Association, AHA-9601457 to QXAS and from National Institutes of Health, CA68064 to YES).

Vascular Endothelium: Mechanisms of Cell Signaling
J.D. Catravas et al. (Eds.)
IOS Press, 1999

Surface Expression of VCAM-1 on Stimulated Human Aortic Endothelial Cells (HAEC) Following Hypoxia / Reoxygenation

Andreina Schoeberlein[1], Gregor Zünd[2], Marko Turina[2]

University Hospital Zurich, Department of Surgery, Research Division' and Clinic for Cardiovascular Surgery', Zurich, Switzerland

Ischemia / reperfusion injury is a critical determinant in many heart diseases and in cardiopulmonary bypass surgery. Compared to other cell adhesion molecules little is known about the role of VCAM-1 in ischemia / reperfusion. This study investigates the role of hypoxia-/-reoxygenation in VCAM-1 cell surface expression on HAEC. Cells were subjected to the following treatments: normoxia 21 h; hypoxia (O_2= 1 %) 3h, 19h, 21h; hypoxia 1 h + normoxia 2h, hypoxia 1h + normoxia 18h and hypoxia 3h + normoxia 18h with and without TNF- (10 ng/ml) stimulation. VCAM-1 expression was assessed by an indirect ELISA. HAEC not stimulated with TNF- expressed low levels of VCAM-1 almost without significant differences between hypoxia / reoxygenation treatments. Stimulation with 1 0 ng/ml TNF- resulted in a 4- to 22-fold increase in VCAM-1 expression ($p < 0.001$) that was hardly altered by hypoxia / reoxygenation. Hypoxia 1h + normoxia 2h lead to lower VCAM-1 expression in both TNF- unstimulated ($p < 0.05$) and stimulated cells ($p < 0.001$). The main ligand of VCAM-1, VLA-4, is expressed on eosinophils and monocytes but not on neutrophils which are mainly responsible for the tissue damage in ischemia / reperfusion injury. This supports our findings that VCAM-1 expression is not influenced by hypoxia / reoxygenation. However, *in vivo* models of ischemia / reperfusion showed an increase in VCAM-1 expression. We postulate that other factors upregulated by ischemia/reperfusion such as cytokines and endotoxin are responsible for the increase in VCAM-1 expression rather than hypoxia / reperfusion per se.

Vascular Endothelium: Mechanisms of Cell Signaling
J.D. Catravas et al. (Eds.)
IOS Press, 1999

Biochemical Evidence of Crossed Cerebellar Diaschisis in Terms of Nitric Oxide Indicators and Lipid Peroxidation Products in Rats During Focal Cerebral Ischemia

Mustafa SERTESER[1], Tomris ÖZBEN[1], Saadet GÜMÜŞLÜ[1], Sevin BALKAN[2], Esor BALKAN[3]

Akdeniz University, School of Medicine, Departments of Biochemistry[1], Neurology[2] and Otorhinolaryngology[3], Antalya, TURKEY
serteser@med.akdeniz.edu.tr

Cerebral hypoperfusion in the contralateral cerebellar hemisphere after stroke is interpreted as a functional and metabolic depression, possibly caused by a loss of excitatory afferent inputs on the corticopontocerebellar pathway terminating in the cerebellar gray matter. This phenomenon is defined as crossed cerebellar diaschisis and can be diagnosed clinically by positron emission tomography, single-photon emission computed tomography, brain magnetic resonance imaging and electroencephalography in terms of regional cerebral blood flow or metabolic rate of oxygen measurements. In the present study, nitric oxide indicators (nitrite and cyclic guanosine monophosphate) and lipid peroxidation products (malondialdehyde and conjugated dienes) were measured in rat cerebral cortices and cerebella after permanent right middle cerebral artery occlusion in order to assess the crossed cerebellar diaschisis. Nitrite values in ipsilateral cortex were significantly higher than those in contralateral cortex at 10 ($p<0.001$) and 60 ($p<0.05$) minutes of ischemia but no significant changes were observed in both cerebellum compared to the 0 minute values. In both cerebral cortex and cerebellum cGMP levels at 10 and 60 minutes were significantly increased ($p<0.001$). This increase was marked in ipsilateral cortex and contralateral cerebellum when compared with opposite cortex and cerebellum ($p<0.001$). MDA values in ipsilateral cortex were significantly higher than those in contralateral cortex at 60 minutes of ischemia ($p<0.05$). Contralateral cerebellar MDA values were found significantly higher than those in ipsilateral cerebellum at 0 ($p<0.001$) and 60 ($p<0.05$) minutes of ischemia. In ipsilateral cortex, conjugated diene values at 0,10,60 minutes of ischemia were higher than those in contralateral cortex. On the other hand 0,10,60 minute conjugated diene levels in contralateral cerebellum were significantly higher than those in ipsilateral cerebellum ($p<0.001$). These findings support the interruption of the corticopontocerebellar tract as the mechanism of the crossed cerebellar diaschisis.

Key words: Diaschisis, rat, nitrite, cGMP, MDA, conjugated diene

Vascular Endothelium: Mechanisms of Cell Signaling
J.D. Catravas et al. (Eds.)
IOS Press, 1999

Binding of Coagulation Factor VIIa to Cell Surface Tissue Factor Induces Signal Transduction via p44/p42 MAPK

B.B. Sørensen, L.K. Poulsen and M. Ezban, L.C. Petersen
FVII/TF RESEARCH, Novo Nordisk A/S, 2820 Gentofte, Denmark

Tissue factor (TF) is a transmembrane protein exposed to the blood upon injury of the vessel wall. Coagulation factor VIIa (FVIIa) circulating in plasma binds to TF and the FVIIa/TF complex initiates the extrinsic pathway of coagulation ultimately leading to thrombin and clot formation. Initiation of coagulation as a result of FVIIa/TF activity is an extracellular event confined to the outer leaflet of the plasma membrane of TF expressing cells.

A number of recent observations also suggest an intracellular function of TF. It was found that TF shows sequence and structural homology to the superfamily of cytokine receptors all involved in signal transduction. Two recent studies [1, 2] reported that FVIIa could induce oscillations in intracellular free calcium in various TF-expressing cells. Other studies have provided evidence that serine residues of the cytoplasmic domain of TF can be phosphorylated in TF-transfected cells [3], and that this domain works as a substrate for protein kinase activity when exposed to cell lysates [4]. Signal transduction was also indicated in studies with cultured human monocytes [5] showing that addition of FVIIa could induce a transient tyrosine phosphorylation of several polypeptides. Finally very recent results suggested that FVIIa induced alteration in gene expression in human fibroblasts [6].

With these diverse observations it was of interest to characterise a putative FVIIa-induced signal transduction pathway in further detail [7]. BHK cells were transfected with human TF (BHK(+TF)) and a gene reporter construction encoding a luciferase gen under transcriptional control of a tandem cassettes of signal transducer and activator of transcription (STAT) elements and one serum response element (SRE). A BHK cell line transfected with the gene reporter construct but without TF served as a control. FVIIa induced a significant luciferase response in cells expressing TF, but not in cells without TF. BHK(+TF) cells responded to FVIIa in a dose-dependent manner, whereas no response was observed with active site-inhibited FVIIa, which also worked as an antagonist to FVIIa-induced signaling. Western blot analysis with phospho specific p44/p42 MAPK antibodies showed a transient phosphorylation when cells were exposed to FVIIa. Induction of p44/p42 MAPK was observed in BHK(+TF), ECV-304, HUVEC, and MDCK-II, but not in LPS-stimulated human monocytes. The proteolytic activity of FVIIa/TF complex was obligatory for activation of the p44/p42 MAPK pathway. Experiments including hirudin showed that thrombin was not involved in FVIIa/TF induced signalling since hirudin did not inhibit FVIIa induced phosphorylation of p44/p42 MAPK.

These results suggest a specific mechanism by which binding of FVIIa to cell surface TF independent of coagulation can modulate cellular functions.

References

[1] Rottingen, J.-A., Enden, T., Camerer, E., Iversen, J.-G., and Prydz, H. (1995) J. Biol. Chem. 270: 4650

[2] Camerer, E., Rottingen, J.-A., Iversen, J.-G., and Prydz, H. (1996) J. Biol. Chem. 271, 29034

[3] Zinocheck, T. F., Roy, S. and Vehar, G. A. (1992) J. Biol. Chem. 267, 3561

[4] Mody, R. S. and Carson, S. D. (1997) Biochemistry 36, 7869

[5] Masuda, M., Nakamura, S., Murakami, S., Komiyama, Y. and Takahashi, H., (1996) Eur. J. Immunol. 26, 2529

[6] Pendurthi, U.R., Alok, D. and Rao, L.V.M. (1997) Proc. Natl.Acad. Sci. USA. 94, 12598

[7] Poulsen, L.K., Jacobsen, N., Sorensen, B.B., Bergenhem, N.C.H., Kelly, J.D., Foster, D.C., Thastrup, O., Ezban, M., Petersen, L.C. (1998) J. Biol. Chem. 273, 6228

Vascular Endothelium: Mechanisms of Cell Signaling
J.D. Catravas et al. (Eds.)
IOS Press, 1999

Induction of Apotosis of Human Endothelial Cells by Proteinase 3 (Pr3): A Possible Mechanism of Vascular Injury in Wegener's Granulomatosis

M.E.J.Taekema-Roelvink, M.C. Janssens, E. Heemskerk,C. van Kooten
and M.R. Daha

Dept. of Nephrology, Leiden University Medical Centre, Leiden, The Netherlands

Introduction: Wegener's granulomatosis (WG) is characterized by necrotizing crescentic glomerulonephritis and systemic vasculitis. PR3, a neutral serine proteinase present in the -granules of neutrophils and the main target antigen of anti-neutrophil cytoplasmic antibodies (ANCA), may play a pathogenic role in inducing endothelial cell injury. In the present study we investigated the effect of PR3 on induction of apoptosis of human umbilical vein endothelial cells (HUVEC).

Materials and Methods: HUVEC were incubated with various concentrations of PR3 in the presence of 0.5% FCS. The presence of apoptosis was assessed morphologically after staining with Hoechst 33258 and confirmed by agarose gel electrophoresis. The effect of PR3 on the induction of apoptosis of HUVEC was quantified using flow cytometry after Annexin V FITC or TUNEL staining.

Results: PR3 induced a dose and time dependent induction of apoptosis of HUVEC. Apoptosis of HUVEC, induced by PR3, was evaluated morphologically by DNA fragmentation and was confirmed by agarose gel electrophoresis. The presence of a high concentration of serum (20%) inhibited PR3-induced apoptosis of HUVEC.

Conclusion: We conclude that PR3 induces apoptosis of human endothelial cells *in vitro* and may thus contribute to vascular injury, as seen in WG.

Vascular Endothelium: Mechanisms of Cell Signaling
J.D. Catravas et al. (Eds.)
IOS Press, 1999

Lipoprotein (A) in Population-Based Samples of South Asian and Europid Adults in Newcastle Upon Tyne, UK

Tavridou A.[1], Unwin N.[2,3], Bhopal R.[2], Laker M.F.[1]
Department of [1]Clinical Biochemistry, [2]Epidemiology and Public Health, and [3]Medicine,
University of Newcastle upon Tyne, UK

There is a higher prevalence of coronary heart disease (CHD) in South Asian subjects living in the UK than European populations. Since elevated lipoprotein(a) [Lp(a)] levels are associated with the presence of CHD, we investigated Lp(a) concentration in 678 South Asian (Indian, Pakistani, Bangladeshi) and 779 European subjects, aged 25-77 yrs, in a cross sectional population based study. The highly skewed distribution of Lp(a) in European subjects was confirmed and a similar distribution was observed in South Asian individuals (163 mg/l [8.5-1280 mg/l] and 190 mg/l [18-876 mg/l], median [2.5-97.5 percentiles] respectively).

Sex	Europids		South Asians	
	n	Lp(a), mg/l	n	Lp(a), mg/l
Male	384	148(132-168)	333	161(144-181)
Female	395	155(135-176)	345	194(174-217)

Values are geometric means (95% CI)

South Asian males had lower serum Lp(a) concentrations than South Asian females (161 vs. 194 mg/l, p= 0.02). South Asian women had also significantly higher serum Lp(a) concentrations than European women (194 vs. 155 mg/l, p=0.009) but there was no significant difference in men. In South Asian females, Lp(a) levels were highest in Pakistani subjects and lowest in Indian subjects (229 vs. 162 mg/l, p= 0.004). In conclusion, there was variation among the three South Asian groups in Lp(a) concentrations. The relative effect of Lp(a) as a risk factor for CHD in South Asian subjects should be considered separately in different ethnic subgroups.

Acknowledgments. *To the British Heart Foundation and the Newcastle Heart Project for their support.*

Vascular Endothelium: Mechanisms of Cell Signaling
J.D. Catravas et al. (Eds.)
IOS Press, 1999

277

Responses of the Pulmonary Capillary Bed to High Blood Flow: A Model for Studying Pulmonary Hypertension

M. J. Theodorakis, J. B. Parkerson, J. D. Catravas
Vascular Biology Center, Medical College of Georgia

Pulmonary hypertension is a restrictive vasculopathy, associated with reduction in the size of the capillary network and may well involve altered or defective capillary responses to various stimuli, such as changing cardiac output. However, the mechanisms underlying recruitment or de-recruitment of the pulmonary capillary bed under conditions of varying blood flow are not well understood.

Objectives: The aim of this study was to assess changes in the extent and functional integrity of the rat pulmonary capillary bed in response to high perfusion flows. In addition, we tested the hypothesis that this method could be of benefit in the evaluation and study of pulmonary hypertension.

Methods: Lung capillary recruitment was assessed from the relative change in the mass of capillary-bound angiotensin converting enzyme (ACE), a protein uniformly distributed throughout the capillary luminal surface. Changes m ACE mass, estimated from the single transpulmonary hydrolysis (v) of the synthetic ACE substrate ^{3}H-bcnzoyl-Phe-Ala-Pro (^{3}H-BPAP), were expressed as CPI (capillary perfusion index). Lungs of male Wistar rats (464-768 gr; N= 23) were perfused *in situ* with 3% dextran (MW=70000) in Kreb's buffer. Flow was adjusted by means of a peristaltic pump and monitored with an acoustic probe connected to an electromagnetic flowmeter. Pulmonary arterial pressure was also recorded continuously. The animals were ventilated mechanically (95% 02 - 5% C02) and arterial blood gases were monitored regularly. Basal cardiac output, in *vivo*, was 26-65 nil/min. Perfusion flow gradually increased, from 5 to 500 ml/min.

Results: CPI increased steadily and pulmonary vascular resistance decreased proportionally to perfusion flow up to ~200 ml/min, after which both parameters reached a plateau. ^{3}H-BPAP-v non-significantly fluctuated around 2.0 for perfusion flows up to 200 ml/min. Beyond this point there was rapid decline, reaching a nadir of 0.7 at 500 ml/min reflecting decreasing capillary transit times of the substrate.

Conclusions: We conclude that at resting cardiac output, the rat lung capillary bed is only partly recruited and that full recruitment is achieved at 3-4 times basal cardiac output. This relationship may be impaired in pulmonary hypertension. Thus, CPI determinations could be used to improve our understanding of mechanisms involved in pulmonary microcirculation responses and would greatly help in delineating aspects of pulmonary hypertension pathophysiology.

(Supported by HL31422 and the "Alexander S. Onassis" Foundation)

Vascular Endothelium: Mechanisms of Cell Signaling
J.D. Catravas et al. (Eds.)
IOS Press, 1999

Physicochemical Aspects of Cardiovascular Calcification

Branko B. Tomazic
Paffenbarger Research Center, American Dental Association Health Foundation (retired)
10814 Beech Creek Drive, Columbia MD, 21044-1023, USA

Pathologic ca I calcification is the major reason for the hardening of arteries. In addition, cardiovascular calcification takes place in heart tissues and in tissue-derived heart valve bioprostheses. The mechanism of cardiovascular calcification is a very complex process governed by many biochemical factors. It is fair to say that at present time the exact mechanism of cardiovascular calcification is not completely known. The objective of this contribution is: 1: to provide a spectrum of physicochemical data that would ascertain the nature of cardiovascular calcified deposits, CCD, retrieved at several different sites of the cardiovascular system; 2: to indicate possible precursor(s) in formation of CCD, and 3: to indicate possible ways to prevent formation of CCD, particularly with emphasis on longevity of heart valve bioprostheses. The CCD have been retrieved from human aortas, carotid arteries, human heart valves, heart valve bioprostheses (human use) and polyurethane total artificial heart (animal use). The comprehensive physicochemical characterization of CCD involved chemical analyses, structural (XRD, FTIR) and optical (SEM, EDX, light microscopy) methods and thermodynamic solubility measurements. These methods prove that CCD are calcium deficient, carbonate/phosphate-substituted bioapatites, with significant sodium, magnesium and fluoride incorporation. Solubility measurements eliminate hydroxyapatite as a valid representative of CCD. The similarity of properties of CCD indicate that these were formed through similar reaction mechanisms, involving hydrolytic transformation of precursors. The combined solubility measurements and *in vitro and in vivo* biomineralization of bovine pericardium, BP, tissue indicates octacalcium phosphate, OCP, as a valid precursor for formation of CCD. This finding is supported by the presence of acidic phosphate as a component of CCD and in the BP biomineralization products. Additional *in vitro* BP biomineralization tests provided very interesting new EDX information that shows that early intrinsic CCD has a high Ca/P ratio > 2. This indicates that early CCD precursor contains a significant biochemical component that may involve proteins. The final task the inhibition of formation of CCD, should be based on the most comprehensive knowledge of mechanisms of *in vitro and in* vivo biomineralization. The most promising strategy is to inhibit the formation of OCP, or acidic phosphate precursor, in the cardiovascular tissue. This may be achieved through the use of polyphosphonates, which are well known to have an inhibitory, while not prolong effect on CCD formation. The application of synergistic mixtures, containing synthetic and natural inhibitors called pharmacologic factors, combined with genetic factors, appears to be a more promising way to counter cardiovascular calcification, with special emphasis on tissue-derived heart valve bioprostheses.

Vascular Endothelium: Mechanisms of Cell Signaling
J.D. Catravas et al. (Eds.)
IOS Press, 1999

Bradykinin Stimulates the Tyrosine Phosphorylation and Bradykinin B2 Receptor Association of Phospholipase Cγ1 in Vascular Endothelial Cells

<u>Virginia J. Venema</u>, Hong Ju, Jimin Sun, Douglas C. Eaton, Mario B. Marrero, and Richard C. Venema
Vascular Biology Center, Medical College of Georgia
Augusta, GA 30912, USA

An early event in bradykinin (BK) B2 receptor signal transduction is activation of phosphoinositide-specific phospholipase C (PLC). Two alternate mechanisms of PLC activation have been reported consisting of either direct allosteric activation of PLCβ isoforms by G-proteins or tyrosine phosphorylation and consequent activation of PLCγ isoforms. Because the B2 receptor is a G-protein-coupled receptor, it has been assumed that the receptor signals exclusively or predominately through the β isoforms of PLC. In the present study, however, we have found that BK stimulation of IP_3 production and the Ca^{2+} signal in cultured endothelial cells is dependent on tyrosine phosphorylation. We have found further that stimulation of B2 receptors in these cells is accompanied by a transient tyrosine phosphorylation of PLCγ1. Phosphorylation is temporally correlated with increased IP_3 production and association of PLCγ1 with the C-terminal intracellular domain of the B2 receptor. The B2 receptor can thus physically associate with intracellular proteins other than G-proteins. Furthermore, it appears that activation of PLCγ isoforms, rather than PLCβ isoforms, may be primarily responsible for BK-stimulated IP_3 generation in endothelial cells.

Vascular Endothelium: Mechanisms of Cell Signaling
J.D. Catravas et al. (Eds.)
IOS Press, 1999

Impaired Nitric Oxide-Mediated Vasodilation in Patients with Autosomal Dominant Polycystic Kidney Disease

Dan Wang[1], J. Iversen[2] and S. Strandgaard[1]
Department of Nephrology[1], Department of Clinical Physiology[2], Herlev Hospital
2370 Herlev, Denmark

We hypothesized that nitric oxide (NO) system is involved in the development of cardiovascular changes in autosomal dominant polycystic kidney disease (ADPKD). Small subcutaneous resistance vessels from predialysis ADPKD patients (n=7) and normal controls (n=9) were mounted in a Mulvany-Halpem myograph. The endothelium-dependent relaxation before and after vessel incubated with L-arginine (a substrate of NO synthase) or N^G-nitro-Larginine methyl ester (L-NAME, an inhibitor of NO synthase), as well as endothelium-independent relaxation were investigated. The results showed: 1) The max relaxation rate of endothelium-dependent relaxation induced by acetylcholine (ACh) was 64,35±21,70 vs. 87,57±6,11(ADPKD vs. control, P<0.05); 2) In the presence of L-arginine, a left-shift of the ACh dose response curves was increased in normals, but not in ADPKD patients. The relaxation rate induced by high concentration of ACh (> 1 0-7 mol/1) were higher in controls than in ADPKD (P<0.05); 3). In the presence of the L-NAME the right-shift of the ACh dose-response curve was slighter in ADPKD than in controls (P<0.05); 4). The max relaxation rate of endothelium-independent relaxation mediated by 3-morphollino-sydnonimine (NO donor) was similar in the two groups.

It was concluded that endothelium-dependent relaxation was impaired in the resistance vessel from ADPKD. The reduced response of the vessel to both the substrate and inhibitor of NO synthase in ADPKD suggested that it is possible that the shortage and/or insufficient activity of nitric oxide synthase is a factor of endothelial dysfunction in ADPKD.

Vascular Endothelium: Mechanisms of Cell Signaling
J.D. Catravas et al. (Eds.)
IOS Press, 1999

TBE Endothelium-Dependent Relaxation and Noradrenaline Sensitivity of Mesenteric Resistance Vessels in Polycystic Kidney (PKD) Rats

Dan Wang[1], J. Iversen[2] and S. Strandgaard[1]

*Department of Nephrology[1], Department of Clinical Physiology[2], Herlev Hospital,
2370 Herlev, Denmark*

Hypertension and vascular disease are common complications in autosomal dominant polycystic kidney Disease (ADPKD). To investigate the function of resistance vessels in polycystic kidney rats, mesenteric resistance vessels dissected from 8, 11 and 14 week old heter'ozygous Han:SPRD rats (polycystic kidney disease rats, PKD, n=12), unaffected Han:SPRD rats (HSPRD, n=11) and normal Sprague Dawley rats (SD, n=12) were mounted in a Mulvany-Halpem myograph. The concentration-contracting to noradrenaline (NA), endothelium-dependent relaxation to acetylcholine (ACh) before and after vessels incubated with N^G-nitro-L-arginine methyl ester (L-NAME, an inhibitor of NO synthase, as well as endothelium-independent relaxation mediated by 3-morphollino-sydnonimine (SIN-1) were carried out. The results show that 1) age, body weight, systolic blood pressure were similar in the three groups. Total kidney weight and serum urea were higher in PKD than HSPRD and control group. 2) Active wall tension and contractile sensitivity to NA were higher in PKD rats than HSPRD rats and control (P<0.05). 3). The max relaxation rate of endothelium-dependent relaxation was 21,52+15, 39,20+11 vs. 78,91+12,12 (PKD, HSPRD vs. control, P<0.05); 4) In the presence of the L-NAME, the right-shift of tire ACh dose-response curve was significant slighter in ADPKD than in controls (P<0.05); 5). Concentration-relaxation curves were similar in three groups. It was concluded that hyperactivity to NA and endothelium-dependent relaxation were impaired in the resistance vessel from Han:SPRD rats, especially in heterozygous Han:SPRD rats. Both abnormalities in the resistance vessel from PKD rats suggest that a functional change occurred in young ADPKD, predisposing to the development of hypertension and vascular disease.

Vascular Endothelium: Mechanisms of Cell Signaling
J.D. Catravas et al. (Eds.)
IOS Press, 1999

Soluble E-Selectin and Hyaluronic Acid as Tumor Markers for Hepatocellular Carcinoma

Wickham N[1], West D[2], Ho S[3], Leung[3] WT and Johnson PJ[3]
*Department of Haematology-Oncology, The Queen Elizabeth Hospital, Adelaide[1],
Australia, Department of Immunology, The Royal Liverpool University Hospital, UK[2] and
Department of Oncology, The Prince of Wales Hospital, Hong Kong[3]*

E-selectin, also known as endothelial-leukocyte adhesion molecule-1 (ELAM-1), is a carbohydrate-binding cellular adhesion molecule which is expressed on activated endothelial cells (EC) following exposure to inflammatory mediators such as lipopolysaccharide (LPS) or interleukin 1 (IL-1) [1]. Soluble E-selectin is shed from the surface of cells and circulates in the plasma at concentrations normally < 65 µg/L. E-selectin is a ligand for sialyl Lewis (a) and Lewis (x) and is involved not only in the adhesion of neutrophils, but also in malignant cell adhesion and metastasis [2].

Hyaluronic acid (HA) is a major polysaccharide component of connective tissues. It is synthesised by fibroblasts and circulates through lymphatics where up to 90% may be cleared by lymph nodes. That, which gains access to the blood, is cleared from the plasma by hepatic sinusoidal cells. There is a normal diurnal variation in the serum of between 10 and 100 µg/L [3]. Levels may be increased by inflammation, sepsis, malignancy (Wilm's tumor, metastatic breast cancer and mesothelioma) and in liver disease such as transplant rejection, primary biliary cirrhosis and alcoholic cirrhosis [4].

HCC is the 7th most common cancer to affect males world-wide. In Hong Kong it has a very high age-specific incidence of 49 per 100,000 males and is the second most common cancer accounting for 8.5% of all new cancers and 12.5% of deaths. Small tumors are amenable to operation and are potentially curative (< 2 cm size - 5 year survival of 85%; 4.1-5 cm - 5 year survival of 60%). However, the majority are more advanced and baseline 3 year survival is only 13%, routine chemotherapy or radiotherapy has little or no effect on survival and transplantation gives disappointing results [5].

Early detection is therefore critical, and the accepted tumor marker is alpha-fetoprotein (AFP), which has an upper limit in normal serum of <25 µg/L. However, as HCC usually arises on the background of cirrhosis which also causes an increase in AFP, there is a grey area, particularly between 100 and 500 µg/L, where the distinction between cirrhosis and HCC is unclear. Furthermore, as many as one third of HCC patients will not have a raised AFP [6], therefore more sensitive and specific markers are needed.

We wondered whether soluble E-selectin and HA, as they are elevated in some other malignancies, might not prove sensitive to the presence of hepatocellular carcinoma (HCC) and, either individually or in combination with AFP, improve the chances of early diagnosis. Stored sera (in the Prince of Wales Hospital serum bank) from 50 patients, 25 with known HCC and 25 with cirrhosis were assayed for AFP, E-selectin and HA. Sera from 25 patients with newly-diagnosed non-Hodgkin's lymphoma served as malignant controls. Samples were assayed blind to the original diagnosis. All 3 tumor markers were assayed in 36 patients -26 with HCC and 15 with cirrhosis. Table 1 gives the initial results for E-Selectin and HA, separately or combined in the three different patient groups. These results show the numbers of sera in each group that had levels raised >1 SD above their respective means (as determined in a normal Caucasian population).

Table 1.

	E-SELECTIN > 65 µg/L	HA > 100 µg/L	E-SEL + HA either/or
HCC	12/25 (48%)	4/14 (28%)	10/13 (77%)
CIRRHOSIS	3/22 (14%)	1/10 (10%)	1/10 (10%)
NHL	5/25 (20%)	1/11 (9%)	1/10 (10%)

E-Selectin and HA were both increased more often in HCC, and the sensitivity in identifying HCC increased if results from both tests were combined. We then asked what were the sensitivity and specificity of these tests, either individually or taken in various combinations with each other and AFP. These results are summarised in Table 2.

Table 2.

	E-SEL > 65 µg/L	HA > 100 µg/L	AFP > 200µg/L	E-SEL + HA	E-SEL +AFP	HA + AFP	E-SEL + HA + AFP
Sensitivity %	48	38	29	71	71	62	86
Specificity %	87	73	87	60	80	60	53

The best overall sensitivity was with the combination of E-selectin and AFP, with a sensitivity of 71% and specificity of 80%. Although all 3 tumor markers together were more sensitive at 86%, specificity was reduced to 53%. Note that if the cut-off for AFP were taken at the lower value of 100 µg/L (not shown), then the combination with E-selectin gives a sensitivity of 100%, but with a specificity of only 40%.

The following conclusions may be drawn from this pilot study:

1) AFP is either sensitive at the expense of specificity or vice versa.
2) Soluble E-selectin and HA are relatively specific but not particularly sensitive by themselves.
3) E-selectin and AFP together produce a "tumor marker profile" that remains sensitive and specific.
4) Addition of HA increases sensitivity, but reduces specificity.
5) Further studies and follow-up of apparent false positives will determine the true benefit of using E-selectin and possibly HA together with AFP to provide an earlier diagnosis of HCC.

Thus, endothelial as well as other vascular and/or intravascular cells shed surface molecules into the circulation that may act as novel markers of inflammation and malignancy, and further studies are warranted to establish their possible role in diagnosis.

References

[1] Groves RW, Allen MH, Barker JNWN, Haskard DO, MacDonald DM. Endothelial leucocyte adhesion molecule-1 (ELAM-1) expression in cutaneous inflammation. Br J Dermatol., 124(2):117-123, 1991.
[2] Irimura T, Izumi Y, Kawamura Y, Nakamori S, Fidler IJ, Cleary KR, Ota DM. Carbohydrate-mediated cell adhesion as a determinant of colorectal metastasis. Cancer Bull., 46 (4):336-343, 1994.
[3] Engstrom-Laurent A. Changes in hyaluronan concentration in tissues and body fluids in disease states. CIBA Foundation Symp., (Netherlands) 143:233-247, 1989.
[4] Laurent TC, Fraser JR. Hyaluronan. FASEB Journal (United States), 6(7):2397-2404, 1992.
[5] Ezaki T. Hepatocellular carcinoma. BMJ., 304:196-197, 1992.
[6] Nomura F, Ohnishi K, Tanabe Y. Clinical features and prognosis of hepatocellular carcinoma with reference to serum alpha-fetoprotein levels. Analysis of 606 patients. Cancer 64:1700-1707, 1989.

Vascular Endothelium: Mechanisms of Cell Signaling
J.D. Catravas et al. (Eds.)
IOS Press, 1999

The Hormone Response Element (HRE) of the Human ApoCIII Enhancer Is Essential for the Intestinal Expression of the Human Apoa-I Gene in Transgenic Mice

Horng Yuan Kan, Spiros Georgopoulos, Eleni Zanni and <u>Vassilis Zannis</u>
Section of Molecular Zenetics, Cardiovascular Institute
Boston University Medical Center
Boston MA 02118

We have generated transgenic mouse lines expressing the human apoA-I gene under the control of a 2.1 kb human apoA-I promoter and 0.89 kb of the apoCIII enhancer. The 8.2 kb transgenic construct contained the entire apoA-I gene and had the apoCIII gene replaced by the CAT cDNA sequence. Mouse lines expressing two similar constructs were generrated. The first line expressed the apoA-I and CAT genes under the control of the wild-type promoter / enhancer; the second expressed a construct mutated in the two HREs present in the apoCIII promoter and enhancer region. The distriibution of apoA-I mRNA was determined by S1 analysis in order to assess the tissue specificity of the wild-type promoter and the effect of the mutations in tissue-specific expression. It was shown that the wild-type promoter / enhancer cluster directed high levels of apoA-I mRNA synthesis in liver and intestine, intermediate levels in stomach and kidney, low levels in heart, spleen and lung, and no expression in muscle and brain. The pattern of apoA-I gene expression in the transgenic mice closely mimics that observed in human fetal tissues. In mice carrying the mutated apoCIII enhancer, the expression of apoA-I m RNA was undetectable in intestine, kidney and stomach, whereas expression in the other tissues was identical to that observed in mice carrying wild-type A-I promoter /CIII enhancer cluster. The findings suggest that a) the 2.1 kb apoA-I promoter, 0.89 kb apoCIII enhancer are required for correct expression of the apoA-I gene in different tissues; b) the apoCIII enhancer is required for the expression of the apoA-I gene in intestine, stomach and kidney; and c) the activity of apoCIII enhancer in specific tissues *in vivo*, is abolished by mutations in the hormone nuclear receptor binding sites.

Vascular Endothelium: Mechanisms of Cell Signaling
J.D. Catravas et al. (Eds.)
IOS Press, 1999

Nitric Oxide Does Not Inhibit Induction of Type II Nitric Oxide Synthase in Rat Aortic Smooth Muscle Cells

Hanfang Zhang, Connie Snead, Michael Gaines, Xingwu Teng and John D. Catravas
Vascular Biology Center, Medical College of Georgia, Augusta, GA 30912

Nitric oxide (NO) is believed to be a negative feedback regulator of INOS in hepatic cells and macrophages. In order to study the potential role of NO on INOS regulation in rat aortic smooth muscle cells (ASMC), we have studied the effects of NOS inhibitor and NO released by NO donors on the inducibility of rat INOS promoter and INOS protein in ASMC. Rat ASMC generated very little NO. However, high-output of NO was generated by SMC in response to cytokine mixture (CM) consisting of IL-lp (350 U/ml), TNF-A (150 U/ml) and IFN-Y (I 50 U/ml), and the activated NO release was effectively blocked by NOS inhibitor, LNAME. A fully functional rat -3.2 kb INOS promoter-luciferase DNA construct was transfected into ASMC. The transfected cells expressed very small amount of basal luciferase activity, and about 20-fold induction of luciferase activity was observed in ASMC in response to CM. NOS inhibitor, L-NAME significantly inhibiting NO release, did not alter the inducibility of the promoter by CM. Exogenous NO released by SNAP and SIN-1, in addition to endogenous NO production, had minimally enhanced basal promoter activity and did not inhibit the induction of INOS promoter by CM. The mass of INOS protein was analyzed by Western blotting. CM significantly induced the expression of INOS protein in ASMC, and the induction was not influenced by NO released by NO donor. However, in lung macrophage cells, NR8383, SNAP produced a concentration-dependent inhibition of INOS protein expression. These data suggest that NO may not regulate INOS at both transcriptional and protein levels in ASMC, and the absence of feedback inhibition on INOS may have important implication in the pathogenesis of septic shock.

Author Index